Ferenc Péter
Wilmar M. Wiersinga
Ulrike Hostalek

The Thyroid and Environment

The Thyroid and Environment

Merck European Thyroid Symposium, Budapest 2000, June 22-25

Chairmen

F. Péter, W. Wiersinga

Editors

Ferenc Péter
Wilmar M. Wiersinga
Ulrike Hostalek

With 35 figures
and 45 tables

Schattauer Stuttgart New York

Editors

F. Péter
Buda Children's Hospital, 23.POB 14-H, 1277 Budapest, Hungary

W. M. Wiersinga
Academic Medical Center, Meibergdreef, 1105 AZ Amsterdam, The Netherlands

U. Hostalek
Merck KGaA, Pharma Strategic Marketing, Frankfurter Strasse 250,
64271 Darmstadt, Germany

Die Deutsche Bibliothek – CIP-Einheitsaufnahme
Ein Titeldatensatz für diese Publikation ist bei Der Deutschen Bibliothek erhältlich.

Besonderer Hinweis:
Die Medizin unterliegt einem fortwährenden Entwicklungsprozeß, so dass alle Angaben, insbesondere zu diagnostischen und therapeutischen Verfahren, immer nur dem Wissensstand zum Zeitpunkt der Drucklegung des Buches entsprechen können. Hinsichtlich der angegebenen Empfehlungen zur Therapie und der Auswahl sowie Dosierung von Medikamenten wurde die größtmögliche Sorgfalt beachtet. Gleichwohl werden die Benutzer aufgefordert, die Beipackzettel und Fachinformationen der Hersteller zur Kontrolle heranzuziehen und im Zweifelsfall einen Spezialisten zu konsultieren. Fragliche Unstimmigkeiten sollten bitte im allgemeinen Interesse dem Verlag mitgeteilt werden. Der Benutzer selbst bleibt verantwortlich für jede diagnostische oder therapeutische Applikation, Medikation und Dosierung.
In diesem Buch sind eingetragene Warenzeichen (geschützte Warennamen) nicht besonders kenntlich gemacht. Es kann also aus dem Fehlen eines entsprechenden Hinweises nicht geschlossen werden, dass es sich um einen freien Warennamen handelt.

Internet http://www.schattauer.de
Printed in Germany

Lektorat: Lektorat durch die Herausgeber
Copy Editors: Dr. Brian Shine, Bucks, United Kingdom; Dr. Thomas Wolffgram, Stuttgart, Germany
Umschlaggestaltung: Ulrike Böge
Satz, Druck und Einband: Gulde-Druck GmbH, Tübingen
Gedruckt auf chlor- und säurefrei gebleichtem Papier.

ISBN 3-7945-2072-6

Preface

The Thyroid and Environment has been selected as the topic for the first symposium in the new millennium for the well-known biennial Merck European Thyroid Symposia on thyroid diseases. At first glance the choice may be a little bit surprising, for iodine intake – one of the environmental factors par excellence in the thyroid field – has been known to modulate the expression of thyroid diseases for more than a century. In addition, the new millennium is about to start with a complete description of the entire human genome. However, the more that is learned about the genotype of specific diseases, the more it becomes evident that interaction with environmental factors may determine the clinical expression of the diseases. This applies in particular to multifactorial conditions such as autoimmune thyroid disease. Studies of the relationship between genotype and phenotype of specific diseases will undoubtedly advance our knowledge of the pathogenesis of a variety of thyroid diseases. It is precisely at this point that environmental factors play an important and often decisive role in the development of disease. Although gene therapy may alter the genotype in the distant future, environmental factors are more accessible to change. Preventive interventions to modulate adverse effects of the environment may have great clinical relevance.

It is against this background that the organizers have arranged the scientific program. We would like to thank Dr. U. Hostalek of Merck KGaA, Darmstadt, Germany, who gave us a free hand in delineating the scientific sessions. Considerable progress has been made in the last decade in unraveling many of the environmental factors involved in thyroid disease. The present meeting will serve to review what is known in this respect, but more importantly will also indicate what is still unknown. We hope that the symposium will generate new studies to close the gaps in our present knowledge on how the environment affects the thyroid. Certainly, the environment in Budapest offers an attractive start.

Amsterdam
and Budapest
June 2000

W. M. Wiersinga

F. Péter

Contents

Contributors

J. M. F. Adam Hasanuddin University, Chairil Anwar 3, 90113 Makassar, Indonesia

M. Adam Children's Hospital, Nicolae Titulescu 38, ap. 5, 3400 Cluj – Napoca, Romania

A. Ametov Dept. of Endocrinology, Russian Medical Academy Postgraduate Education, Chasovaya st. 20, 125315 Moscow, Russia

C. Balazs III Dept Medicine Endocrinology, Teaching Hospital, Bartok B 2–26, 4043 Debrecen, Hungary

Z. Bencsik St. George's Hospital, Seregélyesi st. 3, 8000 Székesfehérvár, Hungary

P. Bodnar Dept. of Endocrinology, National Medical University, T. Sherchenko Blvd. 13, 25 2004 Kiev, Ukraine

P. Bottermann II. Med. Klinik, TUM München, Ismaningerstr. 22, 81675 München, Germany

L. E. Braverman Brigham and Women's Hospital, Boston, MA, USA

T. H. Brix Dept. of Endocrinology, Odense University Hospital, 5000 – C Odense, Denmark

R. Bunevičius Institute of Endocrinology Kaunas Medical University, Eiveniu 2, 3007 Kaunas, Lithuania

J. Cáp 2nd Dept. of Internal Medicine, University Hospital, 500 05 Hradec Králové, Czech Republic

A. Dalea Institute of Endocrinology C. I. Parhon, Doamna Oltea 8, Bucharest, Romania

F. Delange Executive Director of ICCIDD, Avenue de la Fauconnerie 153, 1170 Brussels, Belgium

K. M. Derwahl Department of Medicine, St. Willehad Hospital, Ansgaristr. 12, 26382 Wilhelmshaven, Germany

O. Dohan Dept. of Molecular Pharmacology, Albert Einstein College of Medicine, 1300 Morris Park Avenue, Bronx, NY 10461, USA

A. V. Dreval Moscow Regional Research Clinical Institute, Shchepkinastr. 61/2, 129110 Moscow, Russia

H. A. Drexhage Dept Immunology/Lab Ee 838, Erasmus University, PO Box 1738, 3000 DR Rotterdam, The Netherlands

I. Duncea Dept. of Endocrinology, University of Medicine and Pharmacy, Memorandumului 7, 3400 Cluj-Napoca, Romania

L. H. Duntas Endocrine Unit, „Evgenidion Hospital“, University of Athens, Papadiamantopoulou 20, 11528 Athens, Greece

M. Dvořáková Institute of Endocrinology, Národkí 8, Prague, Czech Republic

E. V. Epshtein Institute of Endocrinology & Metabolism, Vyshgorodska Str. 69, 04114 Kiev, Ukraine

A. P. Farwell Univ. of Mass. Medical Center, Div. of Endocrinology & Metabolism, 55 Lake Avenue North, Worcester, MA 01655, USA

U. Feldt-Rasmussen Division Endocrinology, University Hospital, Blegdamsvej 9, 2100 Copenhagen, Denmark

E. Gaitan P. O. Box 5091, Jackson, MS 39296–5091, USA

M. Ghemigian „C. I. Parhon“ Insitute of Endocrinology, Aviatorilor Blvd. 32 – 36, 71279 Bucharest, Romania

D. Glinoer University Hospital Saint-Pierre, Thyroid Investigation Clinic, 322 rue Haute, 1000 Brussels, Belgium

C. Grossegger Dept. for Nuclear Medicine, Krankenanstalt Rudolfstiftung, Juchgasse 25, 1030 Vienna, Austria

R. Hampel Klinik für Innere Medizin., E.-Heydemann-Str. 6, 18057 Rostock, Germany

L. Hegedüs Department Medicine & Endocrinology, Odense University Hospital, 5000 Odense, Denmark

K. Hristozov Medical University, Dept of Endocrinology, Marin Drinov 55, 9002 Varma, Bulgaria

S. Ismailov Institute of Endocrinological Academy of Sciences, Abdullaeva Str. 56, 700143 Tashkent, Uzbekistan

G. J. Kahaly Depts. of Endocrinology/Metabolism, Gutenberg-University Hospital, Langenbeckstr. 1, 55101 Mainz, Germany

T. S. Kaminina Moscow Regional Clinical Research Clinical Institute, 61/2, Shchepkina str, 129110 Moscow, Russia

E. P. Kasatkina Russian Medical Academy of Postgraduate Education, Chasovaya st. 20, 125315 Moscow, Russia

D. Kirienko City Clinical Endocrinological Hospital, Puschkinskaya Str. 22a, 01004 Kiev, Ukraine

J. Köhrle Klinische Forschergruppe, Medizinische Poliklinik, Röntgenring 11, 97070 Würzburg, Germany

L. Koeva Clinic of Endocrinology, Medical University of Varna, Varna, Bulgaria

A. Konrády „Jávorszky Ödön“ Hospital, Argenti Dömetér 1–3, 2700 Vác, Hungary

D. A. Koutras Athens University Endocrine Unit, Evgenidion Hospital, Papadiamantopoulou 20, 11528 Athens, Greece

A. Kurtaran University of Vienna, Dept. of Nuclear Medicine, Waehringer Gürtel 18 – 20, 1090 Vienna, Austria

P. Langer Institute of Exp. Endocrinology, Vlarska 3, 833 06 Bratislava, Slovakia

P. Laurberg Aalborg Hospital, Department Internal Medicine and Endocrinology, 9000 Aalborg, Denmark

J. Lazarus University of Wales College of Medicine, Heath Park, CF14 4XN Cardiff, Wales, United Kingdom

J. Leclère Service d'Endocrinologie, Centre Hospitalier Universitaire de Nancy, Hopitaux de Brabois, Rue de Morvan, 54511 Vandoeuvre Cédex, France

A. Lewiński Department of Thyroidology, Institute of Endocrinology, Medical University Łodź, Dr. Sterling 5, 91425 Łodź, Poland

C. Liberman University of Chile, Santos Dumont 999, Santiago de Chile, Chile

E. Martino Istituto di Endocrinologica, Università di Pisa, Via Paradisa 2, 56124 Tirrenia – Pisa, Italy

D. Metreveli Center of Endocrinology, Metabolism and Dietology, Tsinandali 9, 380044 Tbilisi, Georgia

V. Mogos University of Medicine and Pharmacy, Bd Independentei 1, 6600 Iasi, Romania

Á. Muzsnai Buda Children's Hospital, Bolyai 5–7, 1023 Budapest, Hungary

O. A. Netchaeva Moscow Regional Research Clinical Institute, Shchepkinastr. 61/2, 129110 Moscow, Russia

H. Niepomniszcze Hospital de Clínicas, University of Buenos Aires, Av. Córdoba 2351, 1120 Buenos Aires, Argentina

Dr. F. Pacini Istituto di Endocrinologica, Università di Pisa, Via Paradisa 2, 56124 Tirrenia – Pisa, Italy

R. Paschke Universitätsklinikum Leipzig, Medizinische Klinik und Poliklinik III, Ph.-Rosenthal-Str. 27, 04103 Leipzig, Germany

L. Persani Institute of Endocrine Sciences, University of Milan, Via Ariosto 13, 20145 Milan, Italy

F. Péter Buda Children's Hospital, Bolyai 5–7, 1023 Budapest, Hungary

M. Petrova Clinic of Endocrinology, Medical University of Varna, Varna, Bulgaria

D. I. W. Phillips MCR Epidemiology Unit, Southampton General Hospital, Tremona Road, Southampton S09 4XY, United Kingdom

C. Poiana Institute of Endocrinology, „C.I.Parhon", Aviatorilor Blvd. 34–36, 79660 Bucharest, Romania

V. Potine The D. O. Ott Research Institute of Obstetrics and Gynocology, Mendeleyevskaya line 3, 199034 St. Petersburg, Russia

Ch. Reiners Klinik u. Poliklinik f. Nuklearmedizin, Josef-Schneider-Str. 2, 97080 Würzburg, Germany

J. Rendl Clinic of Nuclear Medicine, University of Würzburg, Josef-Schneider-Str. 2, 97080 Würzburg; Germany

P. Rodien Medecine C, CHU d'Angers, 4, rue Larrey, 49033 Angers Cédex 01, France

E. Roti Cattedra di Endocrinologia, Università degli Studi di Parma, Via A Gramsci 14, 43100 Parma, Italy

P. Santisteban Instituto de Investigaciones Biomédicas Alberto Sols, CSIC-UAM, Arturo Duperier 4, 28029 Madrid, Spain

L. A. Scheplyagina Research Center of Children's Health, Lomonosovsky pr. 2/62, 117296 Moscow, Russia

M. M. Simescu Institute of Endocrinology, Bul Aviatorilor 34 – 36, Bucharest, Bulgaria

I. Szabolcs Imre Haynal Univ Medical Sciences, Dept Medicine Budapest, H-1389 Budapest, Hungary

E. Toromanyan Republican Endocrinolgy Center, 31 Nalbandian Str., apt. 36, 375001 Yerevan, Armenia

O. Topolčan 2nd Dept. of Internal Medicine, Charles University Hospital, Plzen, Czech Republic

E. A. Troshina Russian Endocrinology Research Center, D. Ulyanova 11, Moscow, Russia

J. Vanderpas Centre Interuniversitaire, Hôpital Ambroise Paré, BD Kennedy 2, 7000 Mons, Belgium

M. P. J. Vanderpump Consulting Physician, Department of Endocrinology, The Royal Free Hospital, Pond street, London, United Kingdom

E. Zbranca Dept. of Endocrinology UMF „Gr. T. Popa", Universitatii Street 16, 6600 Iasi, Romania

G. Zettinig Department of Nuclear Medicine, University Hospital, Währinger Gürtel 18 – 20, 1090 Vienna, Austria

I. Zosin Clinic of Endocrinology, County Hospital N°.1, B – dul Liviu Rebreanu, 1900 Timi soara, Romania

Session I:

Environment, goiter and hypothyroidism

Chairpersons: P. Lind, H. Bürgi

Epidemiology of goiter and hypothyroidism

M. P. J. Vanderpump

Department of Endocrinology, Royal Free Hospital, Pond Street, London NW3 2QG, United Kingdom

Abstract

Thyroid disorders are amongst the most prevalent medical conditions and the limitations of epidemiological studies must be recognized. Their manifestations vary considerably from area to area and are determined principally by the availability of iodine in the diet. Many people within the large industrialized countries of Europe live in areas of low iodine intake.

The most common thyroid disease in the community is simple (diffuse) goiter. Clinical grading of thyroid size is subjective and imprecise, and differences exist in classifying goiter as diffuse or multinodular. Screening by ultrasonography results in much higher estimates of goiter prevalence than reported in studies in which goiter size was assessed by physical examination. In cross-sectional surveys, the prevalence of diffuse goiter declines with age, the greatest prevalence being in premenopausal women, and the ratio of women to men is at least 4:1. This decline in frequency of diffuse goiters with age is in contrast to the increase in frequency of thyroid nodules and thyroid antibodies with age. A higher prevalence of nodular goiter is found in areas of iodine deficiency.

In persons living in iodine-replete areas, the etiology of hypothyroidism is either chronic autoimmune disease (atrophic autoimmune thyroiditis or goitrous autoimmune thyroiditis (Hashimoto's thyroiditis)) or destructive treatment for thyrotoxicosis. The findings of the Whickham survey have a broad application to iodine-replete communities. Spontaneous hypothyroidism has a prevalence of between 1 and 2 %, is more common in older women, and is ten times more common in women than in men. Until recently, there were relatively few prevalence data concerning autoimmune thyroid disease in areas of iodine deficiency where a ten-fold lower prevalence is found. A 20-year follow-up of the Whickham cohort has provided incidence data and allowed the determination of risk factors for hypothyroidism in this period. The annual incidence of spontaneous hypothyroidism in women was 3.5 per 1000, rising to 4.1 per 1000 if all cases including those who had received destructive treatment for thyrotoxicosis were included, and rose with age. Raised serum thyrotropin (TSH) or positive anti-thyroid antibodies alone or in combination are associated with a significantly increased risk of hypothyroidism. Recently a ten-fold lower incidence rate of hypothyroidism in an area with relatively low iodine intake has been observed.

Introduction

Thyroid disorders are amongst the most prevalent medical conditions. Their manifestations vary considerably from area to area and are determined principally by the availability of iodine in the diet.

Thyroid dysfunction can be classified according to the severity of clinical findings, serum hormone levels, the presence or absence of anti-thyroid antibodies, or the biochemical or physiological effect in the target tissues. The problems encountered in epidemiological studies of thyroid disorders are those of definition, for example overt hypothyroidism and subclinical hypothyroidism, the selection criteria used, the influence of age, sex, environmental factors and the different techniques used for the measurement of thyroid hormones (27). The limitations of epidemiological studies of thyroid disorders should therefore be borne in mind when considering the reported frequency of thyroid diseases in different communities.

Almost one third of the world's population lives in areas of iodine deficiency and risk the consequences. Most of these people are in developing countries, but many in the large industrialized countries of Europe are also affected. In areas where the daily iodine intake is below 50 µg, goiter is usually endemic, and when the intake falls below 25 µg a day congenital hypothyroidism is seen (5). The prevalence of goiter in areas of severe iodine deficiency can be as high as 80 %. Iodization programs are of proven value in reducing goiter size and in preventing goiter development and cretinism in children. Autonomy can develop in nodular goiters, leading occasionally to thyrotoxicosis and iodization programs can also induce thyrotoxicosis, especially among those aged over 40 years with nodular goiters. Autoimmune thyroiditis or hypothyroidism has not been reported to complicate salt iodization programs (6). Until recently, there were few data concerning the prevalence of autoimmune thyroid disease in areas of iodine deficiency.

In iodine-replete areas, hypothyroidism is caused by autoimmune disease (either primary atrophic hypothyroidism or Hashimoto's thyroiditis) or is secondary to destructive treatment for thyrotoxicosis (either Graves' disease or nodular goiter). A cross-sectional study performed between 1972 and 1974 in Whickham, a mixed urban and rural area in NorthEast England, has documented the prevalence of thyroid disorders in an iodine-sufficient community (24). The 2779 subjects examined in the survey (82 % of the available sample) represented a one in six sample of the adult population aged over 18 years, and closely resembled the British population as a whole in terms of age, sex and social class. Other cross-sectional studies from Europe have corroborated the findings of the Whickham survey and therefore its findings have a broad application to iodine-replete communities (27, 28). Longitudinal studies are necessary to determine incidence rates, etiological risk factors and the natural history of the disease process. A 20-year follow-up of the Whickham cohort has determined outcomes in terms of thyroid disease in 87 % of the original survey population (26).

Diffuse and nodular goiter

The most common thyroid disease in the community is simple (diffuse) goiter. The clinical grading of thyroid size is subjective and imprecise (22). The World Health Organisation (WHO) grading system recognizes that an enlarged thyroid gland may be palpably but not visibly enlarged. Examiner variation is greatest in deciding whether a thyroid that is palpable but not visible is normal (WHO Stage O-A) or enlarged (WHO Stage O-B). Interexaminer variation may also lead to differences in classifying a goiter as diffuse or multinodular. There is also considerable overlap between the five WHO grades based on clinical criteria compared with thyroid volume estimated by ultrasonography. More recently, ultrasonography has been used in epidemiological studies to assess thyroid size, resulting in much higher estimates of goiter prevalence than in studies in which goiter size was assessed by physical examination (2,11,12).

Most studies define a thyroid that is visible as well as palpable as a goiter (WHO Grade 1 or above). Considerable regional variations exist even in non-endemic goiter areas. In cross-sectional surveys, the prevalence of diffuse goiter declines with age, the greatest prevalence being in premenopausal women, and the ratio of women to men is at least 4:1 (27). In the Whickham survey, 16 % of the cohort had small but easily palpable diffuse or multinodular goiters (24). In men, the prevalence of goiter declined with age from 7 % in those aged less than 25 years to 4 % in those aged 65 to 74 years. No goiters were detected among men aged over 75 years. Among the women, 26 % had a goiter; the frequency ranged from 31 % in those aged less than 45 years (mostly diffuse) to 12 % in those aged over 75 years (who had a higher proportion of nodular goiter) (see Figure 1).

Longitudinal studies confirm the decreasing frequency of diffuse goiter with age (27). In the 20-year follow-up of the Whickham cohort, 10 % of women and 2 % of men had a goiter, compared with 23 % and 5 % respectively among the same subjects at the first survey (26). The presence of a diffuse goiter was not predictive of any clinical or biochemical evidence of thyroid dysfunction. In women, there was no association between goiter and thyroid-antibody status in the initial survey, but at the 20-year follow-up there was a weak association. Although the order in which these events occurred is unknown, it would suggest an autoimmune etiology for some goiters. In this iodine-replete population, thyroid function was similar in the goitrous

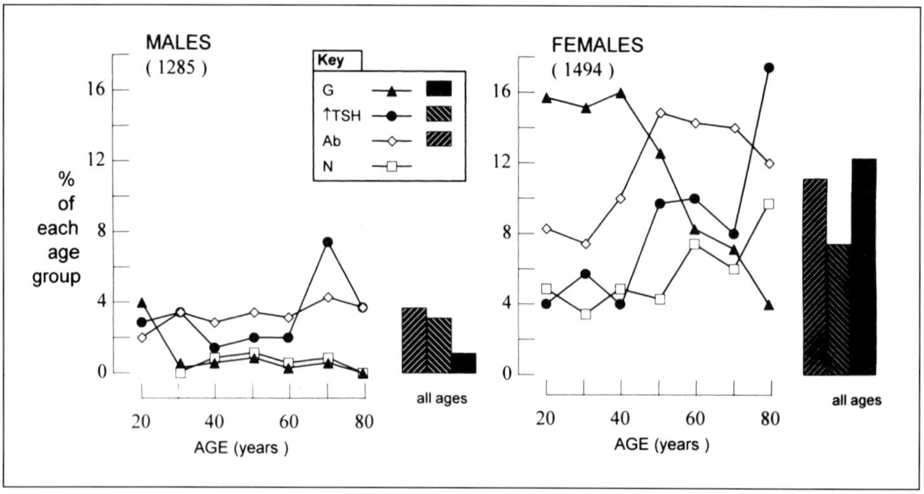

Fig. 1 Age and sex distribution of thyroid microsomal antibodies (Ab), raised serum TSH greater than 6mU/l (↑ TSH), visible diffuse and multinodular goiter (G) and nodules (N) in the Whickham survey (24).

and non-goitrous subjects. Serum TSH concentrations are raised only in very severe iodine deficiency.

This decline in frequency of diffuse goiters with age is in contrast to the increase in frequency of thyroid nodules and anti-thyroid antibodies with age (Figure 1). A nodular goiter may be solitary or part of a multinodular goiter. In the Whickham survey, fewer than 1 % of the men but 5 % of the women had thyroid nodules detected clinically and this frequency increased to 9 % in women aged over 75 (24). Among 5234 subjects aged over 60 years studied over a five-year period in Framingham, USA, the prevalence of single thyroid nodules was 3 % and that of multinodular goiter nodules was 1 % (19). A higher prevalence of nodular goiter is found in areas of iodine deficiency within Europe such as Italy, Germany and Denmark (Table 1). The only available longitudinal data suggest an annual incidence for nodules of 1 per 1000 and that, once formed, they tend to remain present and benign for a long period of time (25). In a survey of 101 women aged 49 to 58 years, thyroid nodules were detected by ultrasonography in 36 % of subjects, of whom less than a third were detected by palpation (2). Other European studies have similar prevalence rates (3, 12, 29). Ultrasonography as a screening tool is too sensitive and will result in unnecessary pursuit of findings so common that they can rarely have pathological significance. However, it may have a place in investigating patients presenting with thyroid nodules to determine whether they are single or multiple.

Table 1 Prevalence of nodular goiter by palpation in epidemiological studies.

Study (Reference)	N	Age (years)	Men		Women
Framingham, USA (20)	5127	30–59	1.5%		6.4%
Whickham, UK (24)	2779	18+	0.8%		5.3%
Pescopagano, Italy (1)	912	15+	58.0%		59.5%
Copenhagen, Denmark (11)	296	13–90		6.1%	
Uusimaa, Finland (2)	253	19–50		5.1%	
Wuppertal, Germany (12)	569	60+		17.6%	
Jutland, Denmark (16)	423	68+	3.2%		12.2%
Reykjavik, Iceland (16)	100	66–70		2%	

Hypothyroidism

The earliest biochemical abnormality in hypothyroidism is a rise in serum TSH associated with normal serum thyroxine (T_4) and triiodothyronine (T_3) concentrations (subclinical hypothyroidism), followed by a fall in serum T_4, at which stage most patients have symptoms and benefit from treatment (overt hypothyroidism). The etiology is rarely discussed in the available studies.

Prevalence of hypothyroidism

In the Whickham survey, the prevalence of newly diagnosed overt hypothyroidism was 3 per 1000 women (24). The prevalence of previously diagnosed and treated hypothyroidism was 14 per 1000 women, rising to 19 per 1000 women when possible but unproven cases were included. The overall prevalence in men was less than 1 per 1000. The mean age at diagnosis was 57 years. One-third had been previously treated by surgery or radioiodine for hyperthyroidism. Excluding iatrogenic causes, the prevalence of hypothyroidism was 10 per 1000 women, rising to 15 per 1000 when possible but unproven cases were included. The diagnosis was based on clinical features and high serum TSH and low free thyroxine index (FT_4I) values in the new cases, and from the original records in the previously diagnosed and treated cases. The figure of 3 new cases per 1000 women in the Whickham survey is comparable to other European studies (See Table 2). The prevalence was higher in surveys of the elderly in the community (4). The overall prevalence of hypothyroidism, including those already taking T_4, in Birmingham of 1210 subjects aged 60 and over was 4 % of women and 0.8 % of men aged over 60 years (18). In a survey in Sweden of 1442

Table 2 Prevalence of previously undiagnosed overt hypothyroidism and incidence of overt hypothyroidism in epidemiological surveys of thyroid dysfunction in Europe

Study Name	N	Age (years)	Test	Prevalence n/1000		Incidence n/1000/year		
				Men	Women	Follow-up	Men	Women
Whickham, UK (24,26)	2779	18+	TSH+T_4	0	3.3	20 years	0.6	3.5
South Finland (10)	3000	18+	TSH	2.0		–	–	–
Mölnlycke, Sweden (7)	2000	18+	TSH	1.3	12.0	–	–	–
Pescopagano, Italy (1)	992	15+	TSH+FT_4	0	0.4	–	–	–
Jutland, Denmark (15)	N/A	0+	TSH+FT_4	–	–	N/A	0.04	0.23
Kisa, Sweden (13)	3885	39–60	TSH+FT_4I	–	0	–	–	–
Göteborg, Sweden (17)	1283	44–66	TSH	–	6.4	4 years	–	1–2
Birmingham, UK (18)	1210	60+	TSH	7.8	20.5	1 year	11.1	
Kisa, Sweden (8)	1442	60+	TSH+FT_4I	-	5.5	–	–	–
Gothenburg, Sweden (23)	1148	70+	TSH	–	–	10 years	–	2

women aged 60 years or over, 6 per 1000 women were detected on the basis of symptoms and signs of hypothyroidism, elevated serum TSH greater than 13 mU/L, and a therapeutic response to T_4. In addition, a further 6 per 1000 were already on T_4 but only two because of primary hypothyroidism (8).

Cross-sectional data for autoimmune thyroid disease in areas of iodine deficiency now exist. In the iodine-deficient community of Pescopagano, Italy, the prevalence of newly diagnosed overt hypothyroidism was 0.3 % of 573 women (autoimmune thyroiditis confirmed as etiology) and none of 419 men (1).

Subclinical hypothyroidism

The term subclinical hypothyroidism is used to describe the finding of a raised serum TSH but a normal free T_4 (FT_4) in an asymptomatic patient. It represents a compensated state in which increased TSH output is required to maintain normal circulating thyroid hormone levels. An elevated serum TSH is a sensitive indicator of some degree of thyroid failure and a clear inverse relationship is found with FT_4 levels. Serum TSH concentrations do not change as a function of age among adult men, but among women over 40 years the concentrations increase markedly. If, however, women with anti-thyroid antibodies are excluded, there is no age-related increase (Figure 1). Nearly all of the older women with elevated serum TSH values have subclinical hypothyroidism. With respect to epidemiological studies, the definition of subclinical hypothyroidism varies from any increase in serum TSH to values greater than 10 mU/L or more stringently, a serum TSH value greater than 10 mU/L and a positive test for circulating thyroid antibodies in serum. It is commonly found either post radioiodine therapy or post surgery in up to 50 % of apparently euthyroid patients. It may be evident for only a few months, but, more often, it represents a stage in the progression towards overt thyroid failure. Less frequent causes include external beam irradiation of malignant tumors of the head and neck, and drugs including lithium and amiodarone. In the community, the most common etiology is chronic autoimmune thyroiditis (27).

In the Whickham survey, 8 % of women (10 % of women aged over 55 years) and 3 % of men had subclinical hypothyroidism (24). Community studies of elderly subjects have confirmed the high prevalence in this age group, approximately 10 % of subjects over 60 years having serum TSH values above the normal range (4, 14).

In iodine-deficient Pescopagano the prevalence of subclinical hypothyroidism was slightly lower at 4 % of women and 3 % of men but the prevalence of anti-thyroid antibodies was similar, although at lower titers, to that in iodine-replete communities (1). There is a higher frequency of subclinical hypothyroidism (18 % in Iceland and 24 % in Hungary) in areas where iodine intake is high but most cases are not of autoimmune origin (16, 21).

Incidence of hypothyroidism

The 20-year follow-up of the Whickham cohort has provided incidence data and allowed the determination of risk factors for hypothyroidism in this period (26). The mean annual incidence of spontaneous hypothyroidism among women surviving over the 20-year follow-up period was 3.5 per 1000 (95 % confidence interval (CI) 2.8 to 4.5). The prevalence rose to 4.1 per 1000 (95 % CI 3.3 to 5.0) if all cases including those who had received destructive treatment for thyrotoxicosis were included. Only 9 % of cases of spontaneous hypothyroidism among surviving women were diagnosed when they were aged less than 45 years, and 51 % were diagnosed between the ages 45 and 64 years. The hazard rate, that is the estimate of the probability of a woman developing hypothyroidism at a particular time, increased with age to 13.7 per 1000 among women aged between 75 and 80 years. The mean annual incidence during the 20-year follow-up period in men (all spontaneous except for one case of lithium-induced hypothyroidism) was 0.6 per 1000 (95 % CI 0.3 to 1.2). The incidence rates for the deceased women and men were similar.

The odds ratios (with 95 % CI) of developing spontaneous hypothyroidism among surviving women in the Whickham cohort are shown in Table 3. Raised serum TSH or positive anti-thyroid antibodies alone or in combination are associated with a significantly increased risk of hypothyroidism. The odds are greatly increased when both risk factors are present and each had a similar effect. The smaller number of ob-

Table 3 Development of spontaneous hypothyroidism in surviving women and men at 20-year follow-up of Whickham survey: odds ratios (with 95 % CI) (26)

Women	
TSH raised, regardless of thyroid antibody status	14 (9–24)
Thyroid antibody + , regardless of TSH status	13 (8–19)
If thyroid antibody – , effect of raised TSH alone	8 (3–20)
If thyroid antibody + , additional effect of raised TSH	5 (2–11)
If TSH normal, effect of thyroid antibody + alone	8 (5–15)
If TSH raised, additional effect of thyroid antibody +	5 (1–15)
TSH raised and thyroid antibody + combined	38 (22–65)
Men	
TSH raised, regardless of thyroid antibody status	44 (19–104)
Thyroid antibody + , regardless of TSH status	25 (10–63)
TSH raised and thyroid antibody + combined	173 (81–370)

served cases in men resulted in wide but highly significant confidence limits and did not allow the independent effects of these risk factors to be calculated. Among surviving women, the annual risk of developing spontaneous hypothyroidism was 4 % in those who had both raised serum TSH values and were thyroid-antibody positive, 3 % if only serum TSH was raised, and 2 % if only anti-thyroid antibodies were positive. At the time of follow-up, the respective rates of hypothyroidism were 55 %, 33 % and 27 %. The probability of developing hypothyroidism in women was plotted against log serum TSH as measured at first survey (Figure 2). The graph indicates that a serum TSH above 2mU/L is associated with an increased probability of hypothyroidism. The probability is further increased anti-thyroid antibodies are positive and decreased if they are negative. The development of hypothyroidism also correlated with the titer of antithyroid microsomal antibodies at first survey. Positive family history of any form of thyroid disease, presence of a goiter at either the first or the follow-up survey, and parity at first survey were not associated with an increased risk of hypothyroidism. These results confirm those from a four-year follow-up of a subgroup of women in the Whickham survey cohort in whom overt hypothyroidism had developed at a rate of 5 % per year in those who initially had a raised serum TSH and a positive test for thyroid antibodies (27). Either alone however, was not associated with an increased risk of hypothyroidism at four years.

The other incidence data for hypothyroidism are from short (and often small) follow-up studies (see Table 2). They show a range dependent on the chosen threshold for serum TSH, thyroid antibody status, the size, age, and sex distribution of the sample, and the number of years of follow-up. A ten-fold lower incidence rate of hy-

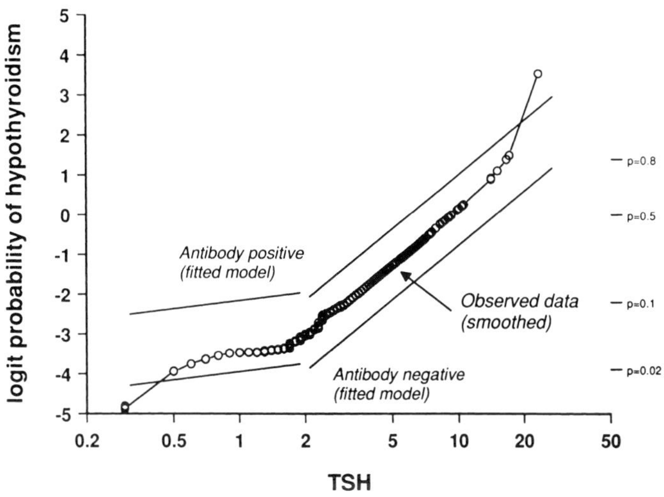

Fig. 2 Probability for development of hypothyroidism within 20 years with increasing values of serum TSH at first Whickham survey in 912 survivors (26).

pothyroidism has recently been reported in an area with relatively low iodine intake (15). In a follow-up study of 437 healthy women aged 40 to 60 years in the Netherlands, 24 % of those who initially had a positive test for anti-thyroid microsomal antibodies and normal serum TSH concentrations had an elevated serum TSH concentration (greater than 4.2mU/L) 10 years later, as compared with 3 % in the antibody-negative group (9). As in the 20-year follow-up of the Whickham cohort, serum TSH concentrations in the upper part of the normal range in this study also appeared to have a predictive value. Among elderly subjects, the annual incidence rate of hypothyroidism varies widely between 0.2 and 7 % in the available studies. In the survey of a Birmingham practice of 1210 subjects aged over 60 years, 18 % of those with high serum TSH on initial testing had proceeded to overt hypothyroidism by one year. Over half of these subjects with elevated serum TSH values were antithyroid microsomal antibody positive initially and they were the more likely to progress (18). The prognostic importance of positive thyroid antibodies has been confirmed in other studies (10, 14, 19).

References

1. Aghini-Lombardi F, Antonangelli L, Martino E et al. The spectrum of thyroid disorders in an iodine-deficient community: The Pescopagano Survey. J Clin Endocrinol Metab 1999; 84; 561–6.
2. Brander A, Viikinkowski P, Nickels J et al. Thyroid gland: US screening in middle-aged women with no previous thyroid disease. Radiology 1989; 173; 507–10.
3. Bruneton J-N, Balu-Maestro C, Marcy P-Y et al. Very high frequency (13MHz) ultrasonographic examination of the normal neck: Detection of normal lymph nodes and thyroid nodules. J Ultrasound Med 1994; 13; 87–90.
4. Chiovato L, Mariotti S, Pinchera A. Thyroid diseases in the elderly. Ballière's Clin Endocrinol Metab 1997; 11(2); 251–70.
5. Delange F. The disorders induced by iodine deficiency. Thyroid 1994; 4; 107–28.
6. Dunn JT. Adverse effects of iodine deficiency and its eradication by iodine supplementation. In: Contemporary endocrinology: diseases of the thyroid. Braverman LE, Ed. Totowa, NJ: Humana Press, Inc. 1997: 349–60.
7. Eggertsen R, Petersen K, Lundberg P-A et al. Screening for thyroid disease in a primary care unit with a thyroid stimulating hormone assay with a low detection limit. BMJ 1988; 297; 1586–91.
8. Falkenberg M, Kågedal B, Norr A. Screening of an elderly female population for hypo- and hyperthyroidism by use of a thyroid hormone panel. Acta Med Scand. 1983; 214; 361–5.
9. Geul KW, van Sluisveld ILL, Grobbee DE et al. The importance of thyroid microsomal antibodies in the development of elevated serum TSH in middle-aged women: associations with serum lipids. Clin Endocrinol 1993; 39; 275–80.
10. Gordin A, Heinonen OP, Saarinen P et al. Serum-thyrotrophin in symptomless autoimmune thyroiditis. Lancet 1972; I; 551–4.
11. Hegedus L, Perrild H, Poulsen LR et al. Determination of thyroid volume by ultrasound and its relationship to body weight, age and sex in normal subjects. J Clin Endocrinol Metab 1983; 56; 260–3.
12. Hintze G, Windeler J, Baumert J et al. Thyroid volume and goiter prevalence in the elderly as determined by ultrasound and their relationships to laboratory indices. Acta Endocrinol 1991; 124; 12–8.
13. Kågedal B, Månson JC, Norr A et al. Screening for thyroid disorders in middle-aged women by computer-assisted evaluation of a thyroid hormone panel. Scand J Clin Lab Invest 1981; 41; 403–8.
14. Lazarus JH, Burr ML, McGregor A et al. The prevalence and progression of autoimmune thyroid disease in the elderly. Acta Endocrinol 1984; 106;199–202.
15. Laurberg P, Bulow Pedersen I, Pedersen KM et al. Low incidence rate of overt hypothyroidism compared with hyperthyroidism in area with moderately low iodine intake. Thyroid 1999; 9; 33–8.
16. Laurberg P, Pedersen KM, Hreidarsson A et al. Iodine intake and the pattern of thyroid disorders: A comparative epidemiological study of thyroid abnormalities in the elderly in Iceland and in Jutland, Denmark. J Clin Endocrinol Metab 1998; 83; 765–9.
17. Nyström E, Bengtsson C, Lindquist O et al. Thyroid disease and high concentration of serum thyrotrophin in a population sample of women. Acta Med Scand. 1981; 210; 39–46.
18. Parle JV, Franklyn JA, Cross KW et al. Prevalence and follow-up of abnormal thyrotrophin (TSH) concentrations in the elderly in the United Kingdom. Clin Endocrinol 1991; 34; 77–83.
19. Sawin CT, Bigos ST, Land S et al. The ageing thyroid. Relationship between elevated serum thyrotropin level and thyroid antibodies in elderly patients. Am J Med 1985; 79; 591–5.
20. Sawin CT, Castelli WP, Hershman JM et al. The ageing thyroid. Thyroid deficiency in the Framingham Study. Arch Intern Med 1985; 145:1386–8.
21. Szabolcs I, Padoba J, Feldcamp J et al. Comparative screening for thyroid disorders in old age in areas of iodine deficiency, long-term iodine prophylaxis and abundant iodine intake. Clin Endocrinol 1997; 47; 87–93.
22. Siminoski K. Does this patient have a goiter? JAMA 1995; 273; 813–7.
23. Sundbeck G, Lundberg P-A, Lindstedt G et al. Incidence and prevalence of thyroid disease in elderly women: results from the longitudinal population study of elderly people in Gothenburg, Sweden. Age Ageing 1991; 20; 291–8.
24. Tunbridge WMG, Evered DC, Hall R et al. The spectrum of thyroid disease in the community: The Whickham Survey. Clin Endocrinol 1977; 7; 481–93.

25. Vander JB, Gaston EA, Dawber TR. The significance of nontoxic thyroid nodules. Final report of a 15-year study of the incidence of thyroid malignancy. Ann Intern Med 1968; 69; 537–40.
26. Vanderpump MPJ, Tunbridge WMG, French JM et al. The incidence of thyroid disorders in the community – A twenty-year follow-up of the Whickham survey. Clin Endocrinol 1995; 43; 55–69.
27. Vanderpump MPJ, Tunbridge WMG. The epidemiology of thyroid diseases. In: Werner and Ingbar's The Thyroid: A Fundamental and Clinical Text. 8th ed. Braverman LE, Utiger RD, Eds. Philadelphia: Lippincott Williams and Wilkins, in press.
28. Wang C, Crapo LM. The epidemiology of thyroid disease and implications for screening. Endocrinol Metab Clin North Am 1997; 26(1);189–217.
29. Woestyn J, Afschrift M, Schelstraete K et al. Demonstration of nodules in the normal thyroid by echography. Br J Radiology 1985; 58; 1179–82.

Genetic predisposition versus iodine deficiency as a risk factor for goiter and hypothyroidism

R. Paschke, S. Neumann

Department of Medicine III, University of Leipzig, Ph. Rosenthal Str. 27, 04103 Leipzig, Germany

Abstract

Iodine deficiency is the most important etiologic factor for euthyroid endemic goiter. However, not all individuals in an iodine deficient region develop goiter, and eradication of iodine deficiency does not result in eradication of goiter in all individuals. Moreover, several family and twin pair studies indicate a genetic predisposition for euthyroid simple goiter. In hypothyroid goiter, several molecular defects in the thyroglobulin (Tg), thyroperoxidase (TPO), and Na^+/I^--symporter (NIS) genes have been identified. The thyroid stimulating hormone receptor (TSHR) with its central role for thyroid function and growth is also a strong candidate gene. In a family with several relapsing euthyroid goiters or thyroidectomies for euthyroid goiter, we recently found evidence for linkage of familial euthyroid goiter to the previously identified locus for familial multinodular nontoxic goiter (MNG-1) on chromosome 14q. The haplotype cosegregates clearly with familial euthyroid goiter. These results provide the first confirmation for MNG-1 as a locus for nontoxic goiter. Together with the results of epidemiological, family and twin studies, these results suggest an underlying genetic predisposition for the development of euthyroid goiters in some patients with euthyroid goiters.

Genetic predisposition as a risk factor for goiter and hypothyroidism

Goiter is prevalent in areas of iodine deficiency. In Germany 52 % of 11 to 17 year-old children suffer from euthyroid endemic goiter due to the alimentary iodine deficiency (1). However, not all individuals in the same iodine-deficient region develop goiter, and iodine supplementation does not prevent goiter development in all treated subjects. Moreover, endemic goiter has also been found in areas with no iodine deficiency or even iodine excess (2). Therefore, a relative defect in secretory processes in response to low TSH stimulation representing a maladaptation to iodine deficiency among patients with large goiters has been suggested (3). Moreover, other etiologic factors are likely to be involved in the pathogenesis of euthyroid goiters. Besides iodine deficiency as the most important etiologic factor (4), and environmental factors, age, and sex, a genetic predisposition for goiter development has been observed. Family studies have shown that children of parents with goiter have a significantly higher incidence of goiter compared with children of healthy parents (5). Moreover, twin pair studies in endemic and nonendemic areas have clearly demonstrated a genetic predisposition for goiter development (6, 7). Furthermore, more rapidly growing goiters in a subgroup of 15–20 % of schoolchildren in spite of iodine supplementation (8) and differences in thyroid volume between adolescent siblings of similar age and adequate iodine intake in Slovakia (9) also support the hypothesis of a genetic influence on thyroid growth. Studies in Greek populations have shown the persistence of endemic goiter in certain regions despite iodine supplementation (10). Familial occurrence of euthyroid goiters in the iodine replete west coast region in Sweden was reported among 41 % of patients with goiter, and the frequency of familial occurrence was even higher among those with prepubertal development of the goiter (11). Therefore, genetic factors most likely play an important role in the development of endemic goiter and, to some extent also, in sporadic euthyroid goiter. The proteins involved in thyroid hormone synthesis, the sodium iodine symporter, thyroglobulin and thyroid peroxidase and the TSH receptor, are obviously the prime candidate genes for familial euthyroid goiters.

In hypothyroid goiters, several molecular defects in the thyroglobulin (Tg) and thyroperoxidase (TPO) genes have been identified. The extent of Tg mRNA expression induced by the different mutations was related to the degree of hypothyroidism (12–17). Recently, two different missense mutations in the Tg gene causing an abnormal three dimensional structure of Tg have been detected among patients whose thyroid function ranged from mildly hypothyroid to euthyroid (18). In a previous study, abnormalities in the degree of glycosylation and iodine content of thyroglobulin have been described among patients with nonendemic simple goiter (19). Some of these cases were associated with a point mutation in exon 10 of the Tg gene (20). The same mutation was observed in only one of 36 patients with endemic goiter (21).

Mutations responsible for dyshormongenesis have also been described in the TPO gene. Abnormal TPO synthesis is caused by a heterogeneous spectrum of TPO mutations (22–28), which lead to complete loss of, or a decrease in, TPO activity resulting in a total iodide organification defect (TIOD), i.e. inability to iodinate thyroglobulin. Most homozygous or compound heterozygous mutations lead to goiter and hypothyroidism. However, compensated thyroid function in adult life has been described for individuals with a TPO mutation in exon 14 resulting in a termination signal. Although this mutation occurred together with a TPO mutation resulting in a Gln660Glu exchange in exon 11, the functional consequences of which are unknown, these data suggest that the exon 11 mutation permits some TPO activity (29). Moreover, given a frequency of TIOD of 1 in 40,000 newborns and its autosomal recessive inheritance, the frequency of heterozygous TPO germline mutations should be about 1 %. It is not known, whether these individuals are at increased of developing goiter. Moreover, the clinical phenotype of the heterozygous parents or siblings of patients with TIOD has not been well characterized.

Since the cloning and molecular characterization of the human Na^+ / I^--symporter gene (NIS) (30), several defects in this gene have been detected in patients with different phenotypes of thyroid diseases (31–36). In contrast to the many homozygous NIS-mutations causing hypothyroidism, only one homozygous mutation in the NIS gene has so far been identified in a patient with euthyroid goiter (33). The subject's daughter with a heterozygous NIS-mutation displayed normal thyroid volume and normal thyroid function. However, the same mutation has also been described in a patient with goiter and congenital hypothyroidism due to a TIOD. Moreover, when expressed in HEK cells the mutated symporter resulted in a complete loss of iodide transport activity (31).

Mutations in the TSHR, which has a central role for thyroid function and growth, have been found in rare cases of congenital hypothyroidism (37, 38). However, the TSHR has been excluded as a candidate gene for familial congenital hypothyroidism (39). It was also excluded as a candidate gene in a family with nontoxic multinodular goiter (MNG) (40). However, MNG-1 on chromosome 14q outside the TSHR locus was established as a susceptibility locus in the same family.

Case studies

Recurrent or relapsing goiter occurring in families represents a phenotype strongly suggesting a genetic etiology. However, few studies have addressed the possible molecular defects. We therefore investigated a patient with euthyroid relapsing goiter and her family, of whom several had goiters (41). The family pedigree is described in Figure 1.

Patient II-2 (51 years)

At the age of 26, euthyroid goiter was identified. Thyroid resection was carried out at the age of 30, followed by postoperative thyroid hormone substitution with 125 µg thyroxine.

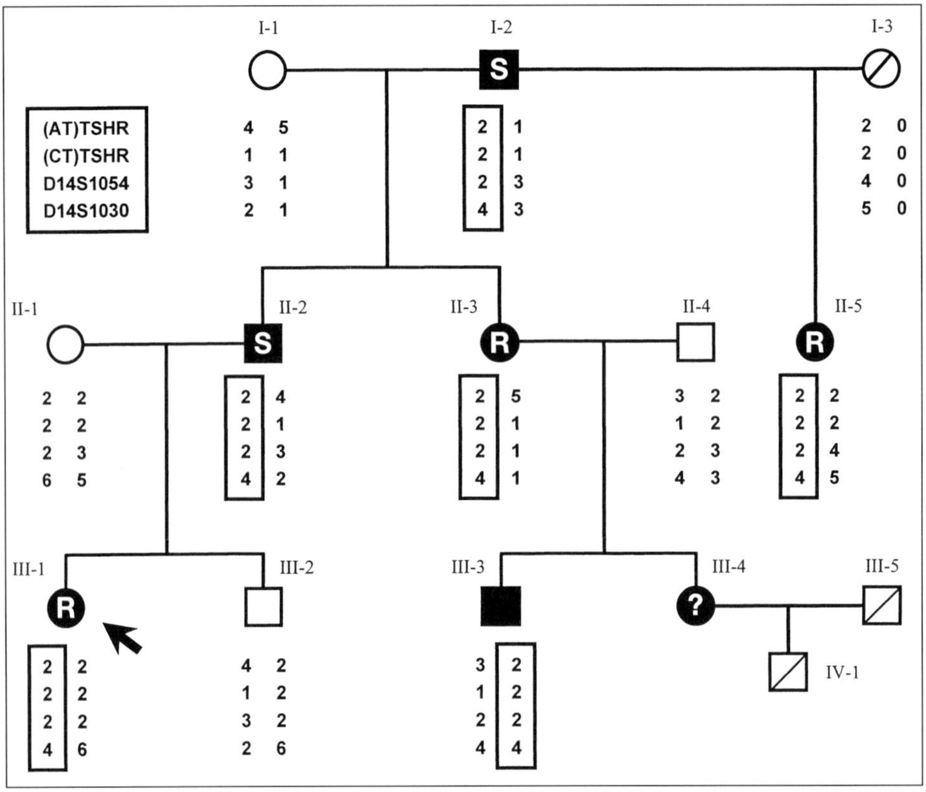

Fig. 1 Family pedigree and results of haplotype analysis.
The proband is patient III-1 (black arrow). The question marks denote individuals not available for testing. The haplotype is shown below each individual. The haplotype that cosegregated with euthyroid simple goiter is shown inside the boxes. The order of the markers is indicated in the box in the upper left corner.
Symbols: ○ = ♀ □ = ♂
● ■ goiter ; ○ □ no goiter; ⊘ ⊠ no examination
R = goiter relapse despite thyroid hormone replacement
S = Surgery < 30 years

Patient II-3 (48 years)

At the age of 19 years, euthyroid goiter was diagnosed. Since treatment with thyroxine did not lead to volume reduction, the patient underwent subtotal thyroidectomy at the age of 22. The goiter recurred while the patient was on postoperative thyroid hormone replacement. She therefore underwent total thyroid resection. At present, the patient is euthyroid on 100 μg thyroxine per day.

Patient II-5 (37 years)

An enlarged thyroid gland was found at the age of 15 years. Because of unsuccessful therapy with thyroxine, the patient underwent resection of the thyroid gland at the age of 16. She experienced a recurrence of goiter on thyroxine replacement. A second thyroidectomy was performed. She currently takes 100 µg thyroxine per day. There is no evidence of thyroid enlargement.

Patient III-1 (18 years, proband)

Euthyroid goiter was identified at the age of six years. Thyroxine treatment was started at a dosage of 100 µg thyroxine per day. During the following year, she presented with increased thyroid volume. She underwent subtotal resection of the thyroid gland followed by therapy with 100/200 µg thyroxine/iodine per day. Subtotal resection was repeated five years later because of recurrent goiter (14 ml). She experienced a second recurrence of goiter at the age of 15 years. She currently takes 125 µg thyroxine per day.

Patient III-3 (23 years) and III-4 (28 years)

Both individuals presented with mild thyroid enlargement and euthyroidism. Thyroxine and iodine were started with 100/200 µg thyroxine/iodine per day.

Further family members

Family members I-1, II-4 and III-2 showed normal thyroid hormones with no sign of thyroid enlargement. Subjects I-3, III-5 and IV-1 could not be investigated.

Results and discussion

Among hypothyroid patients with goiter, mutations in the Tg, TPO, and NIS genes have been detected as a molecular cause. It is likely that development of euthyroid goiter is a compensatory mechanism for genetic defects that are similar to those found in hypothyroid patients, but with minor functional consequences, especially under conditions of iodine deficiency. In order to investigate this hypothesis, we examined a subject with two recurrences of euthyroid goiter and a well documented familial history of euthyroid goiter (see Figure 1). Members of the subject's family were carefully characterized. On collection of clinical data from the family, it was apparent that males were more often affected than females. Since women are usually more commonly affected, this was an unusual finding. This observation together with the family history and the recurrent goiter in the proband suggested the existence of molecular alterations. We therefore investigated the mRNA transcripts of the Tg and TPO genes from the proband's goiter tissue by Northern blot analysis, but could not detect a difference in size and quantity in comparison to control thyroid tissue. Owing to the inherently lower sensitivity of the method, detection of mRNA transcripts of the NIS gene with Northern blot was not possible. We therefore examined the NIS mRNA transcript by RNase protection assay, which is more sensitive than Northern analysis. In contrast to the Tg and TPO gene, the amount of the NIS mRNA transcript was markedly decreased in the goiter tissue compared to normal thyroid tissue. Since no splice variants by RT-PCR and no nucleotide changes could be detected in the NIS cDNA and since the NIS gene was excluded as candidate gene by linkage analysis, the decreased NIS expression is most likely a secondary event. The mechanisms regulating the human NIS gene are largely unknown at present. It is conceivable that downregulation of NIS gene expression in the large goiter maintains euthyroidism in the proband through decreased I^- uptake activity in the goiter tissue with normal Tg and TPO gene expression in spite of thyroid growth. A distinctly higher NIS mRNA transcript level was observed in thyroid tissue from a patient with Graves' disease, which was also used as a control. This observation confirms the findings of Saito et al. (42) who showed that the expression of human NIS is increased in Graves' thyroid tissue compared to normal thyroid tissue.

Since examination of Tg and TPO mRNA expression did not indicate a functionally important genetic alteration, further studies were required. Linkage analysis with microsatellite markers was used to test the hypothesis that the candidate genes Tg, TPO, NIS, and TSHR contribute to the euthyroid goiter disease in this family. On linkage analysis, the polymorphic microsatellite markers for the genes Tg, TPO, and NIS gave two-point and multipoint LOD scores that were negative or below 1 for all assumed recombination fractions. Since no significant evidence for linkage was found on the assumption of either homogeneity or heterogeneity, we conclude that these candidate genes can be excluded as a major cause for the euthyroid goiter disease in this family. By contrast, we found evidence for linkage of familial euthyroid goiter to a locus on chromosome 14q, first described by Bignell et al. (40) as a locus for nontoxic multinodular goiter – MNG-1 – in a large Canadian family. The haplotype clearly cosegregates with euthyroid goiter in our family (Fig. 1). To our knowledge, these results are the first confirmation for the MNG-1 locus as a susceptibility gene locus for nontoxic goiter on chromosome 14q. Using linkage analysis, Tomer et al. (43) identified the GD-1 locus on chromosome 14q31 that was linked to Graves' disease. GD-1 was localized within 2 cM of the MNG-1 locus for nontoxic multinodular goiter. Consequently, our data also support the hypothesis (44) postulating the presence of a thyroid disease gene complex on chromosome 14q, etiologically related to thyroid diseases in general.

In previous studies the TSHR has been excluded as a candidate gene for familial congenital hypothyroidism (39), multinodular nontoxic goiter (40) and Graves' disease (43) by linkage analysis. However, in our family the TSHR gene could not be excluded as a candidate locus by linkage analysis, in particular since for both TSHR microsatellites the haplotype cosegregates with familial euthyroid goiter (Fig. 1). We therefore sequenced the entire TSHR coding region. However, except for a polymorphism, no genetic alteration could be detected. To investigate the relevance of the linkage results in this family we are currently examining further families for linkage to these markers.

Acknowledgement

This work was supported by the Fritz-Thyssen-Stiftung (934 000–89).

References

1. Hampel R, Kulberg T, Klein K, et al. Goiter incidence in Germany is greater than previously suspected. Med Klin 1995; 90; 324–329.
2. Suzuki H, Higuchi T, Sawa K, Ohtaki S, Horiuchi Y. "Endemic coast goitre" in Hokkaido, Japan. Acta Endocrinologica 1965; 50; 161–176.
3. Dumont JE, Ermans AM, Maenhaut C, Coppee F, Stanbury JB. Large goitre as a maladaptation to iodine deficiency. Clin Endocrinol (Oxf.) 1995; 43; 1–10.
4. Eastman CJ, Phillips DIW. Endemic goitre and iodine deficiency disorders: Aetiology, epidemiology and treatment. Bailliere's Clin Endocrinol Metab 1988; 2; 719–735.
5. Malamos B, Koutras DA, Kostamis P, Kralios AC, Rigopoulos G, Zerefos N. Endemic goiter in Greece: epidemiologic and genetic studies. J Clin Endocrinol Metab 1966; 26; 688–695.
6. Greig WR, Boyle JA, Duncan A, et al. Genetic and non-genetic factors in simple goitre formation: Evidence from a twin study. Q J Med 1967; 142; 175–188.
7. Malamos B, Koutras DA, Kostamis P. Endemic goitre in Greece: A study of 379 twin pairs. J Med Genet 1967; 4; 16–18.
8. Tajtakova M, Langer P, Gonsorcikova V, Bohov P, Hancinova D. Recognition of a subgroup of adolescents with rapidly growing thyroids under iodine-replete conditions: seven year follow-up. Eur J Endocrinol 1998; 138; 674–680.
9. Langer P, Tajtakova M, Bohov P, Klimes I. Possible role of genetic factors in thyroid growth rate and in the assessment of upper limit of normal thyroid volume in iodine-replete adolescents. Thyroid 1999; 9; 557–562.
10. Doufas AG, Mastorakos G, Chatziioannou S, et al. The predominant form of non-toxic goiter in Greece is now autoimmune thyroiditis. Eur J Endocrinol 1999; 140; 505–511.
11. Heimann P. Familial incidence of thyroid disease and anamnestic incidence of pubertal struma in 449 consecutive struma patients. Acta Med Scand 1966; 179; 113–119.
12. Ieiri T, Cochaux P, Targovnik HM, et al. A 3' splice site mutation in the thyroglobulin gene responsible for congenital goiter with hypothyroidism. J Clin Invest 1991; 88; 1901–1905.
13. Targovnik HM, Cochaux P, Corach D, Vassart G. Identification of a minor Tg mRNA transcript in RNA from normal and goitrous thyroids. Mol Cell Endocrinol 1992; 84; R23-R26.

14. Targovnik HM, Medeiros-Neto G, Varela V, Cochaux P, Wajchenberg BL, Vassart G. A nonsense mutation causes human hereditary congenital goiter with preferential production of a 171-nucleotide-deleted thyroglobulin ribonucleic acid messenger. J Clin Endocrinol Metab 1993; 77; 210–215.
15. Targovnik HM, Vono J, Billerbeck AE, et al. A 138-nucleotide deletion in the thyroglobulin ribonucleic acid messenger in a congenital goiter with defective thyroglobulin synthesis. J Clin Endocrinol Metab 1995; 80; 3356–3360.
16. Targovnik HM, Frechtel GD, Mendive FM, et al. Evidence for the segregation of three different mutated alleles of the thyroglobulin gene in a Brazilian family with congenital goiter and hypothyroidism. Thyroid 1998; 8; 291–297.
17. Tarkovnik HM, Varela V, Frechtel GD, et al. Molecular genetics of hereditary thyroid diseases due a defect in the thyroglobulin or thyroperoxidase synthesis. Braz J Med Biol Res 1994; 27; 2745–2757.
18. Hishinuma A, Takamatsu J, Ohyama Y, et al. Two novel cysteine substitutions (C1263R and C1995S) of thyroglobulin cause a defect in intracellular transport of thyroglobulin in patients with congenital goiter and the variant type of adenomatous goiter. J Clin Endocrinol Metab 1999; 84; 1438–1444.
19. Mories T, Miralles JM, Reglero A, Felipe S, Corrales JJ, Garcia LC. A study of thyroglobulin and peroxidase activity in the thyroid tissue of patients with non-endemic non-toxic nodular goitre. Clin Sci (Colch.) 1991; 80; 301–307.
20. Corral J, Martin C, Perez R, et al. Thyroglobulin gene point mutation associated with non-endemic simple goitre. Lancet 1993; 341; 462–464.
21. Perez-Centeno C, Gonzalez-Sarmiento R, Mories MT, Corrales JJ, Miralles-Garcia JM. Thyroglobulin exon 10 gene point mutation in a patient with endemic goiter. Thyroid. 1996; 6; 423–427.
22. Abramowicz MJ, Tarkovnik HM, Varela V, et al. Identification of a mutation in the coding sequence of the human thyroid peroxidase gene causing congenital goiter. J Clin Invest 1992; 90; 1200–1204.
23. Bikker H, Vulsma T, Baas F, de Vijlder JJM. Identification of five novel inactivating mutations in the human thyroid peroxidase gene by denaturing gradient gel electrophoresis. Human Mutation 1995; 6; 9–16.
24. Bikker H, Waelkens JJJ, Bravenboer B, de Vijlder JJM. Congenital hypothyroidism caused by a premature termination signal in exon 10 of the human thyroid peroxidase gene. J Clin Endocrinol Metab 1996; 81; 2076–2079.
25. Bikker H, Baas F, de Vijlder JJM. Molecular analysis of mutated thyroid peroxidase detected in patients with total iodide organification defects. J Clin Endocrinol Metab 1997; 82; 649–653.
26. Bikker H, Bakker E, Vulsma T, de Vijlder JJM. Identification of two novel mutations in the TPO gene of patients with severe congenital hypothyroidism due to a total iodide organification defect-frequency of TPO inactivating mutations. J Endocrinol Invest 1998; 21; 82.
27. Bikker H, den Hartog MT, Baas F, Gons MH, Vulsma T, de Vijlder JJ. A 20-basepair duplication in the human thyroid peroxidase gene results in a total iodide organification defect and congenital hypothyroidism. J Clin Endocrinol Metab 1994; 79; 248–252.
28. Pannain S, Weiss RE, Jackson CE, et al. Two different mutations in the thyroid peroxidase gene of a large inbred Amish kindred: power and limits of homozygosity mapping. J Clin Endocrinol Metab 1999; 84; 1061–1071.
29. Santos CL, Bikker H, Rego KG, et al. A novel mutation in the TPO gene in goitrous hypothyroid patients with iodide organification defect. Clin Endocrinol (Oxf.) 1999; 51; 165–172.
30. Smanik PA, Liu Q, Furminger TL, et al. Cloning of the human sodium iodide symporter. Biochem Biophys Res Communications 1996; 226; 339–345.
31. Fujiwara H, Tatsumi K, Miki K, et al. Congenital hypothyroidism caused by a mutation in the Na^+/I^-symporter. Nature Genetics 1997; 16; 124–125.
32. Fujiwara H, Tatsumi K, Miki K, et al. Recurrent T354P mutation of the Na^+/I^- symporter in patients with iodide transport defect. J Clin Endocrinol Metab 1998; 83; 2940–2943.
33. Matsuda A, Kosugi S. A homozygous missense mutation of the sodium /iodide symporter gene causing iodide transport defect. J Clin Endocrinol Metab 1997; 82; 3966–3971.
34. Pohlenz J, Medeiros-Neto G, Gross JL, Silveiro SP, Knobel M, Refetoff S. Hypothyroidism in a Brazilian kindred due to iodide trapping defect caused by a homozygous mutation in the sodium/iodide symporter gene. Biochem Biophys Res Communications 1997; 240; 488–491.
35. Pohlenz J, Rosenthal IM, Weiss RE, Jhiang SM, Burant C, Refetoff S. Congenital hypothyroidism

due to mutations in the sodium/iodide symporter. Identification of a nonsense mutation producing a downstream cryptic 3' splice site. J Clin Invest 1998; 101; 1028–1035.
36. Pohlenz J, Refetoff S. Mutations in the sodium/iodide symporter (NIS) gene as a cause for iodide transport defects and congenital hypothyroidism. Biochimie 1999; 81; 469–476.
37. Abramowicz MJ, Duprez L, Parma J, Vassart G, Heinrichs C. Familial congenital hypothyroidism due to inactivating mutation of the thyrotropin receptor causing profound hypoplasia of the thyroid gland. J Clin Invest 1997; 99; 3018–3024.
38. Krude H, Biebermann H, Gopel W, Gruters A. The gene for the thyrotropin receptor (TSHR) as a candidate gene for congenital hypothyroidism with thyroid dysgenesis. Exp Clin Endocrinol Diabetes 1996; 4;117–120.
39. Ahlbom BE, Yaqoob M, Larsson Agne, Ilicki A, Anneren G, Wadelius C. Genetic and linkage analysis of familial congenital hypothyroidism: exclusion of linkage to the TSH receptor gene. Hum Genet 1997; 99; 186–190.
40. Bignell GR, Canzian F, Shayeghi M, et al. Familial nontoxic multinodular thyroid goiter locus maps to chromosome 14q but does not account for familial nonmedullary thyroid cancer. Am J Hum Genet 1997; 61; 1123–1130.
41. Neumann S, Willgerodt H, Ackermann F, Reske A, Jung M, Reis A, Paschke R. Linkage of familial euthyroid goiter to the multinodular goiter-1 locus and exclusion of the candidate genes thyroglobulin, thyroperoxidase, and Na^+/I^- symporter. J Clin Endocrinol Metab 1999; 84; 3750–3756.
42. Saito T, Endo T, Kawaguchi A, et al. Increased expression of the Na^+/I^- symporter in cultured human thyroid cells exposed to thyrotropin and in Graves' thyroid tissue. J Clin Endocrinol Metab 1997; 82; 3331–3336.
43. Tomer Y, Barbesino G, Keddache M, Greenberg DA, Davies TF. Mapping of a major susceptibility locus for Graves' disease (GD-1) to chromosome 14q31. J Clin Endocrinol Metab 1997; 82; 1645–1648.
44. Brix TH, Kyvik KO, Hegedus L. What is the evidence of genetic factors in the etiology of Graves' disease? A brief review. Thyroid 1998; 8; 727–734.

Selenium and iodine deficiency as risk factors for goiter and hypothyroidism

J. Vanderpas

École de Santé Publique, Campus Erasme, 808 route de Lennick, 1070 Brussels, Belgium

Abstract

Until the end of the eighties, selenium deficiency in humans was associated, mainly in rural villages of People's Republic of China, with an osteoarthropathy named Kashin-Beck disease and a cardiomyopathy named Keshan disease. In parallel with the characterization of iodothyronine 5'-deiodinase I as a selenium-containing enzyme, it was proposed that endemic myxedematous cretinism in endemic goiter areas of northern and eastern Congo (R.D) could be a third geographical disease associated with selenium deficiency. At present, what is the real impact of selenium deficiency on thyroid hormone metabolism in humans, and what is its clinical relevance?

First, when selenium deficiency alone is present (phenylketonuric subjects treated with a low protein diet), basal thyroid function (serum TSH, T_4, T_3 and rT_3) is normal. The correction of selenium deficiency is associated with a significant decrease of T_4 and rT_3, although both parameters remain in a normal range. The relative decrease of hormonal values compared to the basal values is much less pronounced than that of serum selenium or glutathione peroxidase. A biochemical effect of selenium on thyroid hormone concentrations is, then, observed, without clinical evidence of thyroid dysfunction (hypo- or hyperthyroidism).

Second, iodine deficiency is a major health problem in some parts of central Africa. Selenium deficiency could direct the natural course of cretinism towards the myxedematous form – in contrast to the neurological form predominant in most other goiter areas. However, selenium supplementation should not be implemented without concomitant iodine supplementation, at the risk of aggravating hypothyroidism.

Third, in Tibet, iodine deficiency is a public health priority. In a context of extreme selenium deficiency, endemic biochemical hypothyroidism was found to be more severe in Kashin-Beck cases than in age-matched unaffected children. It is not excluded that the correction of iodine deficiency will significantly decrease the incidence of Kashin-Beck disease, as endemic hypothyroidism seems to be associated with it. Recent observations in a rural Chinese villages of Shaanxi province

(Ang'Kan county) show that Kashin-Beck disease has disappeared soon after the introduction of iodized salt.

The epidemiological patterns of iodine- and selenium-deficiencies in the Congo and Tibet are, then, quite different: myxedematous cretinism is frequent and Kashin-Beck osteoarthropathy is absent in the northern and eastern Congo; the opposite pattern is observed in Tibet. A third cofactor such as thiocyanate in northern and eastern Congo and mycotoxins in Tibet has been proposed to explain this difference. Iodine supplementation is sufficient to eradicate goiter and cretinism in central Africa, and its possible preventive role on Kashin-Beck osteoarthropathy is not excluded.

In conclusion, there is an effect of selenium on thyroid hormone metabolism in humans, but it is marginal, even in the most extreme selenium deficient environment (Tibet). The correction of selenium deficiency should not be considered as a public health priority for its role on thyroid hormone metabolism. In humans, its possible preventive action remains limited, up to now, to Kashin-Beck osteoarthropathy and to Keshan cardiomyopathy.

Introduction

Selenium deficiency in humans was associated, until the end of the eighties, with two endemic diseases occurring mainly in a large belt crossing China from the north eastern extremity to the south western extremity, extending to Tibet Autonomous Region. One is a cardiomyopathy occurring in children and in pregnant women named Keshan disease, and the other is a progressive osteoarthropathy beginning in childhood named Kashin-Beck disease. At this point, it should be remembered that selenium deficiency in these geographically affected areas is extreme, with mean serum values below 127 nmol/l (10 ng/ml) (reference range for normal adults in industrialized countries: 762–1390 nmol/l [60–110 ng/ml]).

Besides these very peculiar clinical entities, the role of selenium was known as an essential trace element since 1957 in animal studies (1): deficiency is associated with liver necrosis, and the process is accelerated in case of concurrent vitamin E deficiency. Since then, in industrialized countries, there have been only anecdotal reports of benefits from selenium supplementation in severe malabsorption or in total parenteral nutrition. Actually, there is no clear evidence for selenium supplements in particular clinical entities.

At the end of the eighties, various teams working on thyroid hormone metabolism became interested in selenium for different reasons. In a few years from 1987 to 1990, many data were gathered on the role of this trace element in thyroid biochemistry. In a few words, the Aberdeen group in Scotland (2) was the first to show an effect of selenium deficiency on serum thyroxine and triiodothyronine concentrations in cattle; they invoked a physiological role in deiodination. This was clearly established in 1989–1990 by two independent teams, in Boston (3) and in Germany (4), that showed that at least one of the deiodinases (type I) was a selenium-containing enzyme. In parallel with these experimental studies, physicians in the Free University of Brussels observed that the selenium status was low in an iodine deficient area of eastern Congo (R. D., ex-Zaire) (5) and 2000 kilometers away in the northern part of the same country (6). The work in the Congo was conducted on the hypothesis that the well known effect of selenium deficiency on glutathione peroxidase (a selenium-containing enzyme known since in 1973 (7) might involve thyroid involution by hy-

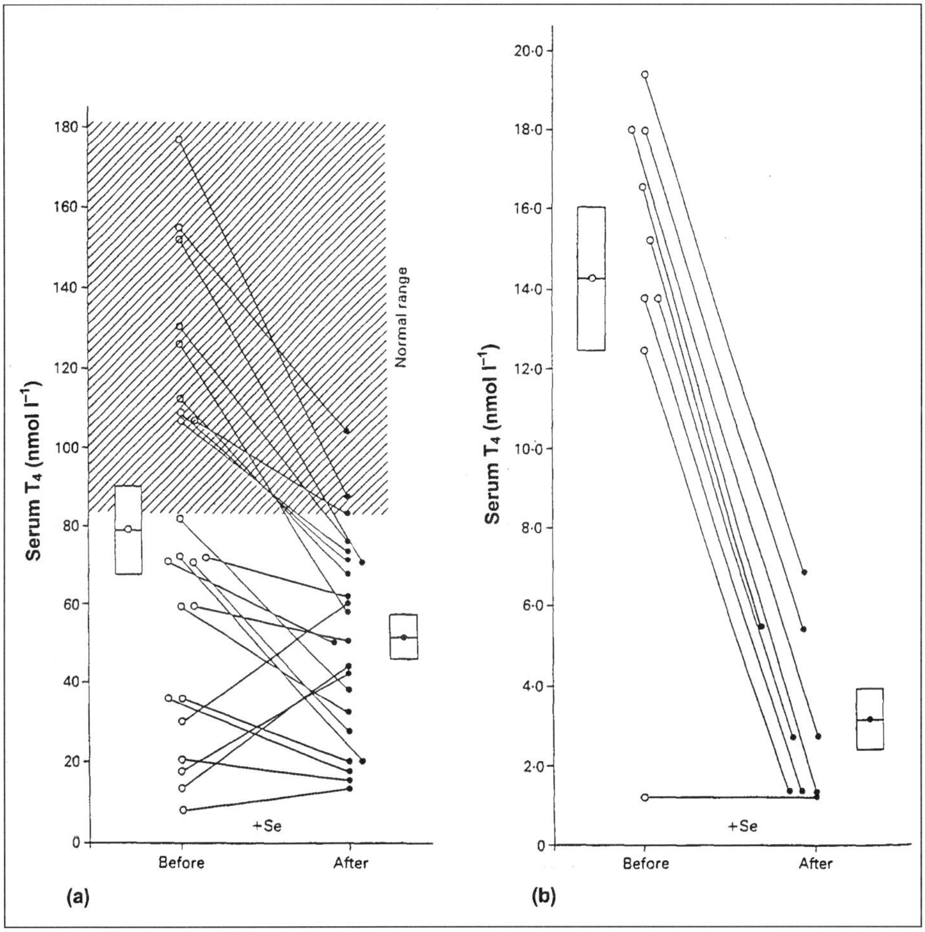

Fig. 1 Effect of 2 months of oral selenium (Se) supplementation (50 µg daily as tablets of selenomethionine) in Se- and iodine-deficient subjects of Congo on serum thyroxine (T_4) concentration. **(a)** Normal schoolchildren, **(b)** myxedematous cretins. Note the different scales of serum T_4.

drogen peroxide toxicity: H_2O_2 synthesis is an essential step in the iodination process of tyrosine in iodoaminoacids within the thyroid. Concurrent selenium deficiency would deplete the gland of antioxidant enzymatic activity mediated by glutathione peroxidase. It was expected that selenium supplementation would improve thyroid functional capacity among iodine- and selenium-deficient children from the Congo by protecting the tissue against oxidative damage. It was paradoxical to observe the reverse (8, 9) selenium supplementation among iodine- and selenium-deficient subjects led to a decrease in serum T_4, much more pronounced in endemic myxedematous cretins among whom thyroid involution has occurred (Fig. 1). The molecular structure of deiodinase as a selenium-enzyme gave theoretical support to the human data. The general concepts available early in the nineties were the following:

- By decreasing deiodinase I activity, selenium deficiency causes metabolic blockade in the conversion of prohormone T_4 to metabolically active hormone T_3 – by analogy, for example, to the metabolic blockade of steroid synthesis in congenital adrenal hyperplasia, with increased concentration of precursors (17-OH-progesterone ↑) and decreased concentration of active hormone (cortisol ↓).
- By decreasing glutathione peroxidase activity, selenium deficiency could be the clue for explaining the thyroid hormone involution in endemic myxedematous cretinism, as explained before.

I shall try to summarize critically the facts obtained during the next decade on selenium and thyroid hormone metabolism, to answer the following question:

"Is there a place for selenium supplementation to improve or establish a functionally normal thyroid hormone metabolism?"

The data will be reviewed in a logical approach – not a chronological one:

- analyzing the data on thyroid hormone metabolism in subjects only deficient in selenium,
- in subjects deficient in iodine and selenium,
- the controversy of iodine versus selenium in Kashin-Beck disease.

When isolated selenium deficiency is present

Phenylketonuria (PKU) is an inherited metabolic disease affecting approximately one in ten thousand children. Profound intellectual impairment has been prevented by the introduction of a low phenylalanine diet beginning as soon as possible after birth. Cases are detected within a few weeks after birth by neonatal screening in most western countries. The restriction of whole protein foods in the diet of treated patients can lead to a low concentration of some trace elements such as selenium. The selenium status of PKU children is similar to that of children living in iodine- and selenium-deficient areas of central Africa, then slightly greater than in rural parts of China endemic for Keshan disease and Kashin-Beck disease.

Still today, correction of selenium deficiency in PKU subjects is not mandatory. No clinical evidence has been reported, so far, of a clear benefit of selenium supplementation on the long-term evolution of this group of patients, despite their profound micronutrient deficiency. In view of the essential role of selenium in thyroid hormone metabolism, a selenium supplementation/depletion study was conducted among PKU children to determine the effect of selenium on thyroid function biological parameters (10).

As shown in the first column of table 1, initially, the mean plasma T_4 concentration was normal (120 nmol/l; reference range: 58–155). It decreased significantly within 3 weeks of selenium supplementation to 102 nmol/l ($p < 0.001$), remained at that level during the whole period of selenium supplementation (until 46 weeks), and returned to initially greater values within three weeks after stopping selenium supplementation.

In the same study, initial plasma reverse T_3 (rT_3) concentration was within the normal range. It decreased in parallel with T_4 to reach a plateau ($p < 0.005$), and remained at that level during the whole period of selenium supplementation. It returned to the initially greater values after stopping selenium supplementation ($p < 0.01$). Serum TSH and T_3 (not shown here) remained stable during both phases of selenium repletion and selenium depletion. Besides the expected change of serum T_4 and reverse T_3, we were surprised by the moderate magnitude of the variation of thyroid hormones compared to that of selenium. If one considers that the biological value attained at full selenium repletion represents 100 %, the serum thyroid hormones de-

Table 1 Ten phenylketonuric subjects were supplemented with selenium for 46 weeks, and then again depleted of selenium until 78 weeks. The table shows the course of selenium status (serum selenium and plasma glutathione peroxidase (GPX)) and of thyroid function parameters (serum T_4 and reverse T_3 (rT_3)). The percentage variation of the biological parameters (Δ) is the difference between the values at 46 weeks (taken as 100 %) and 78 weeks. Compared with the values at 46 weeks, all baseline values and all 78 week values were significantly different ($p < 0.05$). Plasma GPX (plasma glutathione peroxidase): biochemical data should not be compared to those of the other tables and figures, as the methodology of glutathione peroxidase was different (10, 11).

	Basal values	+ Se 46 weeks	Se 78 weeks	Variation 46 wk. vs. 78 wk.	Reference range
Serum selenium, nmol/L	330 ± 152	940 ± 254	368 ± 216	Δ = –61 %	965 ± 165
Plasma GPX, U/L	140 ± 58	312 ± 57	161 ± 48	Δ = –48 %	354 ± 54
Serum T_4, nmol/L	120.4 ± 4.5	101.5 ± 7.8	111 ± 17.8	Δ = 9.3 %	99.7 ± 8.5
Serum rT_3, pmol/L	340 ± 126	259 ± 101	321 ± 92	Δ = 24 %	237 ± 107

creased with a much less pronounced amplitude (T_4: 9 %; rT_3: 25 %) than the increase in parameters of selenium status (serum selenium: minus 61 %; plasma glutathione peroxidase: minus 48 %).

The amplitude of variation of T_4 and rT_3 remained slight, and all values measured in the phenylketonuric subjects were within the normal range – before, during and after selenium supplementation. While this study shows once more that these subjects are selenium deficient, it does not provide clear evidence for convincing pediatricians to supplement systematically. Actually, the therapeutic attitude is variable from one country to the other (northern Europe being more "resistant" to a change in diet) and, within each country, between individual specialists. When discussing with colleagues in charge of phenylketonuria prevention programs, it is apparent that they do not see clinical evidence based argument for selenium supplementation, and their patients grow quite normally – intellectually and physically – without supplementation.

Another question is whether the commercial companies delivering diets for phenylketonuric patients should include some selenium in their food. Even if it is not evidence based medicine, it can do no harm, and, if there is any subtle effect, it should logically be a beneficial one. Maybe one of the difficulties is to define the best selenium preparation: there are two main preparations possible for humans, selenate and selenomethionine. Selenate is an inorganic compound not available in the pharmacopoeia; actually, it is the cheapest way to administer selenium, but we had to buy it from a chemical company and ask the hospital pharmacy to prepare the tablets. Selenomethionine is available in the pharmacopoeia, but it is not a naturally synthesized selenium-amino acid in mammals (its origin is exclusively vegetable). I also do not know of any work that has clearly demonstrated that there is no risk for selenomethionine to be incorporated in place of methionine in some enzymes – as the pKi of the two products differ markedly. If this substitution occurs, it could theoretically modify some biochemical properties of proteins. I should be careful with that product, peculiarly in pregnant women. So, you have Sophie's choice between a harmless product unavailable in the pharmacopoeia (selenate) and a much more expensive, not definitely proven as harmless product largely available (selenomethionine). Sporadically, other selenium preparations have been tested (selenite, selenocysteine, etc.), but their use remains marginal.

When combined iodine and selenium deficiency is present

Table 2 compares the basal values and the epidemiological profile of diseases which have been related to combined iodine and selenium deficiency in two provinces in the northern part and in one province of the eastern part of Democratic Republic of Congo and in Tibet Autonomous Region (6, 11).

Northern and eastern provinces of RD Congo: iodine deficiency with selenium deficiency as cofactor

In severe endemic goiter areas of Congo, epidemiological data collected since the sixties show an extremely elevated prevalence of goiter and cretinism. Goiter affected more than 80 percent of the women of childbearing age and of the children aged more than 5 years. Cretinism was observed in 1 to 10 percent of the child population.

The clinical picture of cretinism was considered peculiar, with a large predominance of myxedematous form compared to the neurological form (12). Myxedematous cretins were dwarf-like, with a disproportionate and symmetrical form of dwarfism (short legs, particularly the long bones), mentally deficient, and definitely hypothyroid. In the adult, the picture is quite similar to that of untreated cases of neonatal hypothyroidism – before the introduction of systematic screening in the middle seventies.

The timing of thyroid involution is mostly postnatal: young children (< 4 yr.) with longstanding hypothyroidism, and then, classified as cretins, regain normal thyroid function after iodine supplementation. This is not the case in older cretins who lose irreversibly their potential to regain normal thyroid function (13). Also, thyroglobulin, a marker of thyroid functional capacity when the gland is stimulated, decreases with age in hypothyroid children (14, 15).

Actually, myxedematous cretinism is the extreme case affecting 1 to 10 percent of the population. Besides these extremes, most children present phases of hypothyroidism of variable severity, variable duration, and variable timing. The spectrum of clinical consequences is, then, also extremely polymorphic.

Why do some subjects evolve to myxedematous cretinism, while others are able to adapt in same environment? Concurrent selenium deficiency offered an interesting hypothesis, as explained in the "Introduction".

On a practical point of view, universal salt iodination programs have now been implemented in most African countries. It is difficult to obtain clear data on the efficiency of this in the field, and things are no easier since the civil war (the northern and eastern provinces are under rebel control, while the universal salt iodination program is managed from the capital Kinshasa). Nevertheless, the informal economy continues to work despite the civil war, and endemic goiter and cretinism are now finally under control, despite the political trouble. In these conditions, selenium supplementation should not be considered a health priority.

Tibet: selenium deficiency with iodine deficiency as a cofactor

The relationship of selenium deficiency with the osteoarthropathy of Kashin-Beck was proposed in the middle seventies, by scientists of the University Medical of Xi'An (16). They observed that cereals of endemic areas were lethal for rats, and pathological examination showed liver necrosis. Selenium deficiency was a known cause of liver necrosis at that time.

Thus, when a Non Government Organisation – Doctors Without Borders – Médecins Sans Frontières, Belgium – decided to intervene with a therapeutic and preventive approach to Kashin-Beck osteoarthropathy in villages around Lhassa, they decided to test the selenium hypothesis. As Tibet is, also, the last province of China to be severely iodine deficient, it was decided to supplement children with iodized oil before supplement of selenium.

From table 2, it can be seen that the clinical expression of endemic diseases is impressively different in Tibet and in the Congo, despite similarly severe iodine deficiency.

In Tibet, the proportion of children in the same age range with endemic goiter is markedly lower, despite a lower urinary iodine excretion. This is a clear demonstration of the influence of other goitrogens besides iodine deficiency in the Congo, which are not present in Tibet. Thiocyanate toxicity resulting from consumption of poorly detoxified cassava is certainly an important factor in the Congo; the staple food in Tibet is barley, and thiocyanate levels in urine or serum are not elevated, excluding this factor.

In Tibet, only 7 cases of cretinism were found on carefully visiting home to home in 13 remote rural villages and examining 575 children. Except in one case, they were typical neurological cretins. This observation shows that, if there is any role of selenium on the clinical expression of cretinism (myxedematous versus neurological), it is not a factor sufficient by itself, when combined with iodine deficiency, to explain the occurrence of myxedematous cretinism in the Congo. Again, thiocyanate overload could be the third factor, which explains the peculiar epidemiological picture of cretinism in central Africa.

At the opposite, Kashin-Beck osteoarthropathy occurs in Tibet and does not occur in the Congo – at least, in its severe forms which do not escape the attention of any medical doctor or physical therapist. More detailed clinical examination in African countries would be necessary to exclude less evident cases who escape a normal clinical examination. If there is any role for selenium in the disease, you have to look for a third factor. Belgian colleagues (17) have corroborated the Chinese data on a possible role of mycotoxins contaminating barley cereals.

In the published report on combined iodine and selenium deficiency in Kashin-Beck disease (11), selenium status (serum selenium concentration and serum glutathione peroxidase activity) was extremely low, but paradoxically lower in unaffected than affected children! This may seem to provide an argument against a causal relationship of the disease with the micronutrient deficiency. When looking to the distributions of both parameters (Fig. 2), 100 % and 89 % of children, respectively, had serum selenium values and serum glutathione peroxidase values below the lower limit of normal adult reference range in occidental selenium sufficient countries (756 nmol/l (60 ng/ml) for serum selenium and 550 U/l for serum glutathione per-

Table 2 Comparison cf thyroid function selenium status in children from endemic villages surrounding Lhassa, Tibet, and in children from endemic villages surrounding Karawa, Ubangi, Northern Congo.

	Tibet children	**Ubangi children (Northern Congo)**	**Reference values for a normal population**
Epidemiological data	N = 575 (ref. 11)	N = 68 (ref. 14)	N = 344 (ref. 14)
Age range – years	5 – 15	5 – 18	1 – 7
Prevalence of goiter – %	46	83	absent
Prevalence of cretinism – ‰	12	88	absent
Prevalence of Kashin-Beck osteoarthropathy – %	49	not described	absent
Thyroid function	N ≥ 530 (ref. 11)	N ≥ 60 (ref.14)	N ≥ 337
Serum TSH – mU/L – geometric mean (Limits[a])	5.8 (2.4 – 13.9)	24.3 (2.5 – 233)	2.0 (0.3 – 4.6) (ref.14)
Serum T4 – nmol/L – mean ± SD	96.5 ± 34.0	60.5 ± 54.2	119 ± 27.1
Serum T3 – nmol/L – mean ± SD	2.55 ± 0.49	2.91 ± 1.20	2.91 ± 0.80
Urine iodine – µg/dl – geometric mean (Limits[a])	1.2 (0.6 – 2.7)	2.06 (0.8 – 8.4)	no data (WHO: >5)
Selenium status	N ≥ 417 (ref. 11)	N ≥ 46 (ref.14)	Personal data in ADULTS
Serum selenium – nmol/L – geom. mean (Limits [a])	124 (64.8 – 225)	not applicable	Not applicable
Serum selenium – nmol/L – mean ± SD	not applicable	344 ± 177	1390 ± 317
Serum GPX – U/L – geometric mean (Limits [a])	202 (110 – 440)	no data	810 ± 130
RBC GPX – U/g Hb – mean ± SD	no data	3.3 ± 2.4	15.0 ± 2.8

[a] Geometric mean and 1 SD-limits are calculated by transforming all data to their log-values; the mean of the log-transformed values is back-transformed to the original scale by taking the base 10 exponent. The lower and upper limits are determined by calculating the mean –1 SD and mean +1 SD of the log-transformed values, and back-transforming the results to the original scale by taking the base 10 exponent.

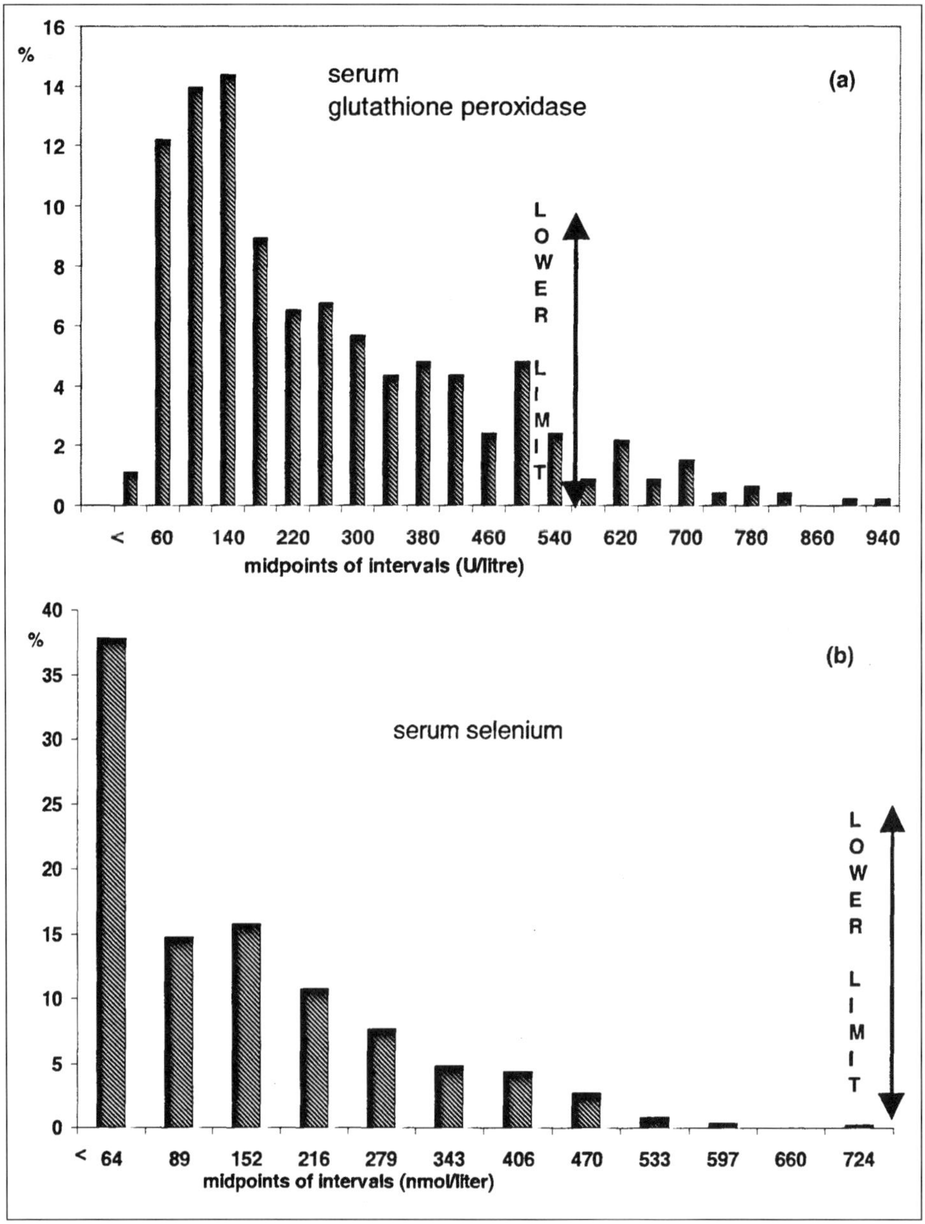

Fig. 2 Distribution of values of serum glutathione peroxidase and serum selenium among children in Tibet. The double-headed arrow represents the lower limit of normal in adults living in Belgium.

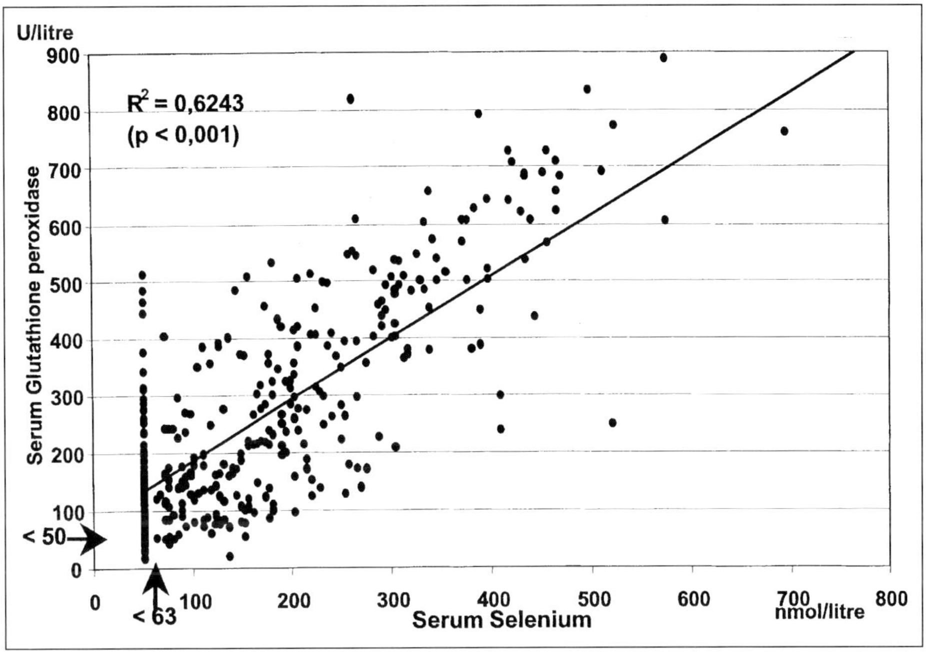

Fig. 3 Variation of serum glutathione peroxidase as a function of serum selenium concentration at baseline, before iodine or selenium supplementation. The arrows represent the limits of analytical sensitivity.

oxidase). The distributions are also asymmetric, with marked skewing to the right; for parametric statistical analysis, the values were, therefore, log-transformed to fit a normal Gaussian distribution better. Thirty-eight percent of subjects were below the functional sensitivity limit[1] for selenium measurement (< 63.5 nmol/l [< 5 ng/ml]) by atomic absorption spectrometry, meaning that the method of measurement was not sensitive enough to give precise results below that threshold. For serum glutathione peroxidase, using the same criteria of functional sensitivity, 11 % of the values were below the analytical threshold (50 U/l) of enzymatic measurement with commercial reagents on a biochemistry analyzer.

Despite the measurements performed at the limit of detection of the methods, the correlation between serum glutathione peroxidase and serum selenium was excellent (Fig. 3), demonstrating the reliability of the analyses. Quality control procedures included, also, serum control samples at various levels of concentrations in each series of measurements. I take the opportunity for a methodological precaution for serum

1 The functional analytical sensitivity limit was defined as the lower value for which between-day analytical coefficient of variation is ≥ 20 percent

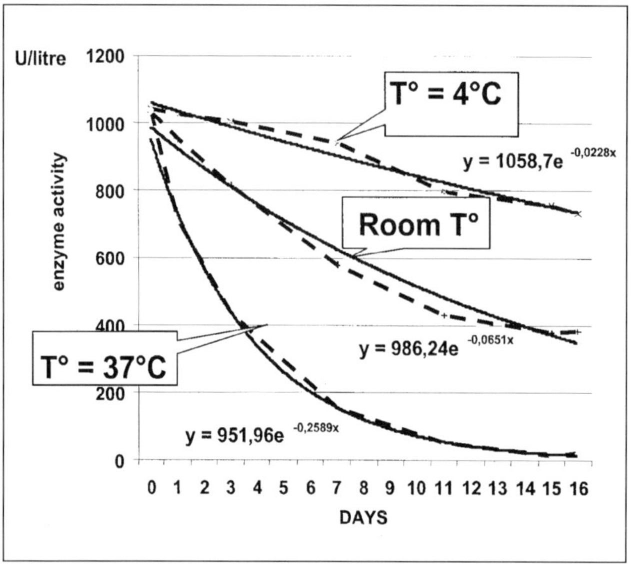

Fig. 4 Serum glutathione peroxidase stability. Pooled human serum was aliquoted in multiple samples and kept at –80 °C. At different intervals, samples were thawed so as to perform all analyses within one run. The experimental points were adjusted to an exponential curve, with the equation indicated for each temperature.

glutathione peroxidase measurement: this enzyme shows poor stability at room temperature, and it should not be refrozen before analysis. Figure 4 shows that its activity decreases by 24% in 24 hrs at 37°C. Every effort should be made to freeze a serum aliquot within one hour of blood collection, and to keep the sample frozen until analysis. These preanalytical procedures are sometimes difficult to respect in remote, rural villages. Besides the usual internal control samples to be included in each run of analysis, it is important to take control samples in the field, and to keep them in the same conditions as blood samples collected from the investigated subjects. This is one way of verifying major preanalytical bias, and is particularly important for plasma or serum glutathione peroxidase measurement. Erythrocyte glutathione peroxidase is apparently much more stable (18).

Actually, as for endemic hypothyroidism and iodine in goiter areas, clinical selenium status in Tibet varies not only from subject to subject, but also within a same subject according to the duration, the severity and the timing during development of selenium deficiency. Within a homogeneously selenium deficient population, the whole population is exposed at some periods of life to extreme deficiency. Figures 5a and 5b substantiate this fact. One protocol consisted of administration of iodine to all children affected by Kashin-Beck osteoarthropathy, followed, four months later, by supplementation with selenium or placebo. This clinical trial was conducted to test the efficacy of selenium supplement in Kashin-Beck osteoarthropathy, and analysis of the data is in preparation (Moreno-Reyes R et al.). Blood samples were taken just before giving iodine and four months later just before giving selenium or placebo. Figures 4a and 4b show the lack of correlation of paired values of serum

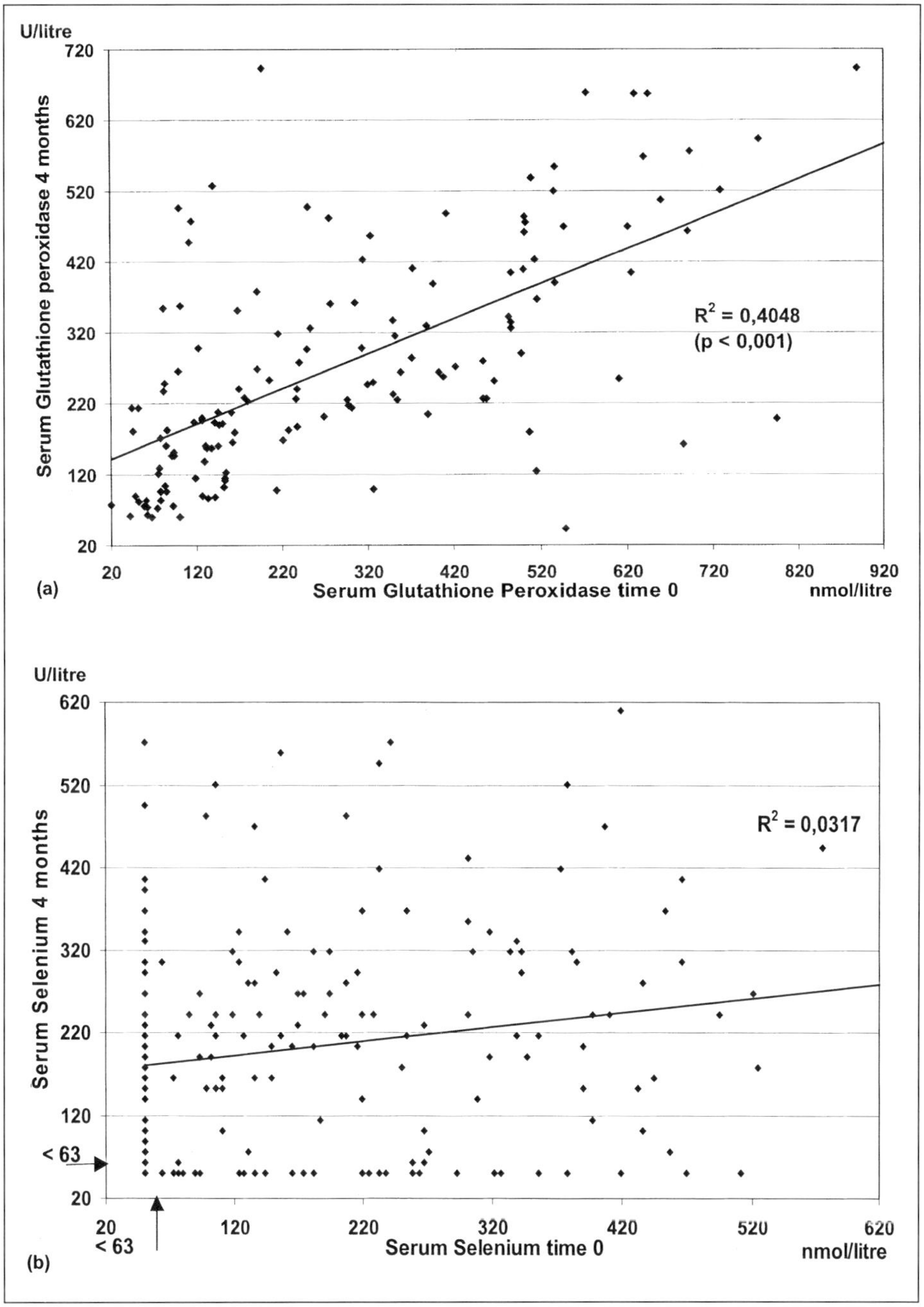

Fig. 5a and **5b** Interday Intra-individual correlation of GPX – Tibet. Paired values of serum glutathione peroxidase and serum selenium are plotted for the same subjects examined at the entry in the study (time 0) and 4 months later (4 months). Iodine supplement was given at time 0 at the entry in the study. No selenium was given at that time.

glutathione peroxidase and serum selenium. Table 3 shows that the pooled variance[2] (which is a good estimate of the intra-individual variance) (19) was of the same order of magnitude as that of inter-individual variance. As stated before, this is not due to a methodological bias (lack of precision of the method at these levels close to the analytical detection limits). At least three control samples at different levels were used, and the quality control assessment shows that, for the lowest values (serum selenium = 6.3 nmol/l (5 ng/ml) and serum glutathione peroxidase = 50 U/l), the between-day coefficient of variation was 20 percent. As classically observed, the between-day coefficient of variation decreases markedly with greater values, and was < 5 percent within the normal range of values. These figures show that within 4 months, a child remains severely selenium deficient, but with an intra-individual variation similar to the inter-individual variation. In these conditions, individual measurements of serum selenium or serum glutathione peroxidase are poor markers of relative risk of developing Kashin-Beck disease. They are epidemiological markers but not individual markers. In order to improve the prognostic value of these biochemical parameters, measurements should be repeated for the same person at various intervals, or other biochemical parameters looking for long term selenium indices should be looked for. Chinese scientists are accustomed to use selenium measurement in the hair, and to obtain excellent correlation with the clinical expression of Kashin-Beck osteoarthropathy. As the hair sample represents the selenium supply during at least 2 months, it may, indeed, be an excellent indicator of selenium status over long periods.

Recently, we had the opportunity to visit remote rural villages of Ang'Kan County, at the North of Shaanxi province, R.R. China, 1600 kilometers east of Lhassa, Tibet. Subjects more than 25-year-old were still affected by Kashin-Beck osteoarthropathy, but no further young cases (< 25-yr-old) were seen. Iodized salt was introduced around 1975, and the program worked very efficiently: we visited some very isolated farms, and found packages of salt adequately wrapped and containing an adequate concentration of iodine – according to the measurements performed on the field with UNICEF kit of reagents (20).

2 In humans, and particularly in developing countries, it is, of course, difficult to determine an intraindividual variance directly, which would require collection of multiple blood samples (at least 12) from the same subject. A good estimate can be obtained by pooling several estimates of variance calculated for duplicates or triplicates.

Conclusions

Selenium interacts with thyroid hormone metabolism, and deficiency leads to an increase in serum thyroid hormones T_4 and reverse T_3. Nevertheless, this biochemical effect is slight, and without any evident clinical effect. When combined with iodine deficiency and other goitrogens such as thiocyanate overload, selenium deficiency might be a third factor that explains the peculiar epidemiological picture of predominant myxedematous cretinism in the northern and eastern Congo. This hypothesis should not modify the present program of universal salt iodination, as this measure is certainly sufficient to eradicate goiter and cretinism.

In Tibet, where people are exposed to extreme selenium deficiency, multiple factors such as iodine deficiency and mycotoxin toxicity may interact to provoke Kashin-Beck osteoarthropathy. While the disease is rapidly regressing in rural China as a result of epidemiological transition and economical development, Tibet remains the last province of China not to benefit from an efficient program of iodine supplementation. This should be the priority. It is not excluded that removing any of the factors related to Kashin-Beck osteoarthropathy (selenium deficiency, iodine deficiency, or mycotoxin exposure) could be sufficient to eliminate the disease. Iodine supplementation is certainly the one for which most experience has been acquired. This is also the number one priority for Tibet.

References

1. Schwarz K, Foltz CM. Selenium as an integral part of factor 3 against dietary necrotic liver degeneration. J Am Chem Soc 1957; 79: 3292–3.
2. Arthur JR, Morrice PC, Beckett GJ. Thyroid hormone concentrations in selenium deficient and selenium sufficient cattle. Res Veterin Sci 1988; 45: 122–3.
3. Berry MJ, Banu L, Larsen PR. Type I iodothyronine deiodinase is a selenocysteine-containing enzyme. Nature 1991; 349: 438–40.
4. Behne D, Kyriakopoulos A, Meinhold H, Kohrle J. Identification of type I 5'-iodothyronine deiodinase as a selenoenzyme. Biochem Biophys Res Comm 1990; 173:1143–9.
5. Goyens P, Golstein J, Nsombola B, Vis H, Dumont JE. Selenium deficiency as a possible factor in the pathogenesis of myxematous cretinism. Acta Endocrinol (Copenhagen) 1987; 114: 497–502.
6. Vanderpas JB, Contempré B, Duale NL, Goossens W, Bebe N, Thorpe R, Ntambue K, Dumont JE, Thilly CH, Diplock AT. Iodine and selenium deficiency associated with cretinism in northern Zaire. Am J Clin Nutr 1990; 52: 1087–93.
7. Flohé L, Günzler WA, Schock HH. Glutathione peroxidase: a selenoenzyme. FEBS Lett 1973; 32: 132–4.
8. Contempré B, Duale NL, Dumont JE, Ngo B, Diplock AT, Vanderpas J. Effect of selenium supplementation on thyroid hormone metabolsm in an iodine and selenium deficient population. Clin Endocrinol 1992: 36: 579–83.
9. Contempré B, Dumont JE, Ngo B, Thilly CH, Diplock AT, Vanderpas JB. Effect of selenium supplementation in hypothyroid subjects of an iodine and selenium deficient area – the possible danger of indiscriminate supplementation of I-deficient subjects with selenium. J Clin Endocrinol Metab 1991; 213–5.

10. Calomme MR, Vanderpas JB, François B, Vancaillie Bertrand M, Herchelz A, Vanovervelt N, Vanhoorbeke C, Van den Berghe DAV. Thyroid function parameters during a selenium repletion/depletion study in phenylketonuric subjects. Experientia 1995; 51: 1208–15.
11. Moreno-Reyes R, Suetens C, Mathieu F, Begaux F, Perlmutter N, Boelaert M, Phelmo D, Nève J, Vanderpas J. Iodine and selenium deficiency in Kashin-Beck disease (Tibet). N Engl J Med 1998; 339: 1112–20.
12. Delange FM. Endemic Cretinism. In: *The Thyroid*, 8th Ed (Braverman LE & Utiger R), under press, chapter 55.
13. Vanderpas J, Rivera MT, Bourdoux P, Luvivila K, Perlmutter-Crener N, Delange F, Lanoie L, Ermans AM, Thilly CH. Reversibility of severe hypothyroidism with supplementary iodine in patients with endemic cretinism. N Engl J Med 1986: 315: 791–5.
14. Vanderpas J. Histoire naturelle de la fonction thyroïdienne de la naissance à 7 ans (chapitre V). In *L'hypothyroïdie juvénile endémique en Ubangi, Zaïre*, Thesis, Université Libre de Bruxelles, 1991: 41–55 (Figure 2).
15. Contempré B, Duale GL, Gervy C, Alexandre J, Vanovervelt N, Dumont JE. Hypothyroid patients showing shortened responsiveness to oral iodised oil have paradoxically low serum thyroglobulin and low thyroid reserve. Tg/TSH ratio as a measure of thyroid damage. Eur J Endocrinol 1996; 134: 342–51.
16. Mo D, Ding D, Wang Z, Zhang J, Bai C. Twenty-five year research on selenium related to Kashin-Beck disease. Xi'An Medical University, Xi'An, People's Republic of China (1996).
17. Chasseur C, Suetens C, Nolard N, Begaux F, Haubruge E. Fungal contamination in barley grains related with Kashin-Beck disease in Tibet. Lancet 1997; 350: 1074–5.
18. Calomme MR. Methodological aspects. In *Selenium supplementation and Lactobacillus biotransformation of inorganic selenium by Lactobacillus species: Development and applications of a bacterial selenium supplement.* Thesis, Universitaire Instelling Antwerp, 1995.
19. Kringle RO, Bogovich M. Statistical procedures (chapter 11). In: *Textbook of Clinical Chemistry,* 3rd edition (Eds Burtis CA, Ashwood ER), WB Saunders Co., 1999: 265–309.
20. Vanderpas J, Nève J. La Maladie de Kashin-Beck en Chine: une ostéochondrodysplasie liée à la nutrition et à l'environnement. Bulletin et Mémoires de l'Académie royale de Médecine de Belgique 1999; 154: 177–89.

Flavonoids as a risk factor for goiter and hypothyroidism

J. Köhrle

Abteilung Molekulare Innere Medizin und Klinische Forschergruppe, Medizinische Poliklinik, Universität Würzburg, Röntgenring 11, 97070 Würzburg, Germany

Abstract

Thyroid function and thyroid hormone (TH) secretion are influenced by several physiological, pharmacological, nutritional, and environmental factors. Among those are secondary metabolites of plants and fungi, especially hydroxylated or phenolic compounds either in their free form or as O- or N-glycosylated conjugates. The most potent natural and synthetic plant derivatives affecting thyroid function and secretion are flavonoids (chalcones, auron(ol)es, flav(a)onon(ol)es, isoflavonoids) comprising several hundred compounds. Our average diet contains up to 2 grams flavonoids per day as constituents of colored fruits, vegetables, plant- or fungus-derived nutrients. The majority of these phenolic hydroxylated compounds is rapidly eliminated after resorption and undergoes first pass metabolism in the liver. However, a significant portion is further activated, deglycosylated or conjugated to yield active metabolites with different kinetic properties. As hydroxylated phenolic compounds affect thyroid function, potential effects of flavonoids on thyroid function and TH metabolism were investigated. Furthermore, many traditional plant extract folk remedies are used for treatment of hyperthyroidism. Several preparations are still in use and available for this purpose.

Several effects of plant extracts containing flavonoids have been documented by in vitro or *in vitro* animal model studies. Plant extracts interfere with pituitary TSH feedback regulation and influence the gonadotropic axis, but the active principle(s) and mechanism(s) of action are not yet established. Oxidized extracts of *Lycopus virg.*, *Melissa off.*, *Lithospermum off.*, and other medical plants act as antagonists of TSH binding to thyroid membranes and suppress basal and TSH-stimulated cAMP production. A series of purified flavonoids and their glycosides interfere with several steps of iodide metabolism in the thyroid of rodents, e.g. iodide uptake, TPO-function, Tg-iodination, and structure-activity and dose-response relationships have been established. In particular, pearl millet, a staple food in many countries, contains potent flavonoids that might contribute to goitrogenesis especially under conditions of inadequate iodide supply or in combination with other goitrogens such as cassava-derived agents. Flavonoids, especially aglycones and monomeric forms, are potent competitors for TH binding to transthyretin, but only weakly interact with TH binding sites of TBG and albumin. Flavonoids elevate free TH levels, and TH are more rapidly transferred to tissues (including pituitary) and eliminated more quickly. Free unconjugated flavonoids inhibit TH deiodination, especially type I 5'-deiodinase in vitro and in vivo. Administration of synthetic flavonoids (F 21388) to animals (rat, mouse, dog, swine) disturbs several pathways of thyroid homeostasis: TSH and TH synthesis and secretion, serum binding to transthyretin, distribution and elimination of TH, TH transfer across the choroid plexus of the blood-CSF barrier and across the placenta, deiodination in mother and fetus, and TH-dependent gene expression. No evidence is available that flavonoids reach the nuclear T_3-receptors and compete for binding of T_3. No clear conclusions on specific anti-thyroid or goitrogenic effects can been drawn due to the multiplicity of actions of flavonoids in the complex TH homeostatic and feedback system which contains fail-safe mechanisms at all levels.

Introduction

Iodine deficiency leads to goiter development and is a risk factor for evolution of thyroid cancer. Apart from iodine deficiency, a series of other factors and processes contribute to goitrogenesis both deteriorating or mitigating the cascade of iodine deficiency-induced growth and proliferation of the thyroid gland. Recently, genetic factors and genes predisposing for hypothyroidism or multinodular goiter have been identified (12). Several nutrients, food additives, chemicals, xenobiotics, and pharmaceuticals are known to interfere with normal thyroid function and to be involved in goitrogenesis (37). Limited knowledge is available on additive, synergistic or antagonistic interaction between goitrogenic and anti-goitrogenic substances and endemic conditions such as iodine or combined iodine- and selenium-deficiency leading to goiter, hypothyroidism, cretinism, or thyroid cancer. In vitro studies using isolated enzymes, disrupted subcellular fractions, cell culture experiments or *in vitro* studies in various animal models and different species as well as epidemiological studies in areas of endemic goiter revealed the contribution of nutrients or food components to goitrogenesis especially in areas of iodine deficiency.

Among the compounds contributing to goitrogenesis are plant derived substances such as C- or N-glycosides which produce cyanate, thiocycanate, isothiocyanate, or other goitrogens (35, 37) known to interfere with thyroid hormone synthesis. The mechanisms are similar to those of thiourea and its congeners, which are established antithyroid drugs such as propylthiouracil (PTU) or methimazole derivatives. The goitrogenic cyanate-related compounds do not occur in free form in the respective plants but are liberated by various glycosidases during processing. Among the goitrogenic plants containing thioglycosides are kale, cabbage, sprouts, broccoli, kohlrabi,

Table 1 Summary of effects of medical plant extracts and flavonoids on the pituitary-thyroid-periphery axis.

Hypothalamus	dopamine-like action?
Anterior pituitary	inhibition of TSH secretion/synthesis
	increased T_4 uptake
Thyroid	inhibition of iodide uptake?
	inhibition of TPO, iodide organification and coupling of iodo-tyrosine residues
	enhanced T_3 secretion
Serum	competition for thyroid hormone binding to transthyretin but not TBG
	increase of free T_4 and free T_3 levels in serum
Liver and other tissues	inhibition of type I 5'-deiodinase activity
	inhibition of thyroid hormone uptake and nuclear transport
	interaction with thyroid hormone conjugating enzymes
Kidney and intestines	enhanced elimination of thyroid hormones

turnips, swedes, rapeseed, and mustard whereas cassava, lima beans, linseed, bamboo shots and sweet potatoes contain cyanogenic glycosides. However, appropriate processing and cooking of food destroys or reduces the content of goitrogenic compounds in most vegetables and plant compounds.

Goitrin (1,5-vinyl-2-thiooxazolidone) has similar actions to thiourea, but its effect cannot be overcome by adequate iodine supply. Goitrin is liberated from progoitrin, contained in turnip, cabbage, and other *Brassicaceae*, by myrosinase in these plants (35). In addition, aliphatic disulfides, contained in high amounts in onions and garlic are potent goitrogens in animal models (35).

Many phenol-derived compounds and agents also interfere with thyroid function both in their free and conjugated form, either as monomeric or as polymeric molecules (Table 1). Serious adverse effects on thyroid function are also exerted by polycyclic aromatic hydrocarbons (PAH), polychlorinated and polybrominated biphenyls (PCB, PBB) and their congeners and metabolites (10, 16, 17, 73). Both short- and long-term effects have been observed on the thyroid axis and thyroid hormone dependent development in animal models. It remains to be established whether these observations can be extrapolated to, and are of significance in humans.

Flavonoids

Flavonoids, ubiquitously distributed polycyclic phenolic secondary metabolites of plants, occur in more than 3000 varieties either in free, conjugated or methylated form (22, 23, 42, 61) (Figure 1). Our average diet contains up to 2 grams of flavonoids, which either are rapidly eliminated if absorbed, metabolized by various enzymes of the host or the gastrointestinal microbial flora, and act either as free compounds, conjugates, complexes, or metabolites on many enzymatic reactions within the body. Whether these actions are of functional, metabolic, pharmaceutical, or pathological relevance is still matter of controversy (81). However, in vitro and animal experiments as well as epidemiological, nutritional, and interventional studies indicate that plant derived flavonoid components interfere especially with the hormone systems of their hosts. As with hormones, low concentrations of potent and abundant natural food-derived compounds and their metabolites lead to marked effects on cellular signal transduction, alterations in gene expression and interference with metabolic reactions and structural remodeling. The most prominent examples are the isoflavonoids acting as phytosteroids or genistein, which interferes with many signal transduction pathways. Flavonoids cannot be synthesized in higher vertebrates. The biological function of flavonoids in plants producing these compounds is still not fully elucidated. They might act as chemical weapons of the 'defenseless' plants against predators or infectious agents and also fulfil a role in light protection and absorption apart from evolutionary advantages related to their coloring properties (22, 23, 61).

Flavonoids exert multiple actions in biological systems depending on their chemical structure. Flavonoids containing at least one free aromatic phenolic group act as antioxidants (66). Many flavonoids interact with nucleotide binding sites in kinases, phosphatases, oxido-reductases (22, 23, 61, 86). Apolar flavonoids are substrates of

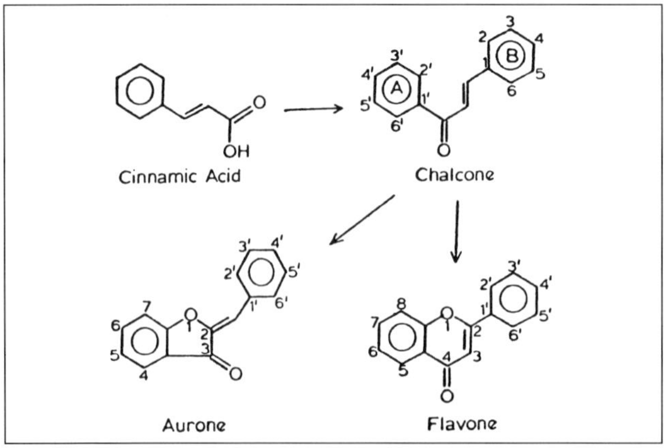

Fig. 1 Structure and biosynthesis of flavonoids

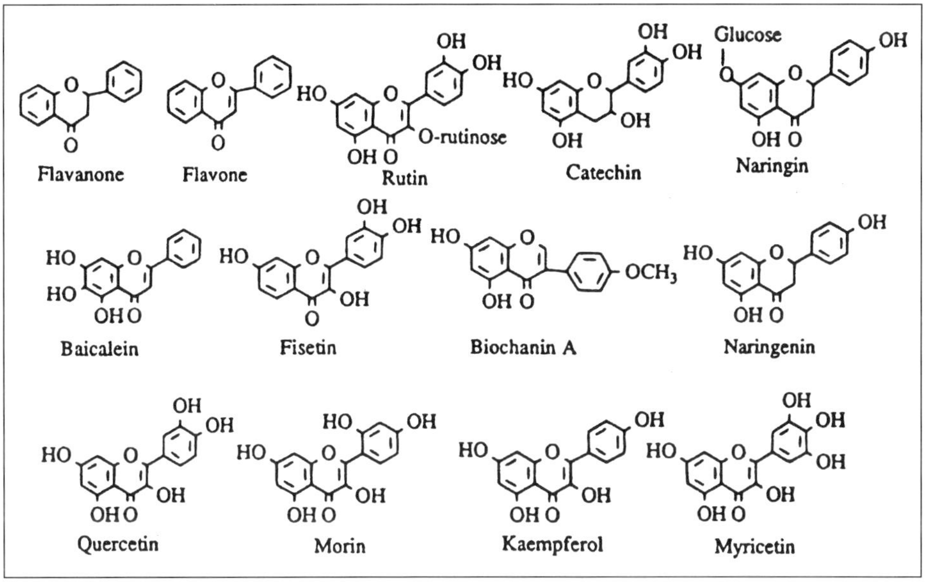

Fig. 2 Structural formulas of representative flavonoids with relevance for thyroid economy (from Divi and Doerge, 1996)

cytochrome p450 enzymes and also hydroxylated flavonoids are readily metabolized by both p450 enzymes and other enzymes involved in phase I or II metabolic reactions (41). As phenolic derivatives they undergo several conjugation and esterification reactions and enzymes of the gastrointestinal microbial flora readily metabolize flavonoids including their β-glycosides, which are not substrate for mammalian enzymes.

Figure 2 summarizes the chemical structures of representative flavonoids that are synthesized from phenolic precursors. Both monocyclic and polycyclic phenolic aromates are known to interfere with the thyroid axis and to contribute to goitrogenesis. Folk medicine has taken advantage of the antithyroid action of flavonoids. They are among the most prominent goitrogens contained in varieties of millet, the staple food in many third world countries in the arid regions. In vitro and animal model studies have contributed to delineate the molecular and systemic mechanisms of flavonoid action on the thyroid. Currently, it is unclear whether interaction of flavonoids with other hormonal or metabolic pathways contributes to their antithyroid action.

Interference with pituitary function and TSH-secretion

Studies on the mode of action of various types of extracts of plants and herbs containing flavonoids administered in folk or herbal medicine and still prescribed or used in 'green or soft medicine' today revealed a potent action of these extracts at the pituitary level. Extracts of *Melissa off., Lycopus virg.* or *europ., Lithospermum off.*, or *Thymus serpyllum* inhibit TSH secretion in the rat (44, 58, 82, 92–94).

Systematic analysis after intraperitoneal injection or oral administration of *Lycopus europ.* extracts to euthyroid male rats revealed suppression of serum TSH at 24 hours and serum thyroid hormone T_3 at 3 to 24 hours, whereas T_4 levels were decreased only more than 24 hrs after oral extract application. A 'reactive' transient TSH elevation was also described at 9 and 12 hrs (93). Apart from alterations in the thyroid axis suppression of LH and testosterone was also found. Analysis of these extracts revealed significant content of luteoline-7-glycoside as well as caffeic and rosmarinic acid (93). TSH suppression was also found after chronic plant extract administration to goitrous rats kept on low iodine diet and PTU treatment (82). These effects were dose-dependent, did not change pituitary TSH content, transiently reduced T_4 and T_3 serum levels, and inhibited thyroid secretion as analyzed by determination of colloid size and colloid droplet number. In addition to effects on the thyrotroph-thyroid axis, suppression of prolactin serum levels and decreased pituitary content of prolactin was also found. The latter observations led the authors to postulate, that hypothalamic action of plant extracts via the dopamine system might be involved, too (82). A combined anti-thyrotropic and anti-gonadotropic action of plant extracts used in herbal medicine had been previously described in rodents, guinea pigs, rabbits, and chicks (15, 30, 58, 92). Analysis of chemical contents of these plant extracts has demonstrated high flavonoid content, assumed to contribute to the anti-hormonal and anti-thyroid action (14, 43). Detailed analysis of pituitary action and inhibition of TSH secretion by the synthetic flavonoid F21388 (3-methyl-4'-6-dihydroxy-3',5'-dibromo-flavone) (Figure 3) is described below.

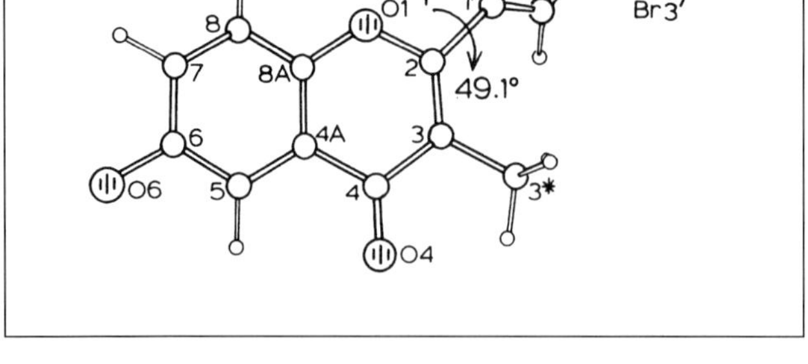

Fig. 3 Structural formula of the synthetic flavonoid F21388, a potent T_4-antagonist

Flavonoid effects on the thyroid

Anti-TSH-action

Suppression of TSH secretion and decreased TSH serum levels result in decreased thyroid hormone secretion. In addition, experimental evidence suggested a direct interaction of TSH and thyroid-stimulating immunoglobulins with constituents of plant extracts, leading to inactivation of circulating TSH-extract complexes (94). Co-administration of TSH with extracts of *Lithospermum off.* resulted in decreased potency of TSH stimulation of thyroid hormone secretion in the rat. In a series of experiments using bovine and human thyroid membranes for determination of binding to and activation of the TSH receptor as well as analysis of basal and TSH-stimulated cAMP production, Auf'mkolk et al. demonstrated that medical plant extracts of the species *Lycopus virg.* and *europ.*, *Melissa off.*, and *Lithospermum off.* inhibit binding of TSH and TSH-receptor-stimulating immunoglobulins to the TSH receptor (5, 6). In addition, these extracts inhibit both basal and TSH-stimulated cAMP production. Mechanistic studies revealed that constituents of these extracts form adducts with bTSH and thus prevent binding to its receptor. Similar interactions of the extracts were also observed for hCG and its binding to rat testis membranes, indicating a further component of antigonadotropic action of plant extracts. Further experiments indicated that oxidation products of 3,4-Dihydroxycinnamic acid (orthoquinones) exert the antithyrotropic activity contained in these extracts (4). Their potency was increased by (auto-)oxidation of the monomeric phenolic precursors. Apparently, these oxidized oligomers form Schiff-base type adducts with thyrotropin and some of the pituitary glycoprotein hormones. The oxidized plant extract compounds also act in vitro by preventing TSH-stimulated release of radioiodide in the mouse McKenzie assay (4). On the other hand, reduced, monomeric flavonoid components or their chalcone precursors do not inactivate TSH and do not inhibit TSH action on thyrocyte membranes or in vitro. These studies indicate a potent inhibitory action of oxidized medical plant constituents on both TSH and TSH-receptor-stimulating immunoglobulins. This might explain the reported antithyroid effect of aqueous or ethanolic extracts of certain plants for treatment of Graves' hyperthyroidism and inhibition of action of elevated TSH levels leading to goiter as reported in early publications (75). As aqueous extracts of phenolic and aromatic compounds tend to oxidize rapidly, the anti-thyrotropin and anti-gonadotropic activity might increase during storage before administration. However, uncertain stability of the active principles contained in the extracts creates problems with reproducible application. Whereas oxidized extracts gain potency with respect to anti-TSH action, they lose activity with respect to the inhibition of other components of the thyroid axis (see below).

One of the potent phenolic compounds interfering with uptake and transport of many solutes is phlorizin and its aglycon phloretin (2,4,6-trihydroxy-β-(4-hydroxy)-

propio-phenone), best known for their inhibitory action on sugar transport. Early work (59) demonstrated potent inhibition of TSH and LATS-stimulated (long-acting thyroid stimulator) thyroid hormone secretion by phloretin phosphate in mice. Phloretin phosphate has been considered to act as prostaglandin antagonist, but in this context a direct interaction of this substance seems to occur with the TSH-receptor. However, subsequent studies did not confirm this mechanism of action and rather favor a direct interaction of TSH with phloretin phosphate similar to the mechanism of action suggested for oxidized herbal plant extracts and orthoquinone compounds (3).

Inhibition of iodide uptake

Certain plant extracts and their constituents also inhibit iodide uptake and subsequent organification.

However, less clear data are available on detailed structure activity relationships or mechanism of action. The recent cloning of the sodium-iodide symporter (NIS) and subsequent analysis of the regulation of its expression revealed a strong TSH-dependent regulation mediated by the cAMP-cascade (for review see (77). Therefore, indirect effects of flavonoids or phenolic oxidized products on TSH action might lead to inhibition of iodide uptake. On the other hand, the function of NIS as symporter offers the possibility that agents affecting Na-transport and interfering with Na-K-ATPase also block iodide uptake. The inhibitory effects on iodide uptake of thiocyanate and isothiocyanate, components released from C- and N-glycosides of *Brassicaceae* are well known. These voluminous anions compete for iodide transport by the NIS.

Flavonoid inhibition of thyroperoxidase (TPO)

The best analyzed effect of flavonoids on the thyroid axis is their potent inhibition of TPO. Here systematic structure-activity and dose-response relationships have been established and *in vitro* data using purified TPO, experiments with intact cells, and *in vivo* analysis in animal models have been reported. Flavonoids are the most potent antithyroid constituents of several species of millet (Pearl millet [*Pennisetum leeke*, also known as *typhoides* or a*mericanum*] or Fonio millet [*Digitaria exilis]*, whose consumption is known to contribute to goitrogenesis in iodine-deficient regions of the third world.

The highest goitrogenic content of millet is contained in the bran fraction, which is also rich in proteins. Three major flavonoids and their C-glycosyl-conjugates have been characterized with respect to their content in millet and action on TPO, vitexin, glycosylvitexin, and glycosylorientin (37–39). TPO inhibition by vitexin and its congeners was demonstrated using porcine thyroid slices, isolated TPO, and *in vivo* animal experiments with potencies approaching those of the classical goitrogens MMI or PTU.

Identification of goitrogenic compounds in Fonio millet failed to demonstrate significant contents of C-glycosylflavones in comparison to Pearl millet. However, large amounts of apigenin and luteolin, and their O-glycosylated forms were found (150 and 350 mg/kg, respectively) and shown to be potent TPO inhibitors (76). In addition, luteolin inhibits cyclic AMP phosphodiesterase, counteracting to some extent the goitrogenic anti-TPO effect. This dual action indicates a multi-faceted antithyroid mechanism similar to that of medicinal plant extracts. Thyroid hormone secretion is inhibited by the flavonoids comparable to thiouracil action with both acute and persisting components of action.

Goitrogenesis combined with enterohepato-nephropathy has also been demonstrated in Nubian goats fed with Pearl millet (0.25 to 1 g/kg body weight for two months) (1). These authors observed major changes in thyroid morphology (follicle size, colloid content, lymphocytic infiltration, iodine and selenium content) and found pathological changes in other tissues and serum parameters after administration of millet in addition to the basal ration. The exact mechanism(s) underlying the goitrogenic effect and the other negative effects is not known, but their study confirms previous observations in animal models.

Inhibition of TPO results in decreased iodination of tyrosine residues in thyroglobulin (Tg), i.e. less MIT and DIT formation. In addition, coupling of MIT and DIT residues is diminished, eventually leading to impaired thyroid hormone synthesis and secretion. No effects of flavonoids on other components involved in synthesis, storage and release of thyroid hormones and their precursors are known.

Systematic structure-activity relationships on inhibition of TPO by flavonoids were performed in comparison to related peroxidase enzymes. Here, IC-50 values ranged from 0.6 to 41 μM and suggested mechanism-based inhibition of TPO similar to previous findings for resorcinol or derivatives (31). Some of the flavonoids act as suicide substrates of TPO forming covalent bonds in the ligand binding site of the compound I complex of TPO (32). The most potent agents were fisetin, kaempferol, naringenin and quercetin, indicating that a free phenolic structure and inhibition mechanism resembling that of resorcinol is active. For some of the compounds tested non-competitive or more complex mechanisms of action were found. Biochanin A even acts as substrate for iodination. With exception of horseradish peroxidase most of the peroxidases tested were also inhibited by the flavonoids tested.

Flavonoid effects on thyrocyte growth

Flavonoids are also known for growth inhibitory effects on several cell lines *in vitro* (13, 22, 23, 28, 33, 86). Most attention has been focused on the inhibition of tumor cell growth exerted by the isoflavonoids genistein and biochanin A, linked to anti-cancer effects in breast and prostate tumors. Moreover, epidemiological data indicate a lower incidence of these tumors in regions of high consumption of plant-derived food and use of soy been products containing high amounts of these phytoestrogens. It is not yet clear if these isoflavonoids act via estrogen receptors or exert direct growth inhibitory effects by inhibition of cellular kinase signaling pathways. Recently, the flavonoids, apigenin and luteolin, were reported to have growth inhibitory effects on thyroid cancer cell lines with IC-50 values around 20–30 μM (97). Biochanin A also was active especially in thyroid tumor cells expressing antiestrogen binding sites. Subsequent studies indicated that most potent inhibition was exerted by flavonoids inhibiting tyrosine kinase, MAP-Kinase and c-myc activation resulting in apoptosis (98). No information is yet available concerning whether flavonoids act also on non-transformed normal thyocytes by activating these pathways. In this case, flavonoid-activated apoptosis would counteract goitrogenesis, well characterized and documented as described above.

Similar to other cell models, flavonoids interact with a series of enzymes involved in cellular signaling. In particular, flavonoid competition for nucleotide binding sites in kinases and phosphatases and binding sites in oxido-reductases has been described (22, 23). Quercetin interacts in a dose-dependent manner with pig thyroid protein kinase C. Stimulation of PKC has been found at low concentrations (10^{-7}M) and inhibition at higher concentrations (72). Whether these mechanisms illustrated *in vitro* in primary culture thyrocytes are involved in goitrogenesis, hormone synthesis, or growth regulation needs to be further investigated

Flavonoid effects on serum thyroid hormone binding and distribution proteins

Rather detailed information is available on specific interaction of flavonoids with thyroid hormone binding and distribution proteins in serum (47, 55). Here systematic structure-activity relationships and dose-response curves have been established *in vitro* using purified thyroid hormone binding proteins. In addition in vivo animal experiments using both acute and chronic administration of naturally occurring and synthetic flavonoids demonstrated marked effects of flavonoids on thyroid hormone homeostasis, metabolism and action. A remarkable general finding from these studies is that the most specific and relevant interaction occurs not with all thyroid hormone binding proteins but preferentially with transthyretin (TTR). Those flavonoids tested in vitro and in vivo seem specifically to displace T_4 and T_3 from TTR but not from TBG or albumin (8, 11, 18, 46, 54, 55, 63). This finding immediately raises the question of whether flavonoid effects are of relevance in humans where TBG is the major thyroid hormone binding protein and whether the marked and rapid effects of flavonoids observed in rat models can be extrapolated to the human situation.

Systematic in vitro studies using purified TTR from several species has revealed a clear pattern of structural requirements of flavonoids for interaction with the T_4 binding site of TTR: presence of one, two or more phenolic aromatic rings, one or more free phenolic groups in positions mimicking the 4'-OH-Group of T_4 and the alanine side chain of T_4, perpendicular orientation of the two aromatic ring systems similar to the skewed or antiskewed orientation of the diphenylether ring system of thyroid hormones, planar ring systems are less avid ligands for TTR, glycosylation of hydroxyl groups is tolerated in some but not all positions of the flavonoid, compatible with the narrow and well defined T_4 binding site of TTR (21, 25, 26, 47, 95).

These in vitro structure activity relationships were confirmed by analysis and evaluation of a series of X-ray structures of complexes of various flavonoids with TTR (20, 21, 24, 25, 27) and confirmed the conclusions delineated from in vitro binding studies in most instances. These studies also allowed to design potent T_4-antagonists such as the synthetic flavonoid F 21388, which mimics the three-dimensional structure of T_4 based on a flavonoid backbone (25, 53, 55). This synthetic flavonoid is relatively stable in vivo, does not undergo first pass metabolism in the liver, and is an potent ligand of both TTR and type I 5'-deiodinase (Figure 4). F21388 has been exploited as a valuable tool to study effects of readily available thyroid hormone bound to TTR, and to analyze the role of TTR bound T_4 for tissue distribution of thyroid hormone, including transfer across the blood-CSF, blood-brain and placental barrier both in the adult rat as well as during pregnancy to the fetus and its

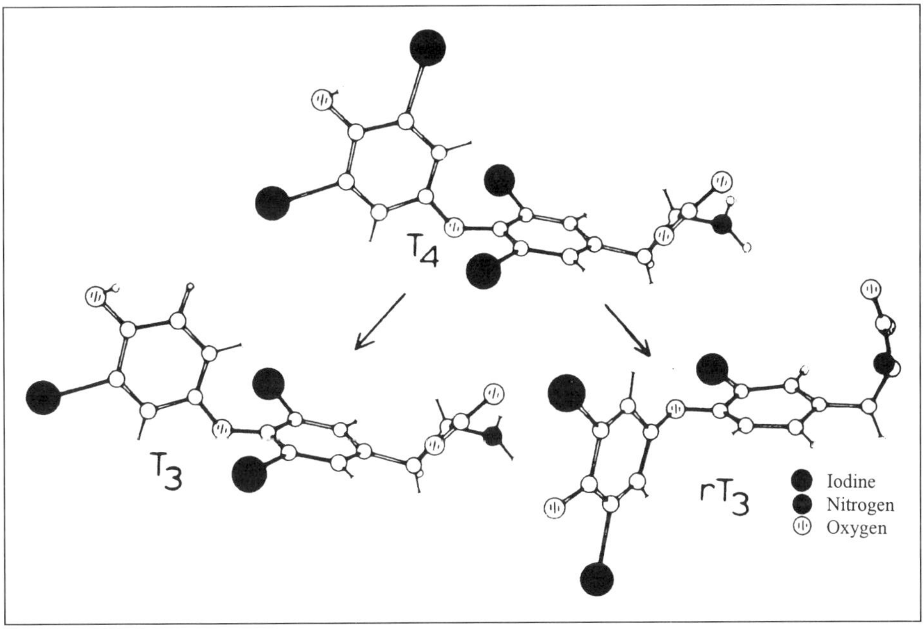

Fig. 4 Schematic presentation of enzymatic 5'- and 5-deiodination of T_4 to T_3 and rT_3

brain. In summary, these in vitro and in vivo studies revealed that only those flavonoids with monomeric, non-oligomeric, reduced and preferentially aglyconic structures are potent ligands for TTR and reversibly displace thyroid hormones from binding to TTR but not from TBG or albumin. Administration of flavonoids rapidly increases free thyroid hormone levels in serum. This elevation of T_4 and T_3 rapidly suppresses TSH secretion and synthesis and leads to alterations of thyroid hormone distribution in extracellular space, tissues, and organs. Furthermore, intracellular thyroid hormone levels are changed both by alterations of thyroid hormone availability and by inhibition of deiodinases (48). The most remarkable alterations occur in tissues expressing type II 5'-deiodinase activity, probably because 5'DII is rapidly inactivated by elevated T_4 (2, 69, 79). In vitro, flavonoids preferentially inhibit 5'DI activity whereas 5'DII and 5-Deiodinase (Type III) is less affected.

Naturally occurring chalcones, including phloretin, aurones and flavonoids, exhibit clear concentration dependent displacement of T_4 from TTR binding *in vitro* with IC-50 values in the range of 0.1 to 50 μM (8, 9, 25, 55). Aurones, also contained in various plant extracts and plant derived dyes, have a five-member C-ring in contrast to flavonoids, and are derived from chalcone precursors (see Figure 2).

The synthetic flavonoid F21388, a potent T_4-antagonist

In vitro effects and acute action of F21388 on the thyroid axis

Modification of the natural flavonoids by introduction of halogen atoms in the phenolic B-ring and restraint of flexibility of the two aromatic ring system by introduction of a methyl group in 3-position revealed the potent inhibitor F 21388 of T_4 binding to TTR with a Ki value of 20 nM (53,55). Relatively weak competition was observed for T_3 binding to nuclear T_3-receptor preparations (55).

In vivo administration of F21388 to intact euthyroid rats immediately (after 3 minutes) but transiently displaced T_4 and T_3 from binding to serum TTR, rapidly increased serum free T_4 and free T_3, decreased circulating total T_4 and T_3 levels and subsequently decreased circulating TSH levels (57). These changes were reversible, indicating that no covalent interaction of F21388 occurred with affected proteins or feedback components. These studies give clear evidence that exogenous compounds are able to rapidly disturb thyroid hormone economy and homeostasis and that F21388 is a valuable tool to study reversible alterations of free thyroid hormone levels and TSH secretion without exogenous thyroid hormone. In hypothyroid rats, no further elevations of TSH levels were achieved after F21388 administration (54).

These transient elevations of free thyroid hormone levels after a single F21338 injection also increased T_4 transfer from the extracellular compartment to the rapidly exchangeable intracellular compartment (e.g. liver and kidney) and the T_4 steady state distribution ratio between these two compartments (60). These data are consistent with the free hormone hypothesis in thyroid hormone transport and distribution.

Injection of F21388 at high doses (2 µmol/100 g body weight) into euthyroid rats decreased percentage T_4 binding to the choroid plexus and reduced CSF T_4 levels with a subsequent decrease in T_4 concentration in cerebral cortex and cerebellum (18). These experiments indicate that serum TTR does not cross the choroid plexus and that free T_4 levels determine transfer of T_4 across the choroid plexus to the CSF. In addition F21388 at these doses appears to reach the CSF and brain structures where it may compete for T_4 binding to TTR secreted by the choroid plexus towards the CSF (18). Transfer of flavonoids to the brain and CNS has also been described for other naturally occurring compounds and synthetic derivatives that act as specific ligands for the GABA-A-receptor or other functional proteins in the CNS (29, 40, 89, 90). In other studies it has been demonstrated that some flavonoids such as naringenin are able to reach the rat brain (70, 71).

More detailed studies on the mechanism of action of F21388 on T_4 transfer across the choroid plexus were performed in an in vitro cell culture model. These revealed that TTR is secreted in a directed manner towards the CSF-oriented lumen and that F21388 competitively inhibits T_4 transfer to the CSF by inhibiting T_4 binding to newly synthesized TTR (83). These findings may have major impact on the biology and pharmacology of thyroid hormone transfer to the brain and its modulation by competitors of T_4 binding to TTR. F21388 effects are not restricted to rat TTR but are also found in other species. F21388 effectively competes for T_4 binding to TTR of humans, dog, rat, pig, and other species with high affinity (34). Therefore, F21388 represents a valuable tool for identification of TTR and related proteins in analysis of evolutionary relationships (74). Whether TTR interaction with naturally occurring flavonoids or their metabolites is of relevance in thyroid hormone physiology remains to be elucidated. TTR is expressed very early in the yolk sac of vertebrates, is synthesized in the choroid plexus in higher vertebrates and is a highly conserved protein throughout the vertebrate kingdom (78). Thus, disturbance of T_4 binding to TTR, at least during development, might have an impact on thyroid hormone dependent development and differentiation of tissues and the brain. Fetal and neonatal disruption of the thyroid hormone system of the maternal-fetal unit has been suggested to be responsible for some of the toxic effects of chlorinated and brominated aromatic and phenolic thyroid disrupters such as PCB, DDT, and related compounds (16, 17, 19, 73, 100). No information is yet available concerning whether flavonoid binding to TTR also interferes with its sandwich-like interaction with retinol-binding protein and Vitamin A binding, another essential functional characteristic of this essential protein complex (74, 78).

Effects of chronic infusion of F21388 in adult rats, pregnant rats, dams and fetuses

Continuous infusion of F21388 (20 µmol/kg body weight per rat per day) for 14 days altered thyroid hormone economy and tissue hormone levels (79). In contrast to acute administration of F21388 (see above), no alterations in serum and pituitary TSH were found: plasma T_4 and T_3 clearance were increased, thyroid T_4 secretion decreased and T_3 secretion elevated. Whereas tissue T_4 was diminished, T_3 tissue levels were lower in those organs where type II 5'-deiodinase is expressed (brain, cerebellum, pituitary, brown adipose tissue), indicating lower local T_3 production from T_4. Whether these alterations result from inhibition of type II 5'-deiodinase activity by transiently elevated T_4 levels (see above) or from decreased systemic and tissue T_4 substrate supply remains to be established. However, a clear alteration of thyroid hormone secretion and metabolism is evident after continuously administered F21388 in the rat model.

Subsequent experiments in MMI-treated pregnant rats, infused with T_4 to minimize thyroid contribution to circulating thyroid hormone levels, showed decreased total T_4 and T_3, and elevated free T_4 and decreased free T_3 after F21388 infusion (69). Furthermore, 21388 reached the fetal circulation and maternal and fetal T_3 formation from T_4 increased, thus mitigating fetal T_3 deficiency. These complex alterations might result from enhanced T_4 transfer to tissues caused by T_4 displacement from TTR and subsequently increased T_3 production via type I 5'-deiodinase. No evidence was found in this setting for in vivo inhibition of type I 5'-deiodinase by F21388 in contrast to in vitro findings (see below). These experiments point to the possibility of enhancing tissue availability of thyroid hormones, especially during fetal development, by administration of drugs like F21388, which displace thyroid hormones from their binding and distributor proteins.

More detailed follow-up studies in pregnant rats and their fetuses with the radiolabeled analogue F49209 of the flavonoid F21388 indicated rapid excretion of F49209 from the intestine (80). Fetal flavonoid content increased with time and F49209 was found by HPLC analysis in all tissues investigated, including the fetal brain. This indicates binding of F49209 to fetal brain TTR, which is highly expressed in the CNS during fetal development. These pilot studies indicate that certain flavonoids rapidly cross the placenta during pregnancy and even reach the fetal brain where they might interact with binding proteins such as TTR and other target molecules. This raises the possibility that nutritional and pharmacological sources of flavonoids might act during fetal development and be involved in differentiation or modulation of the thyroid hormone axis and thyroid hormone dependent processes during differentiation similar to organohalogenic thyroid disrupters.

Flavonoid interference with cellular and nuclear thyroid hormone uptake and T_3-receptor binding

Less clear are the data on flavonoid effects on thyroid hormone uptake. The chalcone, phloretin, a well known inhibitor of solute and glucose transporters also dose-dependently inhibited energy-dependent T_3-uptake in HepG2 human hepatoma cells with a rather high IC 50 of 88 μM (64). Phloretin also reduced nuclear uptake of T_3 in intact hepatocytes and competed for T_3 binding to nuclear T_3 receptors again at rather low affinity (Kd of 43 μM) compared to the potent inhibition of T_4 binding to TTR or deiodinase inhibition which occurs in the low μM range. The β-D-glycoside of phloretin, phlorizin, was inactive. Only sparse data are available concerning inhibition of thyroid hormone uptake and transport by flavonoids. However, compared with competition for TTR binding and in vitro inhibition of type I 5'-deiodinase only a less potent action has been observed (47) (J.K., unpublished data).

At relatively high concentrations (100 μM), the synthetic flavonoid F21388 inhibits T_3 uptake in rat primary pituitary cell cultures (56) and these authors suggested a potential role of flavonoids in TSH release. This T_3-antagonistic effect would, however, result in increased TSH secretion, which is under negative feedback control by T_3. These in vitro data also contradict in vivo findings with F21388, which rapidly suppresses TSH secretion.

Flavonoid inhibition of iodothyronine deiodinases

Ample data are available on the interactions of flavonoids with deiodinase enzymes (7–9, 26, 47, 51–55, 84, 85). Apart from iopanoic acid, which inhibits all three deiodinases, PTU is a potent inhibitor of type I 5'-deiodinase (48). Several drugs and compounds are known to interfere with deiodination metabolism of thyroid hormones (48–50). Extensive structure-activity analysis of more than 100 naturally occurring and synthetic flavonoids allowed delineation of a detailed map of the active site of type I 5'-deiodinase, indicating an extremely close relationship to the binding site of TTR. In contrast, flavonoids are less potent inhibitors of both type II 5'-deiodinase and of 5-deiodinase. The most potent 5'DI inhibitors are the synthetic flavonoids F21388 and its congeners. Aurones and certain chalcones also effectively block 5'DI in vitro in disrupted membrane preparations and intact cells. Most potent inhibition of 5'DI is obtained with those analogues that mimic the 5'DI substrates T_4 and rT_3 but not the products T_3 or 3,3-T2. So far, no evidence for a suicide type interaction between flavonoids and 5'DI, similar to that described for TPO (31) has been found. Among the naturally occurring flavonoids, luteolin and apigenin are the most potent, their glycosides being less active or even inactive. Most of the flavonoids are competitive, reversibly binding inhibitors of 5'DI activity although some act by mechanisms that are more complex.

Inhibition of type I 5'-deiodinase by flavonoids and aurones was observed in intact rat hepatocytes, indicating that the intracellular deiodinase enzyme is reached by the drugs (84). 5'-deiodinase inhibition was effective at concentrations that did not affect cell viability for most analogues tested. Moreover, gluconeogenesis from lactate, a sensitive parameter of metabolic intactness of cells, was only inhibited at concentrations far exceeding that necessary for type I 5'-deiodinase inhibition (45, 47, 84). These studies revealed clear dose-response relationships for deiodinase inhibition by flavonoids and aurones. Furthermore, they present strong evidence, that flavonoids are potent inhibitors of intracellular metabolism of thyroid hormones, provided that flavonoids are not sequestered by serum TTR and provided that their inhibitory effect on intracellular deiodinases is not overcome by increased availability of deiodinase substrate displaced from TTR by the same compound. These findings also indicate that a more detailed analysis of the potential differences in the substrate binding sites of type I 5'-deiodinase versus TTR is still needed in order to achieve selective inhibition of one of the possible thyroid hormone binding site targets.

In vivo administration of F21388 to intact rats has been shown to cause rapid suppression of secretion and serum levels of TSH (54, 57). The displacement of T_4 and T_3 from serum TTR by F21388 increases tissue T_4 content without simultaneously elevating T_3 levels as measured in pituitary and liver (2). Apparently, the transient increase in pituitary T_4 rapidly inactivates pituitary type II 5'-deiodinase. Calculations of the F21388 levels possibly reached in the pituitary revealed that no direct inhibition of 5'DII activity is responsible for decreased T_3 content. However, no direct proof of the complex inhibitory mechanisms involved under these experimental paradigms has been furnished yet. Direct effects of flavonoids on TSH secretion not mediated by the well known negative transcriptional effects exerted by thyroid hormones cannot be excluded.

Whether flavonoids modulate and influence conjugation reactions and elimination processes of thyroid hormones is still an open question. Conjugated thyroid hormones are of major importance in enterohepatic recycling of thyroid hormones (91) and possibly also in maternal-fetal transfer of thyroid hormones during pregnancy (96). Flavonoids are known to interfere with several drug metabolizing and conjugating enzymes (61, 99) and thereby might interfere with thyroid hormone availability and elimination. Increased elimination has been reported after consumption of large amounts of walnut oil or soy beans (92). Whether flavonoids, thiogylcosides, or other components of these nutrients cause these effects is not yet clear.

Antithyroid effects of kojic acid and gugulu

Recently, a series of papers has been published reporting on antithyroid effects and mechanism of action of kojic acid (5-hydroxy-2-(hydroxymethyl)-4-pyrone) (36, 62,

87). This compound is not a flavonoid but is related to these agents. Kojic acid is produced by various fungi (e.g. *Aspergillus* and *Penicillum*), has bacteriostatic activity, is present in fermented traditional Japanese food (sake, soy sauce, miso, etc.), and is used as food additive or for cosmetics. In systematic mutagenicity studies, thyroid hyperplasia and formation of follicular thyroid adenoma were observed in both sexes among mice fed on diets containing this agent (3 %) for 20 months (36). Serum free T_3 was lower and TSH higher than in controls. Follow-up studies showed decreased colloid, follicular cell hypertrophy, and capsular fibrosis in a high dose group of rats fed for 4 weeks on 2 % kojic acid (87). Iodide organification, and serum T_3 and T_4 levels were decreased and TSH was elevated, suggesting TSH-induced alterations of thyroid morphology. In a further mechanistic study, kojic acid was shown to exert promoting effects on thyroid proliferation and carcinogenesis among rats in which tumors were initiated with the nitrosamine derivative BHP (62). Continuous stimulation of the thyroid gland by elevated TSH levels induced by kojic acid inhibition of iodide organification and thyroid hormone synthesis provokes thyroid lesions similar to other models (88).

A furanose-sesquiterpene from Commiphora myrrha, 'gugulu', also has major impact on thyroid physiology. Gugulu increases T_3 formation in mice without affecting T_4 (67). Various extracts and preparations from Commiphora species are used for various diseases, and marketed worldwide as hypolipidemic and hypocholesteremic agents. Fenugreek seed extracts inhibit T_3 production in mice (68) and some of these effects are attributed to altered lipid peroxidation, but compounds exerting these effects have not been isolated yet.

Conclusions

Certain extracts of plants used in folk medicine and phytotherapy, and especially some of their constituents, specifically the flavonoids, are potent antithyroid drugs. Well documented effects include inhibition of TSH secretion, direct inactivation of TSH, inhibition of TPO, competition for thyroid hormone binding to transthyretin (thus increasing free T_4 levels, T_4 transfer to tissues and T_4 elimination), and potent inhibition especially of type I 5'-deiodinase activity. These multifaceted actions might represent the amazing power of the active principles of these plant constituents, but also raises problems of identifying the mechanisms of action and characterizing clear pharmacological profiles. The antithyroid effects can be distinguished from antigonadotropic effects and even more from actions of some flavonoids as phytosteroids or phytoestrogens. In general, most flavonoids have very low toxicity (47, 65, 81) and some of their actions on functional proteins or metabolic pathways are detectable at nanomolar or low micromolar concentrations. Therefore, flavonoids are powerful candidates for innovative drug design. However, their phenolic nature leads to rapid modification by conjugation or oxidation reactions (41) and thus development of derivatives or special galenic properties is mandatory. Whether daily consumption of 1–2 g of flavonoids in our standard diet contributes to goitrogenesis is not clear at the moment. However, high consumption of known goitrogenic flavonoids, as contained in millet bran, will exert antithyroid effects especially under conditions of inadequate iodide supply or in combination with other plant-derived goitrogens such as thioglycosides, gugulu, or phytotherapeutic drugs.

Acknowledgement

This study was supported by grants of the Deutsche Forschungsgemeinschaft (DFG Kö 922/3–3 and Ko 922/7–1).

References

1. Abdel Gadir WS, Adam SEI. Development of goitre and enterohepatonephropathy in Nubian goats fed with pearl millet (*Pennisetum Thyphoides*). Veterinary J 1999;157:178–85.
2. Abend SL, Fang SL, Alex S, Braverman LE, Leonard JL. Rapid alteration in circulating free thyroxine modulates pituitary type II 5'deiodinase and basal thyrotropin secretion in the rat. J Clin Invest 1991;88:898–903.
3. Amir SM, Kasagi K, Corretti M, Blank M, Ingbar SH. Polyphloretin phosphate, an antagonist of thyrotropin action: evidence for an interaction with the hormone rather than the receptor. Endocrinology 1985;117:860–8.
4. Auf'mkolk M, Amir SM, Kubota K, Ingbar SH. The active principles of plant extracts with antithyrotropic activity: Oxidation products of derivatives of 3,4-Dihydroxycinnamic acid. Endocrinology 1985;116:1677–86.
5. Auf'mkolk M, Ingbar JC, Amir SM, Winterhoff H, Sourgens H, Hesch RD, Ingbar SH. Inhibition by certain plant extracts of the binding and adenylate cyclase stimulatory effect of bovine thyrotropin in human thyroid membranes. Endocrinology 1984;115:527–34.
6. Auf'mkolk M, Ingbar JC, Kubota K, Amir SM, Ingbar SH. Extracts and auto-oxidized constituents of certain plants inhibit the receptor-binding and the biological activity of Graves' immunoglobulins. Endocrinology 1985;116:1687–93.
7. Auf'mkolk M, Köhrle J, Gumbinger H, Winterhoff H, Hesch RD. Antihormonal effects of plant extracts. Horm Metab Res 1984;16:136–41.
8. Auf'mkolk M, Köhrle J, Hesch RD, Cody V. Inhibition of rat liver iodothyronine deiodinase: Interaction of aurones with the iodothyronine ligand binding site. J Biol Chem 1986;261:11623–30.
9. Auf'mkolk M, Köhrle J, Hesch RD, Ingbar SH, Cody V. Crystal structure of phlorizin and the iodothyronine deiodinase inhibitory activity of phloretin analogues. Biochem Pharmacol 1986;35:2221–7.
10. Barsano CP. in: Gaitan E, Ed. Environmental goitrogenesis. 1989; chapter. 9, Polyhalogenated and polycyclic aromatic hydrocarbons. p. 115–36.
11. Benvenga S, Cahnmann HJ, Robbins J. Characterization of thyroid hormone binding to apolipoprotein-E: localization of the binding site in the exon 3-coded domain. Endocrinology 1993;133:1300–5.
12. Bignell GR, Canzian F, Shayegi M, Stark M, Shugart YY, Biggs P, Mangion J, Hamoudi R, Rosenblatt J, Buu P, et al. Familial nontoxic multinodular thyroid goiter locus maps to chromosome 14q but does not account for familial nonmedullary thyroid cancer. Am J Hum Genet 1997;61:1123–30.

13. Boege F, Straub T, Kehr A, Boesenberg C, Wachsmut A, Christiansen K, Andersen A, Jakob F, Köhrle J. Selected novel flavones inhibit the DNA binding or the DNA religation step of eukaryotic topoisomerase I. J Biol Chem 1996;271:2262–70.
14. Böhm K. Die Flavonoide. Arzneimittelforschung 1959;9(9):539–44.
15. Breneman WR, Zeller FJ, Carmack M, Kelley CJ. In vivo inhibition of gonadotropins and thyrotropin in the chick by extracts of Lithospermum ruderale. Gen Comp Endocrinol 1976;28:24–32.
16. Brouwer A, Morse DC, Lans MC, Schuur AG, Murk AJ, Klasson-Wehler E, Bergman A, Visser TJ. Interactions of persistent environmental organohalogens with the thyroid hormone system: mechanisms and possible consequences for animal and human health. Toxicology and Industrial Health 1998;14:59–84.
17. Capen CC. Mechanisms of chemical injury of thyroid gland. Prog Clin Biol Res 1994;387:173–91.
18. Chanoine J-P, Alex S, Fang SL, Stone S, Leonard JL, Köhrle J, Braverman LE. Role of transthyretin in the transport of thyroxine from the blood to the choroid plexus, the cerebrospinal fluid, and the brain. Endocrinology 1992;130:933–8.
19. Cheek AO, Kow K, Chen J, McLachlan JA. Potential mechanisms of thyroid disruption in humans: interaction of organochlorine compounds with thyroid receptor, transthyretin, and thyroid binding globulin. Environmental Health Perspectives 1999;107:273–8.
20. Ciszak E, Cody V, Luft J, Kempton RJ, Kesler BS. Flavonoid conformational analysis: comparison of the molecular structure of (Z)-4,4'-6-triacetoxyaurone and (Z)-3',5'-dibromo-2',4,4',6-tetrahydroxyaurone monohydrate by crystallographic and molecular orbital methods. J Mol Struct (Theochem) 1991;251:345–57.
21. Ciszak E, Cody V, Luft JR. Crystal structure determination at 2.3 – A resolution of human transthyretin-3',5'-dibromo-2',4,4',6-tetrahydroxyaurone complex. Proc Natl Acad Sci USA 1992;89:6644–8.
22. Cody V. in: Cody V, Middleton E, Jr., Harborne JB, Eds. Plant Flavonoids in Biology and Medicine – Biochemical, Pharmacological, and Structure-Activity Relationships. New York: Alan R. Liss, Inc. 1986: 1–592.
23. Cody V. in: Cody V, Middleton E, Jr., Harborne JB et al. Eds. Plant Flavonoids in Biology and Medicine II – Biochemical, Cellular, and Medical Properties. New York: Alan R. Liss, Inc.; 1988: 1–461.
24. Cody V. in: Gaitan E, Ed. Environmental goitrogenesis. Boca Raton: CRC Press; 1989; chapter 3, Physical and conformational properties of flavonoids. p. 35–56.
25. Cody V, Köhrle J, Auf'mkolk M, et al. in: Cody V, Middleton E, Harborne JB, Eds. Plant Flavonoids in Biology and Medicine. New York: Alan R. Liss; 1986;Structure-activity relationships of flavonoid deiodinase inhibitors and enzyme active site models. p. 373–82.
26. Cody V, Köhrle J, Hesch RD. in: Gaitan E, Ed. Environmental Goitrogenesis. Boca Raton: CRC Press, Inc. 1989; chapter 5, Structure-Activity Relationships of Flavonoids As Inhibitors of Iodothyronine Deiodinase. p. 57–69.
27. Cody V, Luft J, McCourt M, Irmscher K. Conformational analysis of flavonoids: crystal and molecular structure of 3',5'-dibromo-3-methyl-6,4'-dihydroxyflavone (1:2) triphenylphosphine oxide complex. Struct Chem 1991;2:601–6.
28. Cushman M, Nagarathnam D. Cytotoxicities of some flavonoid analogues. J Nat Prod 1991;54:1656–60.
29. Dekermendjian K, Kahnberg P, Witt MR, Sterner O, Nielsen M, Liljefors T. Structure-activity relationships and molecular modeling analysis of flavonoids binding to the benzodiazepine site of the rat brain GABA(A) receptor complex. J Med Chem 1999;42:4343–50.
30. Dhom G, Wernze H. Zum antithyreotropen und antigonadotropen Wirkunsgmechanismus von Lithospermum officinale. Acta Endocrinol 1963;43:294–304.
31. Divi RL, Doerge DR. Inhibition of thyroid peroxidase by dietary flavonoids. Chem Res Toxicol 1996;9:16–23.
32. Doerge DR, Divi RL. Porphyrin pi-cation and protein radicals in peroxidase catalysis and inhibition by anti-thyroid chemicals. Xenobiotica 1995;25:761–7.
33. Dragsted LO, Strube M, Larsen JC. Cancer-protective factors in fruits and vegetables: biochemical and biological background. Pharmacol Toxicol 1993;72 Suppl 1:116–35.
34. Duan W, Richardson SJ, Köhrle J, Chang L, Southwell BR, Harms PJ, Brack CM, Pettersson TM,

Schreiber G. Binding of thyroxine to pig transthyretin, its cDNA structure, and other properties. European Journal of Biochemistry 1995;230(3):977–86.
35. Ermans A-M, Bourdoux P. in: Gaitan E, Ed. Environmental goitrogenesis. Boca Raton: CRC Press; 1989; chapter 2, Antithyroid sulfurated compounds. p. 15–31.
36. Fujimoto N, Watanabe H, Nakatani T, Roy G, Ito A. Induction of thyroid tumours in (C57BL/6N x C3H/N)F1 mice by oral administration of kojic acid. Food Chem Toxicol 1998;36:697–703.
37. Gaitan E, Ed. Environmental Goitrogenesis. Boca Raton: CRC Press; 1989: 1–250.
38. Gaitan E, Cooksey RC, Legan J, Lindsay RH. Antithyroid effects in vivo and in vitro of vitexin: a C-glucosylflavone in millet. J Clin Endocrinol Metab 1995;80:1144–7.
39. Gaitan E, Lindsay RH, Reichert RD, Ingbar SH, Cooksey RC, Legan J, Meydrech EF, Hill J, Kubota K. Antithyroid and goitrogenic effects of millet: Role of C-glycosylflavones. J Clin Endocrinol Metab 1989;68:707–14.
40. Griebel G, Perrault G, Tan S, Schoemaker H, Sanger DJ. Pharmacological studies on synthetic flavonoids. comparison with diazepam. Neuropharmacology 1999;38:965–77.
41. Hackett AM. in: Cody V, Middleton E, Jr., Harborne JB, Eds. Flavonoids in biology and medicine. New York: Allan R. Liss, Inc. 1986; The metabolism of flavonoid compounds in mammals. p. 177–94.
42. Havsteen B. Flavonoids, a class of natural products of high pharmacological potency. Biochem Pharmacol 1983;32:1141–8.
43. Hoerhammer L, Wagner H, Schilcher H. Zur Kenntnis der Inhaltsstoffe von Lycopus eurepaeus. Arzneimittelforschung 1962;12:1–7.
44. Kemper F. Experimentelle Grundlagen für eine therapeutische Anwendung von Lithospermum officinale zur Blockierung von Hormonen des Hypophysevorderlappens. Arzneimittelforschung 1959;9(6):368–419.
45. Köhrle J. The trace components – selenium and flavonoids – affect iodothyronine deiodinases, thyroid hormone transport and TSH regulation. Acta Med Austriaca 1992;19 Suppl 1:13–7.
46. Köhrle J. Thyroid hormone deiodination in target tissues – a regulatory role for the trace element selenium? Exp Clin Endocrinol 1994;102:63–89.
47. Köhrle J. in: Reinwein D, Weinheimer B, Eds. Schilddrüse 1993. Berlin: W. de Gruyter; 1994;Von Pflanzenextrakten zu Hormonantagonisten – Neue experimentelle Konzepte zur Hyperthyreosetherapie.
48. Köhrle J. The selenoenzyme family of deiodinase isozymes controls local thyroid hormone availability. Reviews in endocrine & metabolic disorders 2000;1:49–58.
49. Köhrle J. Thyroid hormone metabolism and action in the brain and pituitary. Acta Med Austriaca 2000;27:1–7.
50. Köhrle J, Auf'mkolk M, Rokos H, Hesch RD, Cody V. Rat liver iodothyronine monodeiodinase: Evaluation of the iodothyronine binding site. J Biol Chem 1986;261:11613–22.
51. Köhrle J, Auf'mkolk M, Spanka M, et al. in: Cody V, Middleton E, Harborne JB, Eds. Plant Flavonoids in Biology and Medicine. New York: Alan R. Liss; 1986;Iodothyronine deiodinase is inhibited by plant flavonoids. p. 359–71.
52. Köhrle J, Auf'mkolk M, Spanka M, et al. In: Farkas L, Gabor M, Kallay F, Eds. Flavonoids and Bioflavonoids – Proceedings of the International Bioflavonoid Symposium. Budapest: Hungarian Academy of Sciences; 1985;Flavonoids inhibit enzymic thyroid hormone deiodination. p. 411–21.
53. Köhrle J, Fang S-L, Lueprasitsakul W, et al. in: Drexhage HA, de Vijlder JJM, Wiersinga WM, Eds. The Thyroid Gland, Environment and Autoimmunity. Amsterdam: Elsevier; 1990;The Flavonoid EMD 21388, derived from naturally occurring phenolic secondary metabolites of plants, rapidly affects rat serum thyroid hormone binding, metabolism and TSH regulation. p. 121–4.
54. Köhrle J, Fang SL, Yang Y, Irmscher K, Hesch RD, Pino S, Alex S, Braverman LE. Rapid Effects of the Flavonoid EMD 21388 on Serum Thyroid Hormone Binding and Thyrotropin Regulation in the Rat. Endocrinology 1989;125:532–7.
55. Köhrle J, Spanka M, Irmscher K, et al. in: Cody V, Middleton E, Harborne JB, Beretz A, Eds. Plant Flavonoids in Biology and Medicine II: Biochemical, Cellular and Medicinal Properties. New York: Alan R. Liss; 1988;Flavonoid Effects on Transport, Metabolism and Action of Thyroid Hormones. p. 323–40.

56. Lim C-F, Loidl NM, Kennedy JA, Topliss DJ, Stockigt JR. Drug effects on triiodothyronine uptake by rat anterior pituitary cells in vitro. Exp Clin Endocrinol Diabetes 1996;104:151–7.
57. Lueprasitsakul W, Alex S, Fang S-L, Pino S, Irmscher K, Köhrle J, Braverman LE. Flavonoid administration immediately displaces thyroxine (T_4) from serum transthyretin, increases serum free T_4, and decreases serum thyrotropin in the rat. Endocrinology 1990;126:2890–5.
58. Madaus G, Koch FE, Albus G. Tierexperimentelle Untersuchungen über die antithyreoide Wirksamkeit von Lycopus europaeus und Lycopus virginicus (Wolfsfuss). Z Ges Exper Med 1941;109:411–29.
59. Melander A, Sundler F, Ingbar SH. Effect of polyphloretin phosphate on the induction of thyroid hormone secretion by various thyroid stimulators. Endocrinology 1973;92:1269–73.
60. Mendel CM, Cavalieri RR, Köhrle J. Thyroxine (T_4) transport and distribution in rats treated with EMD 21388, a synthetic flavonoid that displaces T_4 from transthyretin. Endocrinology 1992;130:1525–32.
61. Middleton E, Jr. The flavonoids. TIPS 1984;(August):3351–338.
62. Mitsumori K, Onodera H, Takahashi M, Funakoshi T, Tamura T, Yasuhara K, Takegawa K. Promoting effects of kojic acid due to serum TSH elevation resulting from reduced serum thyroid hormone levels on development of thyroid proliferative lesions in rats initiated with N-bis(2-hydroxypropyl)nitrosamine. Carcinogenesis 1999;20:173–6.
63. Miyamoto M, Sugawa H, Mori T, Hase K, Kuma K, Imura H. Epidermal growth factor receptors on cultured neoplastic human thyroid cells and effects of epidermal growth factor and thyroid-stimulating hormone on their growth. Cancer Res 1988;48:3652–6.
64. Movius EG, Phyillaier MM, Robbins J. Phloretin inhibits cellular uptake and nuclear receptor binding of triiodothyronine in human Hep G2 hepatocarcinoma cells. Endocrinology 1989;124:1988–97.
65. Nagao M, Morita N, Yahagi T, Shimizu M, Kuroyanagi M, Fukuoka M, Yoshihira K, Natori S, Fujino T, Sugimura T. Mutagenecities of 61 flavonoids and 11 related compounds. Environmental Mutagenesis 1981;3:401–19.
66. Ng TB, Liu F, Wang ZT. Antioxidative activity of natural products from plants. Life Sci 2000;66:709–23.
67. Panda S, Kar A. Gugulu (Commiphora mukul) induces triiodothyronine production: possible involvement o lipid peroxidation. Life Sci 1999;65:PL137–141.
68. Panda S, Tahiliani P, Kar A. Inhibition of triiodothyronine production by fenugreek seed extract in mice and rats. Pharmacol Res 1999;40:405–9.
69. Pedraza P, Calvo R, Obregón MJ, Asunción M, del Rey FE, de Escobar GM. Displacement of T_4 from transthyretin by the synthetic flavonoid EMD 21388 results in increased production of T_3 from T_4 in rat dams and fetuses. Endocrinology 1996;137:4902–14.
70. Peng HW, Cheng FC, Huang YT, Chen CF, Tsai TH. Determination of naringenin and its glucuronide conjugate in rat plasma and brain tissue by high-performance liquid chromatography. J Chromatogr B Biomed Sci Appl 1998;714:369–74.
71. Picq M, Cheav SL, Prigent AF. Effect of two flavonoid compounds on central nervous system. Analgesic activity. Life Sci 1991;49:1979–88.
72. Picq M, Dubois M, Munari-Silem Y, Prigent A-F, Pacheco H. Flavonoid modulation of protein kinase C activation. Life Sci 1989;44:1563–71.
73. Porterfield SP, Hendry LB. Impact of PCBs on thyroid hormone directed brain development. Toxicology and Industrial Health 1998;14:103–20.
74. Richardson S, Bradley AJ, Duan W, Wettenhall REH, Harms PJ, Babon JJ, Southwell BR, Nicol S, Donnellan SC, Schreiber G. Evolution of marsupial and other vertebrate thyroxine-binding plasma proteins. Am J Physiol 1994;266:R1359–70.
75. Samec V. Die Beeinflussung des Schilddrüsenstoffwechsels und vegetativer Störungen durch Lycopusextrakte. Wiener medizinische Wochenschrift 1961;31:513–6.
76. Sartelet H, Serghat S, Lobstein A, Ingenbleek Y, Anton R, Petitfrère E, Aguie-Aguie G, Martiny L, Haye B. Flavonoids extracted from fonio millet (Digitaria exilis) reveal potent antithyroid properties. Nutrition 1996;12(2):100–6.
77. Schmutzler C, Köhrle J. Implications of the molecular characterisation of the sodium-iodide symporter (NIS). Exp Clin Endocrinol Diabetes 1998;106(Suppl.3):S1-S10.

78. Schreiber G, Richardson SJ. The evolution of gene expression, structure and function of transthyretin. Comp Biochem Physiol B 1997;116:137–60.
79. Schröder-van der Elst J, Van der Heide D, Köhrle J. In vivo effects of flavonoid EMD 21388 on thyroid hormone secretion and metabolism in the rat. Am J Physiol 1991;261:E227–32.
80. Schröder-Van der Elst JP, Van der Heide D, Rokos H, Morreale de Escobar G, Köhrle J. Synthetic flavonoids cross the placenta in the rat and are found in fetal brain. Am J Physiol 1998;274:E253–6.
81. Sheehan DM. Herbal medicines, phytoestrogens and toxicity: risk:benefit considerations. P S E B M 1998;217:379–85.
82. Sourgens H, Winterhoff H, Gumbinger HG, Kemper FH. Antihormonal effects of plant extracts: TSH- and prolactin suppressing properties of Lithospermum officinale and other plants. Planta Med 1982;45:78
83. Southwell BR, Duan W, Alcorn D, Brack C, Richardson SJ, Köhrle J, Schreiber G. Thyroxine transport to the brain: Role of protein synthesis by the choroid plexus. Endocrinology 1993;133:2116–26.
84. Spanka M, Hesch R-D, Irmscher K, Köhrle J. 5'-Deiodination in rat hepatocytes: Effects of specific flavonoid inhibitors. Endocrinology 1990;126:1660–7.
85. Spanka M, Köhrle J, Irmscher K, et al. in: Cody V, Middleton E, Harborne JB, Beretz A, Eds. Plant Flavonoids in Biology and Medicine II: Biochemical, Cellular, and Medicinal Properties. New York: Alan R. Liss; 1988;Flavonoids specifically inhibit iodothyronine-deiodinase in rat hepatocytes. p. 341–4.
86. Suolina E-M, Buchsbaum RN, Racker E. The effects of flavonoids on aerobic glycolysis and growth of tumor cells. Cancer Research 1975;35:1865–72.
87. Tamura T, Mitsumori K, Onodera H, Fujimoto N, Yashuhara K, Takegawa K, Takahashi M. Inhibition of thyroid iodine uptake and organification in rats treated with koijic acid. Toxicol Sci 1999;47:170–5.
88. Thomas GA, Williams ED. in: Capen CC, Dybing E, Rice JM, Willburn JD, Eds. Species differences in thyroid, kidney and urinary bladder carcinogenesis. Lyon: International Agency for Research on Cancer; 1999;Thyroid hormone stimulating hormone (TSH)-associated follicular hypertrophy and hyperplasia as a mechanism of thyroid carcinogenesis in mice and rats. p. 45–59.
89. Viola H, Marder M, Nunez J, Izquierdo L, Wasowski C, Wolfman C, Ardenghi P, Barros D, Medina JH, Paladini AC. 6-Methyl-3'-bromoflavone, a high-affinity ligand for the benzodiazepine binding site of the GABA A receptor with some antagonistic properties. Biochem Biophys Res Commun 1999;262:643–6.
90. Viola H, Wolfman C, Marder M, Goutman JD, Bianchin M, Wasowski C, Calvo DJ, Izquierdo I, Paladini AC, Medina JH. 6-Chloro-3'-nitroflavone is a potent ligand for the benzodiazepine binding site of the GABA(A) receptor devoid of intrinsic activity. Pharmacol Biochem Behav 2000;65:313–20.
91. Visser TJ. Pathways of thyroid hormone metabolism. Acta Med Austriaca 1996;23:10–6.
92. Winterhoff H. Arzneipflanzen mit endokriner Wirksamkeit – Auswirkungen auf Schilddrüsen- und Ovarfunktion. Zeitschrift für Phytotherapie 1993;14:83–94.
93. Winterhoff H, Gumbinger H-G, Vahlensiek U, Kemper FH, Schmitz H, Behnke B. Endocrine effects of Lycopus europaeus L. following oral application. Arzneimittelforschung 1994;44(I):41–5.
94. Winterhoff H, Sourgens H, Kemper FH. Antihormonal effects of plant extracts – Pharmacodynamic effects of Lithospermum officinale on the thyroid gland or rats; comparison with the effects of iodide. Horm Metab Res 1983;15:503–7.
95. Wojtczak A, Luft JR, Cody V. Structural aspects of inotropic bipyridine binding. Crystal structure determination to 1.9 A of the human serum transthyretin-milrinone complex. J Biol Chem 1993;268:6202–6.
96. Wu S-Y, Polk DH, Chen W-L, Fisher DA, Huang W-S, Yee B. A 3,3'-diiodothyronine sulfate cross-reactive compound in serum from pregnant women. J Clin Endocrinol Metab 1994;78:1505–9.
97. Yin F, Giuliano AE, Van Herle AJ. Growth inhibitory effects of flavonoids in human thyroid cancer cell lines. Thyroid 1999;9:369–76.
98. Yin F, Giuliano AE, Van Herle AJ. Signal pathways involved in apigenin inhibition of growth and induction of apoptosis of human anaplastic thyroid cancer cells. Anticancer Res 1999;19:4297–303.
99. Zhu BT, Taneja N, Loder DP, Balentine DA, Conney AH. Effects of tea polyphenols and flavonoids

on liver microsomal glucuronidation of estradiol and estrone. J Steroid Biochem Molec Biol 1988;64:207–15.
100. Zoeller RT, Dowling ALS, Vas AA. Developmental exposure to polychlorinated biphenyls exerts thyroid hormone-like effects on the expression of RC3/Neurogranin and myelin basic protein messenger ribonucleic acids in the developing rat brain. Endocrinology 2000;141:181–9.

Short communication:

The volume of the thyroid gland in girls and boys of age 6, 10, 13 in Czech Republic

M. Dvořáková, J. Čeřovská, V. Zamrazil

Institute of Endocrinology, Prague, Czech Republic

Ultrasonography is a safe noninvasive technique that provides precise and objective method for determining thyroid volume. During years 1991–1999 we investigated more than 1500 children randomly selected from 9 areas of the Czech Republic. Thyroid volume was calculated according to Brunn's formula, i.e. a x b x c x 0,479.

The results were compared according to age and the body surface of the examined children. The thyroid volume is more directly a function of total body surface area.

In comparison with the European "Thyromobil" study in school children (1997) – the upper limits of normal thyroid volume from which have been recommended as standards of WHO and ICCIDD – , our results show lower values for upper limits of the normal thyroid volume related to body surface in boys and girls. This finding is surprising since our study many children had urinary iodine levels below 100 µg/l (approximately 46 % of girls and 41 % of boys).

The work was supported by Grant No. 5393–4 of the Internal Grant Agency of the Czech Ministry of Health.

Short communication:

Thyroid volumes and urinary iodine in German school children with optimal iodine supply

J. Rendl, N. Juhran, Chr. Reiners, [1]U. Hostalek

Clinic of Nuclear Medicine, University of Würzburg, Würzburg; [1]Merck KGaA, Darmstadt, Germany

According to WHO/UNICEF/ICCIDD school children, particularly those aged 8–10 years, are one of the best target groups for surveillance of iodine deficiency disorders (IDD). The aim of this study was to evaluate the current status of iodine nutrition and its effect on thyroid gland volume of school children in the city of Würzburg, previously considered to be an area of borderline iodine deficiency (median urinary iodine 75 µg/L).

Thyroid volume was measured by ultrasonography in 266 (137 female, 129 male) school children aged 7–10 years attending a primary school. A mobile unit (Thyro-Mobil van, Merck KGaA) equipped with a sonographic device and facilities for collection of urine samples was used for this study. Ultrasonography and urinary iodine determinations were performed by two investigators. The results from this study compared with reference values proposed by WHO/ICCIDD are summarized in the tables below.

	Age (years)			
Girls	7	8	9	10
No.	27	35	43	32
Thyroid volume (median), mL	2.0	2.5	2.7	2.8
WHO reference (median), mL	3.4	3.9	4.4	5.0
Maximum of thyroid volume, mL	3.8	4.1	6.6	7.2
WHO 97th percentile volume, mL	5.9	6.9	8.0	9.2
Urinary iodine (median), µg/L	198.8	178.5	195.0	188.7

	Age (years)			
Boys	7	8	9	10
No.	34	33	37	25
Thyroid volume (median), mL	2.2	2.6	2.8	2.6
WHO reference (median), mL	3.4	3.7	4.1	4.5
Maximum of thyroid volume, mL	3.0	4.8	5.3	6.1
WHO 97th percentile volume, mL	5.7	6.1	6.8	7.8
Urinary iodine (median), µg/L	229.9	214.8	233.2	243.4

These data show that the status of iodine nutrition in school children of Würzburg has markedly improved with an urinary iodine concentration in all age groups of about 200 µg/L. The improvement is due to regular use of iodized salt in households and by local food industries (butchers and bakers) and to taking iodine containing tablets (25 % of all children). Because of the high iodine intake, the thyroid volumes (median and even maximum values) of these children are significantly lower than the corresponding WHO/ICCIDD reference data.

Environmental natural goitrogens

E. Gaitan

Endocrinology Section, VA Medical Center, University of Mississippi Medical School, Jackson, Mississippi, USA

Abstract

A large number of natural agents in the environment are known to affect thyroid gland morphology and function. Goiter is the most prominent effect of these agents. Iodine deficiency (ID) is an established cause of goiter. Even in the presence of extreme ID, however there is unequal geographical distribution of goiter, reflecting exposure to goitrogens in staple foods. Best examples are those of people living in Zaire, Sudan, Guinea and Northern Brazil, where thiocyanate from linamarin (a cyanogenic glucoside in cassava), flavonoids in millet and phenolic agents in babassu, respectively, are consumed in large amounts as part of these staple foods. Flavonoids are polyhydroxyphenols with a C_6-C_3-C_6 structure. Demonstration that vitexin, one of the three major flavonoids in Pearl millet, exerts clear in vivo antithyroid effects provided direct evidence that flavonoids are the goitrogens in this staple food of people with goiter living in the semiarid tropics. Flavonoids which are present in a large number of food plants are an obligatory step and integral part of the biogeochemical cycle of organic goitrogens in nature. Coal is also a source of a large variety of antithyroid and goitrogenic compounds contamining water supplies. The most abundant of these pathogenic organic compounds are phenol and dihydroxyphenols-resorcinol, thiocyanate, disulfides, hydroxypyridines, substituted dihydroxybenzenes, phthalate esters, phthalic acids, and halogenated and polycyclic aromatic hydrocarbons. Many of these organic polutants which are present in drinking water from iodine-sufficient goitrous areas, form dissociable complexes with large organic molecules called humic substances (HS). Decaying organic matter – plants and animals – become the substrate of lignin and flavonoid types of HS during fossilization – or coalification. Thus, flavonoid structures are the link between phenolic goitrogens in foodstuffs and those present in coals, shales, soils and water. Finally, microorganisms in soils and water, as well as in the gastrointestinal tract, play an important role in the process of biomagnification or activation of many food and coal-derived organic goitrogens. These observations emphasize the importance of our environment in the etiology of this disease, and provide basic information to develop cost-effective medical and/or public health measures to prevent and/or treat goiter and its associated disorders.

Introduction

A large number of natural agents in the environment are known to affect thyroid gland morphology and function. Goiter is the most prominent effect of these agents. They may cause the goitrous condition by acting directly on the thyroid gland (Figure 1) but also indirectly by altering the regulatory mechanisms of the thyroid gland and the peripheral metabolism and excretion of thyroid hormones (1,2). Figure 1 illustrates the three main steps in thyroid gland function, showing the environmental agents that act directly on the gland by interfering with the process of hormone synthesis. However, the mechanism that induces the trophic changes leading to goiter formation is not well understood, because besides thyrotropin or thyroid stimulating hormone (TSH), other humoral, paracrine, and autocrine growth factors appear to be involved in the process (3). These agents may enter into the food and water exposure pathways, becoming an important environmental antithyroid and/or goitrogenic factor in humans (1,2). Their effects may be additive to those of iodine deficiency (ID), making the intensity of the manifestations of goiter, hypothyroidism and iodine deficiency disorders (IDD) (cretinism, congenital hypothyroidism, and various degrees of impairment of growth and mental development) more severe. In iodine-sufficient areas, these compounds may be responsible for the development of 'sporadic' goiters or the persistence of the goiter endemia with its associated disorders, namely, au-

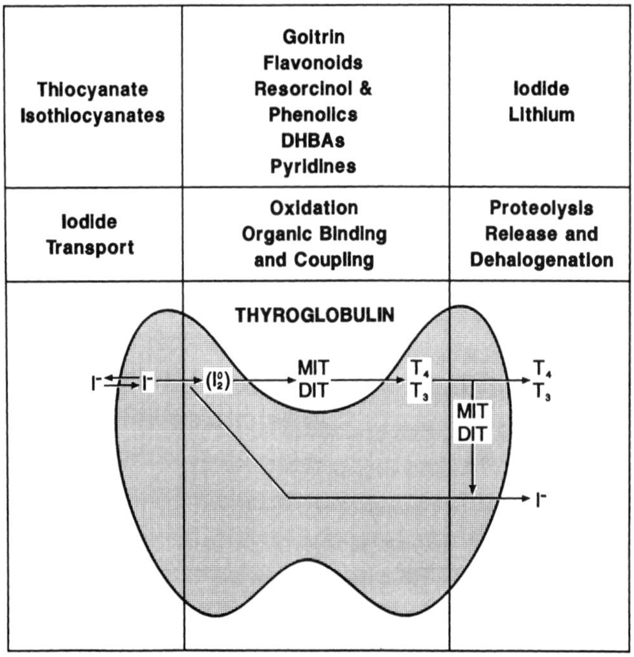

Fig. 1 Environmental antithyroid/goitrogenic compounds and their site of action in the thyroid gland. Abbreviations: goitrin, L,5-vinyl-2-thio-oxazolidone; DHBAs, dihydroxy-benzoic acids; I^-, iodide; MIT, monoiodotyrosine; DIT, diiodotyrosine; T_4, thyroxine; T_3, triiodothyronine.

toimmune thyroiditis, hypothyroidism, hyperthyroidism, and, probably, thyroid carcinoma (4,5).

Naturally occurring goitrogens

Sulfurated organics

Thiocyanate, isothiocyanates and thio-oxazolidone (Goitrin)

Thiocyanates and isothiocyanates are goitrogenic principles in plants of the Cruciferae family. The potent antithyroid compound L-5-vinyl-2-thio-oxazolidone or 'goitrin' was isolated from yellow turnips and from brassica seeds. Cyanogenic glycosides (thiocyanate precursors) are also present in several staple foods (cassava, maize, bamboo shoots, sweet potatoes, lima beans) from the Third World. After ingestion, these glycosides can be readily converted to thiocyanate by widespread glycosidases and the sulfur transferase enzyme. Isothiocyanates not only use the thiocyanate metabolic pathway but react with amino groups forming derivatives with thiourea-like antithyroid effects. Thus, the actual concentration of thiocyanates or isothiocyanates in a given foodstuff may not represent its true goitrogenic potential, nor does the absence of these compounds negate a possible antithyroid effect, because inactive precursors can be converted into goitrogenic agents both in the plant itself or in the animal after its ingestion. Thioglycosides undergo a rearrangement to form isothiocyanate derivatives and, in some instances, thiocyanate. Therefore, the amount of thiocyanate in the urine is a good indicator of the presence of thioglycosides in food. Ingestion of progoitrin, a naturally occurring thioglycoside, elicits antithyroid activity in rats and humans because of its partial conversion by intestinal micro-organisms into the more potent antithyroid compound 'goitrin'. This ability of plants and animals readily to covert inactive precursors into goitrogenic agents must be considered when the possible etiological role of dietary elements in endemic goiter is being investigated (1,2).

Several goiter endemias have been attributed to the presence of these sulfurated organic compounds in foodstuffs (1,2,5). The best documented is that in some areas of Zaire, where as many as 60 % of the population are affected by goiter. Cassava, a staple food in these areas, has definite antithyroid effects in humans and experimental animals. Thus, daily consumption of cassava, in the presence of severe iodine deficiency, is thought to be the cause of endemic goiter and cretinism in these areas of Zaire. The goitrogenic action of cassava is due to endogenous release of thiocyanate from linamarin, a cyanogenic glucoside present in cassava, particularly in the tuberous roots. Thiocyanate is also present in Pearl millet (Pennisetum [L] leeke, also known as typhoides or americanum), the staple food of people living in iodine-deficient endemic goiter areas of western Sudan. Pearl millet is rich in C-glycosylflavones which in combination with thiocyanate exert additive and complementary antithyroid and goitrogenic effects (1,2).

Thiocyanate is also found in high concentrations (1g/L) in wastewater effluents of coal conversion processes (6). This goitrogenic effect of thiocyanate is more evident in the presence of iodine deficiency. Several observations suggest that thiocyanate crosses the human placenta and may cause both goiter and neonatal hypothyroidism (7).

Thiocyanate. Thiocyanate or thiocyanate-like compounds primarily inhibit the iodine concentrating mechanism of the thyroid, and their goitrogenic activity can be overcome by iodine administration (Fig. 1). Thiocyanate at low concentrations inhibits iodide transport by increasing the velocity constant of iodide efflux from the thyroid gland. At high concentrations, the iodide efflux is greatly accelerated while the unidirectional iodide clearance into the gland is inhibited. Thiocyanate at these high concentrations also inhibits the incorporation of iodide into thyroglobulin by competing with iodide at the thyroid peroxidase (TPO) level (1). Thiocyanate is rapidly converted to sulfate in the thyroid gland. Administration of thyroid-stimulating hormone (TSH) increases the intrathyroidal catabolism of thiocyanate and is capable of reversing the block of iodide uptake produced by this ion.

Isothiocyanates. The isothiocyanates and cyanogenic glycosides act on the thyroid mainly by their rapid conversion to thiocyanate. However, isothiocyanates also react spontaneously with amino groups to form thiourea derivatives, which produce a thiourea-like antithyroid effect. Isothiocyanates also possess intrinsic antithyroid activity as demonstrated by in vitro inhibition of iodide uptake in the case of methyl- and allyl-isothiocyanates and of both, iodide uptake and organification in the case of butyl-isothiocyanate (1).

Thio-oxazolidone (goitrin). The thionamide or thiourea-like goitrogens interfere in the thyroid gland with the organification of iodide and formation of the active thyroid hormones, and their action usually cannot be antagonized by iodine. Naturally occurring goitrin is representative of this category (Figure 1). Long-term administration of goitrin to rats results in increased thyroid weight and decreased radioactive iodide uptake and hormone synthesis by the thyroid gland (1). Actually, goitrin possesses 133 % of the potency of propylthiouracil in humans. Goitrin is unique in that it is not degraded like thioglycosides. Additive antithyroidal effects of thiocyanate, isothiocyanate, and goitrin also occur with combinations of these naturally occurring goitrogens (1).

Disulfides. The small aliphatic disulfides (R-S-S-R; R = methyl- ethyl-, *n*-propyl, phenyl-), the major components of onion and garlic, exert marked thiourea-like antithyroid activity (1,2,6). None of these disulfides inhibits in vitro the thyroid peroxidase enzyme (11), but fractions with sulfur-bearing organic compounds, possibly aliphatic disulfides from the goitrogenic well supplying a Colombian district with endemic goiter, inhibited in vitro ^{125}I-organification (7). Disulfides are also present in high concentration (0.3 to 0.5 g/L) in aqueous effluents from coal-conversion processes and they have also been identified as water contaminants in the U.S.A. (1,2,6,7). The most frequently isolated compounds in the U.S.A. are dimethyl, diethyl, and diphenyl disulfides.

Flavonoids

Flavonoids are important stable organic constituents of a wide variety of plants. Flavonoids are universally present in vascular plants and in a large number of food plants. Because of their widespread occurrence in edible plants such as fruits, vegetables, and grains, flavonoids are an integral part of the human diet (1,8,9). They are present in high concentrations in polymeric (tannins) and oligomeric (pigments) forms in various staple foods of the Third World, such as millet, sorghum, beans and ground nuts.

Flavonoids are polyhydroxyphenolic compounds with a C_6-C_3-C_6 structure (1,8,9). Mammalian organisms are unable to synthesize the flavone nucleus. Flavonoids are strictly exogenous food components of exclusively vegetable origin. They have high chemical reactivity with multiple important biological implications (8,9). Flavonoids are quickly metabolized in higher organisms and that is the reason why they are not found in normal tissue constituents (1). Most flavonoids are present as β-glucosides which cannot be absorbed in tissues. No mammalian enzymes have been found which deglycosylate these compounds to their bioactive aglycone species. Following ingestion by mammals, flavonoid glycosides are hydrolyzed by intestinal microbial glycosidases to flavonoid aglycones. These may be absorbed and undergo metabolism by mammalian tissues or be further metabolized by intestinal micro-organisms to undergo B-ring hydroxylation and middle ring fission, with production of various metabolic monomeric compounds, including phenolic acids, phloroglucinol, resorcinol, and gallic acid (1). Each metabolic step is characterized by a marked increase in antithyroid effects (1). Flavonoid aglycones, such as apigenin and luteolin present in Fonio millet (Digitaria exilis) (10), and a variety of flavonoid metabolites (phloroglucinol, resorcinol, phenolic acids) are several times more potent than the parent glycosides glucosylvitexin, glucosylorientin and vitexin present in Pearl millet (Pennisetum [L] leeke, also known as typhoides or americanum) (1,2,7,10), as inhibitors of thyroid peroxidase (TPO), the enzyme catalyzing iodide oxidation and hormone synthesis in the thyroid gland. This greater inhibitory effect is further enhanced by the additive effects exerted by mixtures of flavonoid aglycones and flavonoid metabolites which are formed after ingestion of mixtures of flavonoid glycosides present in many plant foodstuffs. In addition, these metabolic products may produce adverse effects on other parameters of thyroid function not observed with the glycosides. As a result, the antithyroid effects of flavonoid glycosides in foodstuffs may be greatly enhanced by metabolic alterations after ingestion by mammals, as in the case of the flavonoids present in the Pearl millet grain, the staple food of people living in iodine-deficient endemic goiter areas of western Sudan, which make a major contribution to and are primarily responsible for its antithyroid and goitrogenic effects (1,7,10). Furthermore, antithyroid effects in vivo of vitexin, one of the three major flavonoids in Pearl millet, has been demonstrated (7) providing direct experimental evidence that C-glycosylflavones are the goitrogens in this cereal grain. It is of interest that a significant portion of the flavonoids isolated from Fonio millet (10), the staple food of people living in the severely affected endemic goiter area of Guinea in west Africa, are already present as the aglycones apigenin and luteolin, with more potent antithyroid activity than their parent glycosides.

Flavonoids not only inhibit TPO but, acting on iodothyronine deiodinase enzymes, also inhibit the peripheral metabolism of thyroid hormones. Flavonoids also affect serum thyroid hormone binding and thyrotropin (TSH) regulation (1,8,9). Thus, this class of compounds alter thyroid hormone economy in a complex manner.

At this point, there is substantial evidence indicating: first, that various millet species used as staple food by the populations in the semiarid tropics, are rich in flavonoids; second, that flavonoids have potent and diverse antithyroid properties; and third, that under the appropriate environmental dietary conditions of low iodine and protein-calorie intakes, which are prevalent in most countries of the Third World, flavonoids become an important etiologic determinant of endemic goiter and hypothyroidism (1,5,7,10).

Polyhydroxyphenols and phenol derivatives

Coal is a source of a large variety of antithyroid and goitrogenic compounds, such as, phenol, dihydroxyphenols (resorcinol), substituted dihydroxybenzenes, thiocyanate, disulfides, phthalic acids, pyridines, and halogenated and polycyclic aromatic hydrocarbons (PAH) (1,2,6,7). Most of these compounds have been identified in drinking water from the iodine-sufficient goitrous areas of Kentucky (U.S.A.) and Colombia (S.A.) (1,7). Phenolics are the major organic pollutants in wastewater effluents from various types of coal treatment processes. Resorcinol, substituted resorcinols, and other antithyroid phenolic pollutants are present at levels of as much as 5g/L in coal derived effluents. Up to 8 % of shale bitumen is also composed of phenols. Phenol, dihydroxyphenols, trihydroxyphenols, and halogenated phenols are readily absorbed from the gastrointestinal tract (1). A major route of metabolism of polyhydroxyphenols, polyhydroxyphenolic acids, and halogenated phenols is by conjugation to glucuronic or sulfuric acids. The major route of excretion of these compounds is the urinary tract and various amounts of the free parent compound and its monoglucuronide and monosulfate conjugates are excreted in the urine (1).

Resorcinol, the prototype of this group of compounds, is antithyroid and goitrogenic both in man and experimental animals (1,2,6). Several observations suggest that resorcinol crosses the human placenta and may cause both goiter and neonatal hypothyroidism (7). Resorcinol has been shown both in vivo and in vitro to inhibit thyroidal organification of iodide (1). A comparison of the antiperoxidase activity of resorcinol (1,3-dihydroxybenzene), catechol (1,2-dihydroxybenzene), and hydroquinone (1,4-dihydroxybenzene) indicates the importance of hydroxyl groups in the meta position for maximal activity (11). Furthermore, the net antiperoxidase effects of mixtures of dihydroxyphenols, as well as dihydroxyphenols and thiocyanate, also a coal derived pollutant, are equivalent to or greater than the sum of the effects produced by individual compounds, indicating that the true goitrogenic potential of the major water soluble compounds present in coal and shales are due to the combined effects of the individual constituents rather than to any single compound (11).

Demonstration in vivo and in vitro of antithyroid and goitrogenic activities of coal-water extracts from iodine-sufficient goiter areas (7) indicate that shale and coal derived organic pollutants appear to be a major factor contributing to the high goiter prevalence and associated disorders observed in certain areas with aquifers and watersheds rich in these organic rocks (1,2,6,7).

Studies of the physical state of organic goitrogens in water indicate that the active compounds form dissociable complexes and that they are part of larger organic molecules, possibly humic substances (HS) (1,2,6,7). Furthermore, resorcinol and other parent antithyroid phenolic and phenolic-carboxylic compounds are degradation monomeric by-products of reduction, oxidation, and microbial degradation of HS. HS, high molecular weight complex polymeric compounds, are the principal organic compounds of soils and waters. More than 90 % of total organic matter in water consists of HS, which are also present in coals and shales. Decaying organic matter becomes the substrate of lignin and flavonoid types of HS during the process of fossilization (or coalification). Actually, cyanidin, a naturally occurring flavonol used as the model subunit of flavonoid-type HS, yields by reductive degradation the antithyroid compounds: resorcinol, phloroglucinol, orcinol and 3,4-dihydroxybenzoic acid (DHBA) (6). Demonstration in vivo and in vitro of antithyroid effects of vitexin (10), a major C-glucosylflavone in Pearl millet, provide evidence that flavonoid structures are the link for phenolic goitrogens in foodstuffs (e.g., millet) and those present in coals, shales, soils and water, all of which are an obligatory step and integral part of the biogeochemical cycle of organic-phenolic goitrogens in nature (1,2) (Figure 2).

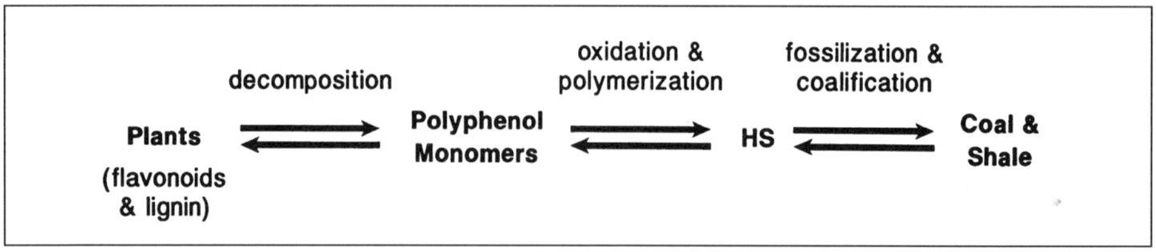

Fig. 2 Simplified scheme of the biogeochemical cycle of phenolic goitrogens and interrelationships among plant flavonoids (e.g. millet), polyhydroxyphenols, humic substances (HS), coals, and shales.

Pyridines

Hydroxypyridines also occur in aqueous effluents from coal conversion processes (2,6,7,11). Dihydroxypyridines and 3-hydroxypyridine are potent inhibitors of thyroid peroxidase (TPO), producing effects comparable to or greater than those of propylthiouracil (11). After ingestion, mimosine, a naturally occurring amino acid in the seeds and foliage of the tropical legume Leucaena leucocephala, is metabolized to 3,4-dihydroxypyridine (3,4-DHP), a potent antithyroid agent that produces goiter in mammals (1,2,6). 3,4-DHP crosses the placenta barrier producing goitrous offspring. The phenolic properties of the 3-hydroxy group in various hydroxypyridines are reflected in the metabolism of these compounds in vivo. 3-hydroxypyridine fed to rabbits is converted to ethereal glucuronide and sulfate conjugates. 3,4-DHP glucuronide and sulfate conjugates account for the majority of 3,4-DHP in the blood of cattle grazing on leucaena. The ring structure of dihydroxypyridines does not appear to be broken down in the body and also appears to be relatively stable to bacterial degradation (1).

Phthalate esters and metabolites

Phthalic acid esters, or phthalates, are ubiquitous in their distribution and have been frequently identified as water pollutants (1,2,6). Dibutyl (DBP) and dioctyl phthalates (DOP) have been isolated from water supplying areas of endemic goiter in western Colombia (S.A.) and eastern Kentucky (U.S.A.) (1,2,6). Although, phthalate esters are most commonly the result of industrial pollution they also appear naturally in shale, crude oil, petroleum, plants and fungal metabolites, and as emission pollutants from coal liquefaction plants (1,2,6).

Phthalate esters are well absorbed from the gastrointestinal tract. Prior to intestinal absorption there is hydrolysis to the corresponding monoester metabolite. This is particularly true of the longer chain derivatives such as DOP. Phthalates are widely distributed in the body; the liver being the major, initial repository organ. Clearance from the body is rapid. Short-chain phthalates can be excreted unchanged or following complete hydrolysis to phthalic acid. Prior to excretion most longer-chain compounds are converted, by oxidative metabolism to polar derivatives of the monoesters. The major route of phthalate esters elimination from the body is urinary excretion (1).

Although phthalate esters and phthalic acids do not possess intrinsic antithyroid activity, they undergo degradation by Gram-negative bacteria to form dihydroxybenzoic acid (DHBA) (1,2,6). DHBAs are known to possess antithyroid properties (1,6). The 3,4- and 3,5-DHBAs also inhibit in vitro TPO and the incorporation of iodide into thyroid hormones. The proven effective role of Gram-negative bacteria in phthalate biodegradation may explain in part the relationship established between frequency of goiter and bacterial contamination of water supplies (1,2,6). Furthermore, marked ultrastructural changes of the thyroid gland, similar to those seen after administration of TSH, and decreased serum T_4 concentration, have been observed in rats treated with phthalic acid esters (7). Thus, phthalates may become goitrogenic under appropriate conditions; they are also actively concentrated and metabolized by several species of fish. Whether these widely distributed pollutants exert deleterious effects on the thyroids of humans has not been investigated.

Polycyclic aromatic hydrocarbons (PAH)

PAHs have been found repeatedly in food and domestic water supplies, and in industrial and municipal waste effluents (1,2,6). They also occur naturally in coal, soils, ground water and surface water, and in their sediments and biota. One of the most potent of the carcinogenic PAH compounds, 3,4-benzpyrene (BaP), is widely distributed and, as in the case of other PAHs, is not efficiently removed by conventional water treatment processes.

The PAH carcinogens, BaP and 3-methylcolanthrene (MCA) by enhancement of hepatic UDP-glucuronyltransferase and glucuronidation, accelerate T_4 metabolism and excretion of T_4-glucuronide, resulting in decreased serum T_4 concentrations, activation of the pituitary-thyrotropin-thyroid axis, and eventually in goiter formation (1,2,6).There is also indication that MCA interferes directly with the process of hormonal synthesis in the thyroid gland. Furthermore, MCA, as well as 7,12-dimethylbenzanthracene, also induces goitrous thyroiditis in the BUF rat (12). Thus, MCA exerts its deleterious effects on the thyroid gland by at least three different mechanisms. Finally, the coal derived PAH methylanthracene (MA), which has been identified in drinking water from the goitrous coal rich district of eastern Kentucky (U.S.A.) (1,2), was found to produce goiter in the BUF rat without alteration of hormone synthesis or lymphocytic infiltration of the thyroid gland (2).

References

1. Gaitan E, ed. Environmental Goitrogenesis. Boca Raton: CRC, 1989.
2. Gaitan E. Goitrogens in food and water. Annual Review of Nutrition 1990;10: 21–39.
3. Dumont JE, Lamy F, Roger P, Maenhaut C. Physiological and pathological regulation of thyroid cell proliferation and differentiation by thyrotropin and other factors. Physiological Reviews 1992;72:667–97.
4. Gaitan E, Nelson NC, Poole GV. Endemic goiter and endemic thyroid disorders. World Journal of Surgery 1991;15:205–15.
5. Gaitan E, Dunn JT. Epidemiology of iodine deficiency. Trends in Endocrinology and Metabolism 1992;3:170–75.
6. Gaitan E. Goitrogens. Bailliere's Clinical Endocrinology and Metabolism 1988;2: 683–702.
7. Gaitan E. Environmental Goitrogens. In: Braverman LE, ed. Diseases of the Thyroid. Totowa: Humana Press 1997: 331–48.
8. Cody V, Middleton E Jr, Harborne JB, eds. Plant Flavonoids in Biology and Medicine: Biochemical, Pharmacological and Structure-Activity Relationships. New York: Liss 1986.
9. Cody V, Middleton E Jr, Harborne JB, Beretz A, eds. Plant Flavonoids in Biology and Medicine II: Biochemical, Cellular and Medicinal Properties. New York: Liss 1988.
10. Gaitan E. Flavonoids and the thyroid. Nutrition 1996;12:127–29.
11. Lindsay RH, Hill JB, Gaitan E, Cooksey RC, Jolley RL. Antithyroid effects of coal-derived pollutants. Journal of Toxicology and Environmental Health 1992;37: 467–81.
12. Weetman AP, McGregor AM. Autoimmune thyroid disease: Further development in our understanding. Endocrine Reviews 1994;15:788–830.

Industrial pollution by polychlorinated biphenyls and the thyroid status of adult and adolescent populations

P. Langer, [1]M. Tajtáková, [2]A. Kočan, [2]J. Petrík, [3]G. Fodor, [2]J. Chovancová, [2]B. Drobná, [2]S. Jursa, [2]M. Pavúk, P. Bohov, [3]J. Michálek, [3]A. Kreze, E. Šeboková, I. Klimeš

Institute of Experimental Endocrinology, Slovak Academy of Sciences, Bratislava; [1]First Clinic of Internal Medicine, Faculty of Medicine, P.J. Šafárik University, Košice; [2]Gas Chromatography/Mass Spectrometry Laboratory, Institute of Preventive and Clinical Medicine, Bratislava; [3]Institute of Clinical Endocrinology, Ĺubochňa, Slovakia

Abstract

Objective was to evaluate the thyroid status among the adult and adolescent population of an area that was heavily polluted by polychlorinated biphenyls (PCB) between 1955 and 1985.

Thyroid volume (ThV) was measured by ultrasound in 238 employees of a factory formerly producing PCB and 486 controls. Serum TSH and TT_4, and antibodies to thyroperoxidase (TPOab), thyroglobulin (TGab) TSH receptor (TSHRab) were estimated by specific RIA or IRMA. The level of PCB and other chlorinated organic substances (see below) in human adipose tissue, serum and milk was estimated by congener specific analysis. Urinary iodine was estimated by mild acid digestion followed by Sandell-Kolthoff reaction.

In 1990–94 high average levels of PCB in adipose tissue (6870 ng/g lipids), serum (2890 ng/g) and human milk (1320 ng/g) were found among adults from the polluted area compared with controls from much less polluted areas (1528, 1122 and 762 ng/g, respectively).

ThV (mean ± SE) was higher among employees (EMPL) of the factory formerly producing PCB (18.85 ± 0.69 ml, n = 238) than among controls (13.47 ± 0.48 ml, n = 486, $p < 0.001$). Moreover, the prevalence of positive thyroid antibodies was higher among EMPL than among adult controls, e.g. TPOab among all women 54/190 vs. 99/482 ($p < 0.05$), TGab among women aged 31–60 years 36/169 vs. 50/342 ($p < 0.05$) and TSHRab 25/238 vs. 6/238 ($p < 0.001$). The prevalence of arbitrarily defined normal thyroids (1. negative personal history, routine clinical and ultrasound examination; 2. normal plasma TSH and FT_4 level; 3. negative TPOab, TGab and TSHRab; 4. ThV < 22.0 ml) among EMPL working in the factory for 21–35 years (43/128 = 33.6 %) was lower than among EMPL working for 11–20 years (36/73 = 49.3 %, $p < 0.05$) or that in twice the number of matched controls (118/256 = 46.1 %; $p < 0.025$).

Urinary iodine was in the optimal range and similar in both groups.

Introduction

During the past five to six decades the global environment has been polluted by several organochlorinated substances including pesticides and insecticides (e.g. DDT, DDE, hexachlorobenzene, chlorophenoxy herbicides etc.), industrial chemicals of great commercial value (e.g. polychlorinated biphenyls – PCB) and some toxic compounds formed as byproducts in large scale chemical syntheses (e.g. polychlorinated dioxins and furans, the most toxic of which is 2,3,7,8-tetrachlorodibenzo-p-dioxin – TCDD).

In the late eighties, it was hypothesized that alterations of reproduction in wildlife might result from pollution by such chemicals, which were labeled "endocrine disrupters". Later, the US Environment Protection Agency defined the endocrine disrupter as *"an exogenous agent that interferes with the production, release, transport, metabolism, binding, action or elimination of natural hormones in the body responsible for the maintenance of homeostasis and the regulation of developmental processes"* (22).

Biochemical and toxic effects of organochlorinated aromatic hydrocarbons are mediated by aryl hydrocarbon (Ah) receptor, which functions as a ligand-activated transcription factor (32) via a mechanism that is superficially similar to that of members of the steroid/thyroid/retinoid receptor superfamily (53), although no endogenous ligand has yet been identified. However, there still remains a possibility that some effects of organochlorines are not linked to the Ah-receptor (Okey et al., 1995) and may be linked directly to the steroid/thyroid/retinoic receptor. Thus, binding of some industrial chemicals with estrogenic activity to the newly identified estrogen receptor beta was recently reported (31; 41). Nevertheless, there are still several non-receptor mediated effects, e.g. displacement of thyroid hormone from plasma protein binding (see Section 2).

Besides endocrine disruption, the main toxic and biochemical responses to organochlorines observed in wildlife and laboratory animals include carcinogenicity, dermal, immuno- and hepatotoxicity, teratogenicity, neurobehavioral effects, numerous biochemical responses, induction of several drug metabolizing enzymes and numerous biochemical responses (1).

Experimental studies on PCBs and the thyroid

One well known effect of PCB on thyroid function is a decrease in plasma T_4 level due to displacement of T_4 from plasma protein carriers (36; 11). This has also been observed in the case of the plasma transport protein complex for vitamin A (5). Recent reports have shown that hydroxylated PCBs have an affinity similar to thyroid hormone for transthyretin (10). It has also been demonstrated that methylsulfonylated PCB (which have been detected in human serum, milk and adipose tissue) cause a decrease in serum T_4 and T_3, an increase in TSH and increase in thyroid weight among rats (23). It should be mentioned that such metabolites are less lipophilic than CBs and thus enter the metabolic processes more actively. The reduction in plasma T_4 level further results from increased hepatic metabolism of T_4 due to the induction of UDP-glucuronyltransferase by PCB (52). Such reductions in plasma T_4 levels due to both displacement from protein binding and increased hepatic conjugation apparently resulted in increased TSH level in rats (37; 29).

Thyroid ultrastructural alterations have been found in rats after PCB feeding, suggesting a specific effect on the thyroid, since the changes were distinct from those observed after short- and long-term TSH stimulation and feeding low iodine diet (9). Direct effects of PCB on the thyroid are further supported by the decreased effect of TSH on T_4 and T_3 release from the thyroid in rats pretreated with PCB compared with controls (7).

Because of a structural similarity to T_4, PCBs may also interfere with transport of T_4 into the cell and with T_4 to T_3 conversion. It was thought that PCBs may also mimic thyroid hormone action and even modulate the mechanism of T_3 binding to its nuclear receptor and resulting gene expression (49). However, it has recently been reported that hydroxylated PCBs undergo only negligible binding to recombinant thyroid receptors (10).

Epidemiological studies on the effects of organochlorinated substances on the human thyroid

Since concern has been mostly focused on gonadal disruption, the thyroid has received little attention. It may be concluded from the reviews by *Nicholson and Landrigan* (40) and *Swanson* (54) that several previous epidemiological surveys on the effects of PCB did not pay attention to the thyroid.

For this reason, there are relatively few data from epidemiological studies concerning possible interrelations between exposure to PCB or other toxic organochlorinated substances and the human thyroid. Thus, *Bahn et al.* (1980) found 4 cases of primary hypothyroidism with high antimicrosomal antibody titer among 35 workers in a factory making polybrominated biphenyls (2). *Zober et al.* (58) observed that, 30 years after the uncontrolled escape of fumes containing TCDD in a chemical factory, 7 % of 158 exposed workers had thyroid disease compared to only 1.2 % among 161 controls.

Saracci et al. (51) reported 4 thyroid cancer deaths among 13,482 workers from 10 countries exposed to organic chlorinated substances with an average follow-up of 17 years. *Grimalt et al.* (1991) found 3 cases of thyroid cancer during a 10-year period (1980–1989) among 5003 inhabitants (about 50,000 person-years) of a Spanish village located close to a factory producing organochlorinated compounds (20). *Bertazzi et al.* (1997) reported 4 thyroid cancer deaths during a 15-year follow-up (about 260,000 person-years of subjects > 30 years) of the population of Seveso (3), Italy exposed to TCDD after the accident in 1976. In a 28-year follow-up of 81 patients with Yusho disease (after consumption of PCB contaminated rice oil) in Japan, *Tsuji et al.* (56) found 3 cases of thyroid cancer, 7 cases of elevated TSH level; among 41 patients with high serum PCB levels, 8 cases had high thyroglobulin antibodies. Although the findings described above of thyroid cancer were not significant, they at least merit some attention. It should be also noted that in those reports only cases of overt thyroid cancer were listed, while a number of latent cases possibly remained undetected.

In a 14-year follow-up of 795 Yucheng patients in Taiwan (similar to those with Yusho in Japan), 22 cases of goiter were reported (18 treated with medication or surgery) compared with 7 cases (4 treated) among 693 age and sex matched controls (21). *Calvert et al.* (1999) reported the levels of FT_4 of 27.8 ± 0.27 nmol/L (mean ± SE) among 278 workers employed for > 15 years in the manufacture of 2,4,5-trichlorophenol contaminated with TCDD (8). Surprisingly, these were significantly higher ($p < 0.02$) than levels found among 257 controls adjusted for race, sex, age, and current medication (26.8 ± 0.28 nmol/L). Among several hundred second-grade schoolchildren exposed to toxic waste from an incineration plant in Germany, *Osius et al.* (42) recently found a significant positive correlation between the serum level of the congener PCB 118 and FT_3. They also found a negative correlation between the sum of congeners PCB 138, 153, 180, 183 plus 187 and FT_3.

Of special interest is a recent study showing a significantly higher incidence of thyroid cancer among Norwegian women married to fishermen and fishery workers based on 2409 thyroid cancer cases among women during the period 1969–92 according to the Cancer Registry of Norway (17). Although this is a purely statistical analysis, it gives rise to speculation concerning the interrelations with possible increased levels of organochlorinated substances in fish. This is in agreement with several recent papers concerning saltwater fish as dietary predictor of plasma organochlorine concentrations (14; 50; 16; 48).

Among the most heavily exposed humans are the fetuses, neonates, and nursing infants of mothers with high blood levels of organochlorinated substances. Thus, perinatal exposure to maternal milk containing polychlorinated dioxins and furans resulted in increased TSH levels among nursing infants after 11 weeks (46) and decreased total and free thyroxine levels (30) or total thyroxine and triiodothyronine levels (Nagayama et al., 1998) in blood among breast-fed infants. Also irreversible neurological damage resembling that seen in those exposed to thyroid hormone deficiency in utero and/or in infancy was observed (47).

Studies on possible effects of PCB on the thyroid status in the polluted area in East Slovakia

Environmental pollution level

Although various harmful effects have been found even in human subjects after accidental or occupational exposure, recent reviews concluded that little is known about the effects from chronic environmental exposure, and that further epidemiological studies should be undertaken (22; 40). For these reasons, we decided to study the thyroid status among the adult and adolescent population living in an area heavily polluted by PCB. This became possible only after the change of regime in this country in 1989/90.

The chemical factory in Strážske (East Slovakia) manufactured more than 22,000 tons of PCB closely resembling the well-known Arochlor 1242 in the period 1955–85. Solid wastes of about 900 tons of PCB polluting the surrounding area still exist near the factory. The liquid wastes, which were dumped directly into the river without any protective treatment, resulted in heavy contamination of underground sources of drinking water and of superficial waters in the vicinity of the river (including a large artificial resort lake and an artificial fish pond) with resultant contamination of the food chain.

Although production was terminated in 1985, very high levels of total PCBs in environmental and human samples from the polluted area were still found by congener specific analysis (43) in preliminary surveys in 1990–94 (25, 27). Thus, the mean total PCB (congeners IUPAC No. 28, 52, 101, 138+163, 152, 180, 105, 118 and 156) concentration in 12 samples of human adipose tissue from that area was 6870 ng/g lipids (range 2560–16930 ng/g), about 4 times higher than in 57 samples from 5 control areas of Slovakia (mean 1528 ng/g, range 363–5180 ng/g). Similarly, in 15 samples of blood serum from polluted areas, the total PCB concentration was 2890 ng/g (range 1150–9200 ng/g), more than twice as high as in 81 samples from 5 control areas (mean 1122 ng/g, range 450–4350 ng/g). Finally, in 12 samples of human milk from polluted area the total PCB concentration of 1320 ng/g (range 610–2790 ng/g) was about twice as high as in 55 samples from 5 control areas (average 762 ng/g, range 300–1420 ng/g).

In that preliminary survey no samples from employees of the chemical factory were used in this series of examinations. However, the concentration of polychlorinated dibenzodioxines (PCDD), dibenzofurans (PCDF) and toxic mono/ortho PCB (congeners IUPAC No. 77, 81, 126 and 169) in 3 samples from employees and 30 samples from 4 control areas was estimated in the Centers for Disease Control and Prevention in Atlanta, Georgia (26). In this survey, in three employees of the chemical factory, the level of total toxic equivalency factor (TEF) for PCDD+PCDF was 137.74 and that for mono/ortho PCB was 238.59, while that in 30 control subjects was 22.12 and 38.39, respectively. A later group of employees had a serum TEF for PCCC+PCDF+mono/ortho PCB of about 600 pg/g (26).

Population and methods

Thyroid volume was measured by ultrasound in two groups of adults (34), 238 employees (EMPL) of the chemical factory formerly manufacturing PCB and 572 controls from control areas. The data on smoking and alcohol consumption obtained by questionnaire did not reveal any significant differences between those two groups.

Urinary iodine in 170 samples was kindly estimated by Prof. F. Vertongen (Department of Clinical Chemistry, University of Brussels, Brussels, Belgium) by the colorimetric ceric ion arsenious acid wet ash method using a Technicon auto-analyzer (15).

In serum aliquots obtained from the majority of examined subjects the concentration of TSH, total T_4 and autoantibodies to thyroid peroxidase (TPOab), thyroglobulin (TGab) and TSH receptor (TSHRab) were measured using appropriate commercial kits manufactured by Brahms Diagnostica GmbH (Berlin, Germany).

Differences between groups of exposed and control subjects were evaluated using the non-parametric Mann-Whitney test. Differences in the prevalence of thyroid disorders, individual thyroid antibodies or abnormal TSH levels were evaluated with the Chi-square test using the following cut-off points: 70 U/ml for TPOab, 150 U/mL for TGab and 10 U/mL for TSHRab), > 4.5 mU/L or < 0.1 mU/L for TSH.

Results

Urinary iodine: The median values of spot urine samples were in optimal range of 100 to 200 μg/L and did not differ significantly (median in μg/L per number of estimations) between EMPL (126/90) and adults from the pooled control areas (141/80).

Thyroid volume (ThV): Figure 1 shows the distribution of ThV, which was significantly higher ($p < 0.001$) among 238 EMPL than among 486 controls. The most remarkable difference was found in the number of values above the cut-off level of 22.0 ml (65/238 = 27.3 % among EMPL vs. 32/486 = 6.6 % among controls; $p < 0.02$).

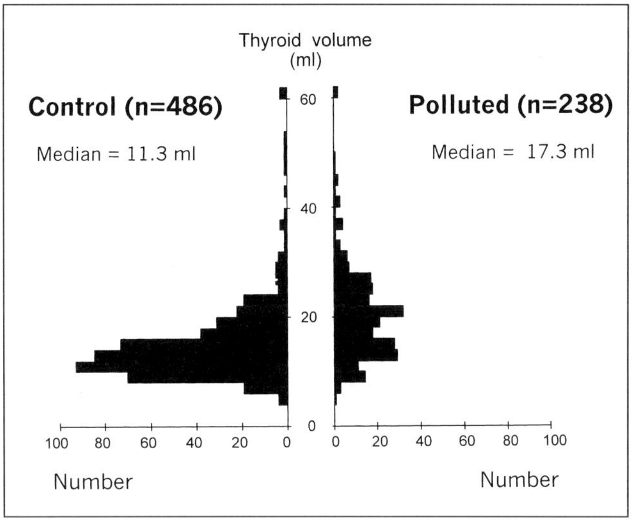

Fig. 1 Thyroid volume (ml) in the employees of a formerly PCB producing factory (right panel, n=238) and control adults (left panel, n=486)

Thyroid antibodies: The prevalence of TPOab was significantly higher ($p < 0.05$) among all women from the chemical factory compared with controls (54/190 = 28.4 % vs. 99/482 = 20.5 %), while the difference for TGab was significant ($p < 0.05$) only among women aged 31–60 years (36/169 = 21.3 % vs. 50/342 = 14.6 %). The most significant difference ($p < 0.001$) was found in the prevalence of TSHRab among all EMPL (25/238) compared with sex and age matched control subjects (6/238).

Hormone levels: The level of total T_4 (mean ± S.D.) among all EMPL (116.1 ± 31.2 nmol/L, n = 238) was similar to that among 498 controls (112.2 ± 37.0 nmol/L). No significant difference was found in the prevalence of TSH levels > 4.5 mU/L between EMPL (14/238 = 5.9 %, 6/14 TPOab negative) and controls (28/498 = 5.6 %). The prevalence of TSH < 0.1 mU/L was also about the same among EMPL (5/238 = 2.1 %, 2/5 TSHRab negative) and controls (10/498 = 2 %, 6/10 TSHR Ab negative). Among the remaining EMPL (mean ± S.D. = 1.56 ± 0.86 mU/L, n=219) and controls (1.51 ± 0.84 mU/L, n=460) no significant difference in TSH level was found.

Prevalence of normal thyroids and thyroid disorders: For the purpose of epidemiological evaluation of the prevalence of thyroid disorders vs. normal thyroid, the latter was arbitrary defined as: 1. Negative personal history; 2. Negative routine clinical examination; 3. Negative ultrasound examination; 4. Normal plasma TSH and total thyroxine concentration; 5. Negative thyroid antibodies (TPOab, TGab, TSHRab), 6. ThV < 22.0 ml.

The prevalence of such normal thyroids among the EMPL who had worked in the factory for 21–35 years (age 49 ± 8 years, mean ± S.D.) was 43/128 (33.6 %). This was significantly lower ($p < 0.05$) than among EMPL who had worked there for 11–20 years (36/73 = 49.3 %, age 43 ± 8 years)) and in double the number of age- and sex-matched controls (118/256 = 46.1 %, $p < 0.025$).

Significant differences between the EMPL working in the factory for 21–35 years (N=128) and double the number of age and sex matched controls (N=256) were found for prevalence of ThV > 22.0 ml (13/128 = 10.2 % vs. 6/256 = 2.3 %; p < 001), at least one positive out of three antibodies (18/128 = 14.1 % vs. 16/256 = 6.2 %; $p < 0.01$) and overt plus subclinical hypothyroidism (15/128 = 11.7 % vs. 14/256 = 5.4 %, $p < 0.025$).

Discussion

ThV was significantly higher among employees occupationally exposed to PCB and adolescents from the polluted area compared to the control groups. There was also an increased prevalence of total thyroid disorders among exposed employees. Since the level of urinary iodine was sufficient in all areas examined, the differences in ThV do not appear to be caused by regional differences in iodine intake.

The assumption of a sufficient iodine intake in Slovakia since early fifties is based on mandatory and well monitored consumption of iodized salt and on the embargo of importing any other salt. In addition, Slovakia was recently evaluated by the European ThyroMobil Study as a country with sufficient iodine intake and low ThV in schoolchildren (12). Finally, the low ThV and optimal urinary iodine observed in this study also supports the view of life-long sufficient iodine intake.

It should be noted that, because of global pollution, even the control population may have been exposed to PCB and other organochlorines (e.g. pesticides). However, since levels of PCB in human samples from the polluted area were at least 3–4 times higher than those from control areas (see Section 5), it may be concluded that PCB played a prominent role among the variety of organochlorines. Nevertheless, our recent survey (35) showed that even the other organochlorines, e.g. hexachlorobenzene and DDE (1,1-[dichloroethynylidene]bis[4-chlorobenzene]), might participate in the antithyroid action, since the frequency of thyroids with volume greater than 20.1 ml (15/46 = 32.6 %) in the upper decile of 46 subjects with the highest serum level of the sum of organochlorines (15,643–64,376 ng/g lipids) was significantly higher ($p < 0.001$) than that in lower 8 deciles of 368 subjects (31/368 = 8.4 %) with low levels (1016–11,664 ng/g lipids).

The mechanism by which PCB produced an increase in thyroid volume and increased prevalence of thyroid disorders remains to be explained. Such changes presumably resulted from long-term multiple effects on the thyroid including possible deterioration of cell membranes, interference with peripheral thyroid hormone metabolism, immunomodulatory, and other non-specific effects. It should be emphasized that more than four decades of exposure to the toxic effects resulted in a new steady state of pituitary-thyroid function which might not be manifested by persistently detectable abnormalities in hormone levels or thyroid function. This view is partly supported by the similar levels of TSH and thyroxine among employees and controls. For such reasons, it is not surprising that Triebig et al. (55) did not find any decrease in serum T_4 and T_3 among 250 workers exposed to dioxin when employed for up to 40 years in thermal metal recycling manufacture. It may be suggested that such long-term development of a new steady state results in a dichotomy between the levels of T_4 and TSH, which appear to be normal, and the consequences of such a long process, e.g. thyroid volume and antibody level which remain increased.

Some effects on the thyroid might even result from multiple non-specific toxicity, since PCBs are not typical thionamide like antithyroid substances. Among their primary effects on the pituitary-thyroid axis is displacement of thyroid hormones from plasma protein binding, an increase in their conjugation in the liver, and interference with their intracellular metabolism (7; 36; 47; 49; 52).

Highly lipophilic organochlorines are bound to plasma lipids and they are stored for decades in adipose tissue. They may also accumulate in cell membranes and damage their fluidity, as shown in renal tubules (Lopez-Aparicio et al., 1997), and stimulate free radical toxicity to destroy cellular structures, as shown in the testis (44). Similar changes in the thyroid, if any, may facilitate the communication between thyroid autoantigens and circulating immunocompetent cells. This possibility is supported by our preliminary findings (unpublished) that PCB are detectable in human thyroids from a polluted area (25–45 ng/g wet weight, the most abundant congeners being PCB IUPAC No. 108, 138, 153 and 180).

One of the most significant general effects of organochlorines may be immunomodulation (13; 4; 24). Evidence in support of this includes the increased prevalence of anti-myelin, anti-smooth muscle and other autoantibodies in exposed groups (57) and the increased prevalence of autoimmune diabetes mellitus and high fasting serum glucose level in Agent Orange sprayers among Vietnam veterans (39) and as well as in the cohort involved in the dioxin accident in Seveso, Italy (45). The increased prevalence of thyroid antibodies (e.g. TPOab, TGab and TSHRab) found in the present study might result from similar effects of PCB and other organochlorines. This view is in agreement with the findings of increased prevalence of antiperoxidase antibodies in the areas of Kentucky contaminated by polycyclic hydrocarbons (19). The participation of immunomodulatory effects of organochlorines is also supported by our previous finding of a highly significant decrease in β_2-microglobulin level among chemical factory employees (33).

Even estrogen-like effects on the thyroid cannot be ruled out, since several PCB congeners show estrogenic effects, estrogen receptors are present in human thyroid tissue (Valle et al., 1998), and striking estrogen receptor-mediated potencies of PCB including xenobiotics combinations have recently been described (Arnold et al., 1996). A role of estrogens in the stimulation of thyroid growth is also suggested by the inhibitory effect of tamoxifen on the growth of human cancer cells (Hoelting et al., 1996) and by the increased proliferation of FRTL-5 cells after estradiol (18).

Although our main aim was to study the population in an exceptionally PCB-polluted area and to evaluate some possible effects of organochlorines on the thyroid, the majority of questions remain unanswered.

Acknowledgements

This work was mainly supported by Merck Spol. sr.o. (Bratislava), Merck KgaA, Darmstadt, Germany, Ministry of Environment (Slovak Republic), Brahms Diagnostica (Berlin) and partly supported by Ministry of Education (grant No. 1/2293/95/0195/1297) and Grant Agency for Science, Slovak Republic (grant GAV No. 2/543/93). Some results presented (References by Kočan et al., 25–28) are based on work sponsored by the U.S.-Slovak Science and Technology Joint Fund in co-operation with the Ministry of Health (Slovak Republic) and the U.S. Department of Health and Human Services under the Project Number 94022.

References

1. Ahlborg UG, Brouwer A, Fingerhut MA et al. Impact of polychlorinated dibenzo-p-dioxins, dibenzofurans, and biphenyls on human and environmental health, with special emphasis on application of the toxic equivalency factor concept. Eur J Pharmacol 1992; 228; 179–199.
2. Bahn AK, Mills JL, Snyder PJ et al. Hypothyroidism in workers exposed to polybrominated biphenyls. New Engl J Med 1980; 302; 31–33.
3. Bertazzi PA, Zocchetti C, Guercilena S et al. Dioxin exposure and cancer risk: a 15-year mortality study after the "Seveso accident". Epidemiology 1997; 8; 646–652.
4. Birnbaum LS. Workshop on perinatal exposure to dioxin-like compounds. V. Immunologic effects. Environ Health Perspect 1995; 103,Suppl 2; 157–169.
5. Brouwer A. The role of enzymes in regulating the toxicity of xenobiotics. Biochem Soc Transact 1991; 19; 731–737.
6. Brunn J, Block U, Ruf G et al. Volumetrie der Schilddrüsenlappen mittels real-time Sonographie. Dtsch Med Wschrift 1981; 106; 1138–1140.
7. Byrne JJ, Carborne JP, Hanson EA. Hypothyroidism and abnormalities in the kinetics of thyroid hormone metabolism in rats treated chronically with polychlorinated biphenyl and polybrominated biphenyl. Endocrinology 1987; 21; 520–527.
8. Calvert GM, Sweeney MH, Deddens J et al. Evaluation of diabetes mellitus, serum glucose, and thyroid function among United States workers exposed to 2,3,7,8-tetrachlorodibenzo-p-dioxin. Occup Environ Med 1999; 56; 270–276.
9. Capen CC, Martin SL. The effects of xenobiotics on the structure and function of thyroid follicular and C-cells. Toxicol Pathology 1989; 17; 266–293.
10. Cheek AO, Kow K, Chen J et al. Potential mechanisms of thyroid disruption in humans: interaction of organochlorine compounds with thyroid receptor, transthyretin, and thyroxine-binding globulin. Environ Health Perspect 1999; 107; 273–278.
11. Darnerud PO, Morse D, Klasson-Wehler E et al. Binding of a 3,3',4,4'-tetrachlorobiphenyl (CB-77)

metabolite to fetal transthyretin and effects on fetal thyroid hormone levels in mice. Toxicology 1996; 106; 105–114.
12. Delange F, Benker G, Caron Ph et al. Thyroid volume and urinary iodine in European schoolchildren: standardization of values for assessment of iodine deficiency. Eur J Endocrinol 1997; 136; 180–187.
13. Devailly E, Ayotte P, Bruneau S et al. Inuit exposure to organochlorine through the aquatic food chain in arctic Quebec. Environ Health Perspect 1993; 101; 618–629.
14. Devoto E, Kohlmeier L, Heeschen W. Some dietary predictors of plasma organochlorine concentrations in the elderly German population. Arch Environ Health 1998; 53; 147–155.
15. Dunn JT, Crutchfield HE, Gutekunst R et al. Methods for measuring iodine in urine. ICCIDD, 1993
16. Fitzgerald EF, Hwang SA, Bush B et al. Fish consumption and breast milk PCB concentration among Mohawk women at Akwesasne. Am J Epidemiol 1998; 148; 164–172.
17. Frich L, Akslen LA, Glattre E. Increased risk of thyroid cancer among Norwegian women married to fishery workers – a retrospective study. Brit J Cancer 1997; 76; 385–389.
18. Furlaneto TW, Nguyen LQ, Jameson JL. Estradiol increases proliferation and down-regulates the sodium/iodide symporter gene in FRTL-5 cells. Endocrinology 1999; 140:5705–5711.
19. Gaitan E, Cooksey RC, Gaitan D et al. Goiter and autoimmune thyroiditis in iodine-sufficient areas. In Autoimmune Thyroiditis. Schernbaum WA, Bogner U, Weinheimer B, Botazzo GF, eds. Berlin: Springer, 1991; 175–181.
20. Grimalt JO, Sunyer J, Moreno V et al. Risk excess of soft-tissue sarcoma and thyroid cancer in a community exposed to airborne organochlorinated compound mixtures with a high hexachlorobenzene content. Internat J Cancer 1994; 56; 200–203.
21. Guo YL, Yu ML, Hsu CC et al. Chloracne, goiter, arthritis, and anemia after polychlorinated biphenyl poisoning: 14-year follow-up of the Taiwan Yucheng cohort. Environ Health Perspect 1999; 107; 715–719.
22. Kavlock RJ, Daston GP, DeRosa C et al. Research needs for the risk assessment of health and environmental effects of endocrine distruptors: A report of the U.S. EPA-sponsored workshop. Environ Health Perspect 1996; 104; 715–740.
23. Kato, Y, Haraguchi K, Shibahara T. et al. Reduction of thyroid hormone levels by methylsulfonyl metabolites of tetra- and pentachlorinated biphenyls in male Sprague-Dawley rats. Toxicol Sci 1999; 48; 51–54.
24. Kerkvliet NI. Immunological effects of chlorinated dibezo-p-dioxins. Environ Health Perspect 1995; 103,Suppl 9; 47–53.
25. Kočan A, Petrík J, Drobná B et al. Levels of PCBs and some organochlorine pesticides in the human population of selected areas of the Slovak Republic. I. Blood. Chemosphere 1994; 29; 2315–2325.
26. Kočan A, Patterson DG, Jr, Petrík J et al. PCDD, PCDF and coplanar PBC levels in blood from the human population of the Slovak Republic. In: Human Exposure-Human Health Risk Assessment. van den Berg M, ed. Amsterdam: University of Amsterdam, 1996: 137–142.
27. Kočan A, Patterson DG, Jr, Petrík J et al. Research Report 1997 (in Slovak). Institute of Preventive and Clinical Medicine, Bratislava 1997.
28. Kočan A, Petrík J, Turner WE et al. Research Report 1997 (in Slovak). Institute of Preventive and Clinical Medicine, Bratislava 1998
29. Kolaja KL, Klaasen CD. Dose-response examination of UDP-glucuronosyltransferase inducers and their ability to increase both TGF-beta expression and thyroid follicular cell apoptosis. Toxicol Sci 1998; 46; 31–37.
30. Koopman-Esseboom C, Morse DC, Weisglas-Kuperus N et al. Effects of dioxins and polychlorinated biphenyls on thyroid hormone status of pregnant women and their infants. Pediatric Research 1994; 4; 468–473.
31. Kuiper GGJM, Lemmen JG, Carlsson B et al. Interaction of estrogenic chemicals and phytoestrogens with estrogen receptor beta. Endocrinology 1998; 139; 4252–4263.
32. Lai ZW, Pineau T, Esser C. Identification of dioxin-responsive elements (DREs) in the 5·regions of putative dioxin-inducible genes. Che-Biol Interact 1998; 100; 97–112.
33. Langer P, Kaušitz J, Tajtáková M et al. Decreased blood level of β_2-microglobulin in the employees of a factory which produced polychlorinated biphenyls. Chemosphere 1997; 34; 2595–2600.

34. Langer P, Tajtáková M, Fodor G et al. Increased thyroid volume and prevalence of thyroid disorders in an area heavily polluted by polychlorinated biphenyls. Eur J Endocrinol 1998; 139; 402–409.
35. Langer P, Tajtáková M, Koçan A et al. Thyroid status and blood level of polychlorinated biphenyls and pesticides in exposed and control population (abstract), this book, page 335.
36. Lans M, Klasson-Wehler E, Willemsen M et al. Structure-dependent, competitive interaction of hydroxy-polychlorobiphenyls, -dibenzo-p-dioxins and -dibenzo-furans with human transthyretin. Chem-Biol Interact 1993; 88; 7–21.
37. Liu J, Liu Y, Barter RA et al. Alteration of thyroid homeostasis by UDP-glucuronotransferase inducers in rats: a dose-response study. J Pharmacol Exper Ther 1995; 273; 977–985.
38. López-Aparicio O, Merino MJ, Sánchez E et al. Effect of Aroclor 1248 and two pure congeners upon the membrane fluidity of rat renal tubular cultures. Pesticide Biochem Physiol 1997; 57; 54–62.
39. Michalek JE, Akhtar FZ, Kiel JL. Serum dioxin, insulin, fasting glucose and sex-hormone binding globulin in veterans of operation Ranch Hand. J Clin Endocrinol Metab 1999; 84; 1540–1543.
40. Nicholson WJ, Landrigan PJ. Human health effects of polychlorinated biphenyls. In: Dioxins and Health. Schecter A, ed. New York: Plenum Press 1994; 487–524.
41. Ogawa S, Inoue S, Watanabe T et al. The complete primary structure of human estrogen receptor ß (hERß) and its heterodimerization with ERa in vivo and in vitro. Biochem Biophys Res Commun 1998; 243; 122–126.
42. Osius N, Karmaus W, Kruse H, Witten J. Exposure to polychlorinated biphenyls and levels of thyroid hormones in children. Environ Health Perspect 1999:843–849,1999
43. Patterson DG, Jr, Isaacs SG, Alexander LR et al. Method 6: Determination of specific polychlorinated dibenzo-p-dioxins and dibenzofurans in blood and adipose tissue by isotope dilution-high-resolution mass spectrometry. In: Environmental carcinogens. Methods of analysis and exposure measurements. Vol. 11. Polychlorinated dioxins and dibenzofurans. Rappe C, Buser HR, Dodet B, O'Neill IK, eds. Lyon:IARC Scientific Publications No. 108,1991:299–342.
44. Peltola V, Mantyla E, Huhtaniemi I et al. Lipid peroxidation and antioxidant enzyme activities in the rat testis after cigarette smoke inhalation or administration of polychlorinated biphenyls or polychlorinated naphthalens. J Andrology 1994; 15; 353–361.
45. Pesatori AC, Zocchetti C, Guercilena S et al. Dioxin exposure and non-malignant health effects: a mortality study. Occup Environ Med 1998; 55; 126–131.
46. Pluim HJ, de Viljder JJM, Olie K et al. Effects of pre- and postnatal exposure to chlorinated dioxins and furans on human neonatal thyroid hormone concentrations. Environ Health Perspect 1993; 101; 504–408.
47. Porterfield SP. Vulnerability of the developing brain to thyroid abnormalities: environmental insults to the thyroid system. Environ Health Perspect 1994; 102,suppl 2; 125–130.
48. Rylander L, Stromberg U, Dyremark E et al. Polychlorinated biphenyls in blood plasma among Swedish female fish consumers in relation to low birth weight. Am J Epidemiol 1998; 147; 493–502.
49. Safe S. Modulation of gene expression and endocrine response pathways by 2,3,7,8-tetrachlorodibenzo-p-dioxin and related compounds. Pharmacol Ther 1995; 67; 247–281.
50. Salama AA, Mohamed MAM, Duval B et al. Polychlorinated biphenyl concentration in raw and cooked North Atlantic bluefish (Pomatomus saltatrix) fillets. J Agric Food Chem 1998; 46; 1359–1362.
51. Saracci R, Kogevinas M, Bertazzi PA et al. Cancer mortality in workers exposed to chlorophenoxy herbicides and chlorophenols. Lancet 1991; 338; 1027–1031.
52. Schuur AG, Boekhorst FM, Brouwer A et al. Extrathyroidal effects of 2,3,7,8-tetrachlorodibenzo-p-dioxin on thyroid hormone turnover in male Sprague-Dawley rats. Endocrinology 1997; 138; 3727–3734.
53. Sogawa K, Fujii-Kuriyama Y. Ah-receptor, a novel ligand-activated transcritpion factor. J Biochem 1997; 122; 1075–1079.
54. Swanson GM, Ratcliffe HE, Fischer LJ. Human exposure to polychlorinated biphenyls (PCBs): A critical assessment of evividence for adverse health effects. Regul Toxicol Pharmacol 1995; 21; 136–150.
55. Triebig G, Werle E, Päpke O. Effects of dioxins and furans on liver enzymes, lipid parameters, and thyroid hormones in former thermal metal recycling workers. Environ Health Perspect 1998; 106,suppl.2; 697–700.

56. Tsuji H, Sato K, Shimono J et al. Thyroid function in patients with Yusho: 28 year follow-up study (in Japanese). Fukuoka Igaku Zasshi 1997; 88; 231–235.
57. Vial T, Nicolas B, Descortes J. Clinical immunotoxicity of pesticides. J Toxicol Environ Health 1996; 48; 215–229.
58. Zober A, Ott MG, Messerer P. Morbidity follow up study of BASF employees exposed to 2,3,7,8-tetrachlorodibenzo-p-dioxin (TCDD) after a 1953 chemical reactor incident. Occup Environ Med 1994; 51; 479–486.

Effects of low level environmental perchlorate exposure on thyroid function

J. E. Lawrence, S. H. Lamm, S. Pino, K. Richman, **L. E. Braverman**

Section of Endocrinology, Diabetes and Nutrition; Boston Medical Center, and The Brigham & Women's Hospital; Boston, MA, USA

Abstract

Perchlorate (ClO_4) salts are found in rocket fuel, fireworks and fertilizer. Due to ground water contamination, ClO_4 has recently been detected in large public water supplies in several states in the 4–15 µg/l (ppb) range. The potential adverse effect of chronic low level ClO_4 ingestion on thyroid function is of concern to the EPA. The daily ingestion of ClO_4 at these levels would be magnitudes below the therapeutic effect level of hundreds of mg ClO_4 used in treating hyperthyroidism.

Studies in 9 healthy male volunteers were carried out to determine whether the ingestion of 10 mg ClO_4 daily (approximately 300 times the estimated maximum amount of ClO_4 consumed from the affected water supplies) would affect any aspect of thyroid function. They ingested the 10 mg ClO_4 dissolved in a liter of spring water during waking hours for 14 days. Baseline serum TSH, FTI, TT_3 and thyroid Ab, 4, 8 and 24h thyroid ^{123}I uptakes (RAIU), serum and 24 h urine ClO_4, 24 h urine iodine, CBC, and chemistry profile were determined. All blood and urine tests were repeated on days 7 and 14 of ClO_4 administration and thyroid RAIU on day 14 of ClO_4 administration. All tests were repeated 14 days after ClO_4 was discontinued. No effect of ClO_4 on serum thyroid hormone or TSH concentrations, urinary iodine excretion, CBC or blood chemistry was observed. Urine and serum ClO_4 levels were appropriately elevated during the course of ClO_4 ingestion in all subjects, demonstrating compliance. By day 14 of ClO_4 administration, the 4, 8 and 24 h thyroid RAIU values decreased in all subjects by a mean value of 38 % from baseline and rebounded above baseline values by 25 % at 14 days after ClO_4 withdrawal ($p < 0.01$, ANOVA and Tukey).

The present study demonstrates the sensitivity of the thyroid iodide (NIS) trap to ClO_4 since a low dose of 10 mg daily significantly decreased the thyroid RAIU without affecting circulating thyroid hormone or TSH concentrations. However, it is now of interest to determine a no effect level for ClO_4 on the inhibition of the thyroid RAIU and to carry out another study to determine whether thyroid function could be affected by a more prolonged exposure to low level ClO_4.

Introduction

Perchlorates have been used for over 50 years as oxidizers in solid propellants for rockets and missiles in the space program. In addition, perchlorates have been used in fireworks, and more recently, in road flares and air bag inflation systems and have been found in some commercial fertilizers. Perchlorate salts are highly soluble in water and have been detected as contaminants in surface and ground waters in several states. Surveys of wells and drinking waters found that levels rarely exceeded 18 ppb or 18 μg/l (1). In California, wells exceeding this level were closed, or their waters were diluted before public use. Assuming a daily water consumption of approximately two liters per person per day, the consumption of water containing up to 16 ppb perchlorate would result in the ingestion 36 μg perchlorate daily.

The major pharmacological effect of the perchlorate anion is to decrease the active transport of iodide into the thyroid. Perchlorate is a competitive inhibitor of the sodium / iodide symporter (NIS), the thyroid cell surface protein responsible for transporting iodide from the plasma into the thyroid. The rat symporter was first cloned by Dai et al. in 1996 (2) and the human NIS by Smanik et al. (3). In view of its antithyroid action, perchlorate was used in large doses up to 2,000 mg daily to treat hyperthyroid Graves' disease in the 1950s and early 1960s (4). This practice was abandoned because of a concern for a toxic effect on the bone marrow at high doses that resulted in aplastic anemia and agranulocytosis (5–9). However, in 1984, Wenzel and Lente reported the successful use of perchlorate as therapy of hyperthyroid Graves' disease with daily doses of 900 mg or less for up to 1 year (10). No serious side effects were reported. Shortly thereafter, perchlorate was also employed in doses of up to 1000 mg daily for 4 weeks or longer as adjunctive therapy of iodine-induced hyperthyroidism secondary to the iodine rich antiarrhythmic drug, amiodarone (11). More recently, perchlorate (900 mg daily) has also been reported to be useful in preventing iodine-induced hyperthyroidism following the administration of iodine rich x-ray contrast agents used in coronary angiography (12). In these more recent studies, no serious toxic effects were observed. Perchlorate has also been given to euthyroid volunteers. Bürgi et al. reported in 1974 that the daily administration of 600 mg perchlorate to 5 normal volunteers over the course of a week increased non-thyroxine iodine release by 65 %, suggesting that iodine uptake might have been completely blocked (13). In 1992, Brabant et al. treated 5 healthy males with 900 mg potassium perchlorate daily for 4 weeks and were unable to induce thyroid iodine depletion (14). Both of these studies were conducted in moderately iodine deficient regions and not in an area where ambient iodine intake is adequate, as in the United States.

We recently studied workers in the only U.S. industrial site currently manufacturing ammonium perchlorate (American Pacific Corporation Cedar City, Utah) and found no adverse effects (15). Airborne exposures ranged from 0.004 to 167 mg total particulate perchlorate daily and urinary perchlorate was readily detected in the exposed workers. Serum perchlorate ranged from zero to 1.6 μg/ml. No thyroid abnormalities were found on physical exam and no differences in thyroid function (serum TSH, FT_4 index, TT_3 and TPO antibodies) were detected. Finally, neither hematologic nor blood chemistry abnormalities were present in these workers chronically exposed to perchlorate.

The present study was carried out to determine whether the ingestion of perchlorate enriched water (10 mg / daily) would affect thyroid function in normal male volunteers. The most sensitive effect of perchlorate is on the thyroid iodine uptake. Therefore, thyroid ^{123}I uptakes (RAIU) before, during, and after perchlorate ingestion were also determined. The daily 10 mg dose of perchlorate is approximately 300 times greater than potential exposure from the consumption of drinking waters known to contain perchlorate. A no-observed-adverse-effect-level (NOAEL) of perchlorate was sought to evaluate potential human health risks from environmental perchlorate contamination.

Materials and methods

This study was carried out in 9 euthyroid male volunteers ages 22 to 30 years after approval by the Institutional Review Board. Blood was obtained for baseline measurement of thyroid function tests and TPO antibodies. All baseline thyroid function tests were normal and the 9 volunteers were enrolled in the study. A baseline 24 hour urine was collected, and baseline thyroid RAIUs were measured at 4, 8, and 24 hours after the ingestion of 150 μCi ^{123}I.

Ten mg perchlorate as potassium perchlorate was dissolved in 1 liter bottles of spring water. Each subject was asked to consume one liter per day intermittently during waking hours for 14 days in order to simulate how the general public ordinarily drinks water. Blood specimens were drawn between 8 and 9 am, and 24 hour urines were obtained on days 7 and 14 during perchlorate ingestion and again 2 weeks after perchlorate was discontinued. The 4, 8, and 24 hour thyroid ^{123}I uptakes were repeated on the final day of perchlorate consumption (exposure day 14) and again 2 weeks later.

CBC and routine blood chemistries were measured on all samples drawn during the course of the study to identify any potential perchlorate-induced abnormalities. Twenty-four hour urine collections were measured for iodine, perchlorate and creatinine. Thyroid function tests were measured on blood drawn throughout the study and were measured after completion of the study, in duplicate, in the same assay, and in random order. Serum iodine and perchlorate levels were measured in the blood samples.

Statistical analysis for the thyroid RAIU values was carried out by Analysis of Variance (ANOVA) with post-hoc pairwise comparisons using Tukey's method. Statistical analyses of the thyroid function tests and urine and serum perchlorate and iodine values were carried out by ANOVA and SNK. Values are reported as the mean ± standard error (SE).

Results

No adverse effects of perchlorate were noted on hepatic, renal, or hematologic parameters. Throughout the study, the volunteers remained asymptomatic and had no changes in their normal physical exams.

Thyroid function tests (Table 1)

Baseline thyroid function tests were normal and remained unchanged during and after perchlorate administration. TPO antibodies were negative in all subjects.

Urine and serum perchlorate levels (Table 2)

Eighteen samples of the perchlorate drinking water were analyzed for perchlorate content and found to contain 10.8 ± 0.6 mg per liter bottle which was almost identical to the amount of perchlorate added to the bottles. No perchlorate was detected in the urine samples collected before perchlorate exposure or two weeks after perchlorate had been discontinued. During perchlorate administration, urinary perchlorate markedly increased, reaching levels of 7.7 ± 0.8 mg / 24 hr and 7.5 ± 1.0 mg/ 24 hr at 7 and 14 days, respectively. Perchlorate was not detected in the serum before and 2 weeks after perchlorate ingestion. During perchlorate administration, serum levels were markedly elevated to 0.61 ± 0.02 and 0.59 ± 0.02 μg/ml on days 7 and 14, respectively.

Table 1 The effect of perchlorate (ClO_4) administration (10 mg daily) for 14 days on thyroid function tests.

Time	T_4 (μg/dl)	THBR	FTI	T_3 (ng/dl)	TSH (μU/ml)
Baseline	6.6 ± 0.4*	0.96 ± 0.02	6.3	136 ± 6	1.05 ± 0.14
7 Days ClO_4	6.7 ± 0.4	0.94 ± 0.02	6.2	140 ± 8	1.00 ± 0.17
14 Days ClO_4	6.6 ± 0.5	0.96 ± 0.03	6.3	151 ± 6	0.96 ± 0.12
14 Days after ClO_4	6.5 ± 0.5	0.97 ± 0.02	6.3	157 ± 9	1.23 ± 0.17

* Mean ± SE

Table 2 Urine and serum perchlorate (ClO_4) values before, during, and after the ingestion of 10 mg of ClO_4 daily for 14 days.

Time	Urine perchlorate (mg/24hrs)	Serum perchlorate (µg/ml)
Baseline	< 0.5	0
7 Days ClO_4	7.7 ± 0.8*	0.61 ± 0.02
14 Days ClO_4	7.5 ± 1.0	0.59 ± 0.02
14 Days after ClO_4	< 0.5	0

* Mean ± SE

Table 3 Urine and serum iodine values before, during, and after the ingestion of 10 mg ClO_4 daily for 14 days.

Time	Urine iodine (µg/24hrs)	Serum iodine (µg/dl)
Baseline	254 ± 69	6.5 ± 0.42 *
7 Days ClO_4	233 ± 49	6.2 ± 0.34
14 Days ClO_4	385 ± 123	6.4 ± 0.37
14 Days after ClO_4	208 ± 42	6.3 ± 0.57

* Mean ± SE

Urine and serum iodine levels (Table 3)

There were no significant changes in urinary iodine excretion during or 2 weeks after perchlorate administration whether values were expressed as µg/dl, µg/total volume, or µg/gm creatinine. Values were variable throughout the study as iodide ingestion was not controlled in the volunteers' diet. Serum total iodine values remained normal and unchanged during and 2 weeks after perchlorate ingestion.

Thyroid ^{123}I uptakes (Table 4 and Figure 1)

Baseline 4, 8, and 24 hr thyroid RAIUs were normal. During perchlorate ingestion, there was a highly significant decrease in the thyroid RAIUs at all 3 time points. The average decrease below baseline values over all 3 time points was 38 %. Two weeks after perchlorate was discontinued, the thyroid RAIUs were significantly higher than baseline at 4, 8, and 24 hours, averaging 125 % of baseline values.

Table 4 Thyroid ^{123}I uptakes before, during and after the ingestion of 10mg ClO_4 daily for 14 days.

Time	Thyroid ^{123}I uptake (% dose)		
	Baseline day	on 14 ClO_4	14 days after ClO_4
4 Hours	12.5 ± 1.3	8.2 ± 0.7*	16.6 ± 2.4**
8 Hours	17.3 ± 1.9	10.6 ± 1.0*	21.9 ± 2.8**
24 Hours	23.6 ± 2.6	14.0 ± 1.6*	27.1 ± 3.3***

* p <0.01 vs. Baseline and after ClO_4
** p <0.01 vs. Baseline
*** p <0.05 vs. Baseline

Discussion

The present study demonstrates that low doses of perchlorate (10 mg daily) administered for 14 days did not affect circulating thyroid hormone and TSH concentrations but did significantly decrease the thyroid ^{123}I uptake. This finding was not unexpected since the major effect, and almost certainly the only effect, of perchlorate on the thyroid is a decrease in the thyroid iodide trap by competitive inhibition of NIS (2). Since the thyroid has large stores of iodine, T_4, and T_3, the observed decrease in the thyroid iodide trap would not be expected to have resulted in changes in the circulating levels of thyroid hormones and TSH over a 2 week period. This modest reduction in the thyroid RAIU would have decreased the entrance of stable iodide into the thyroid in these subjects, but dietary iodine was more than adequate (approxi-

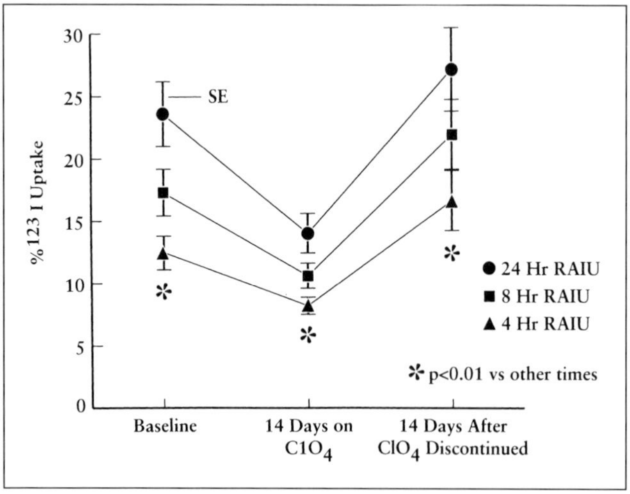

Fig. 1 The effect of low dose perchlorate on the 4, 8, and 24 hour thyroid ^{123}I uptakes.

mately 250 μg daily). Over 2 weeks this modest decrease in iodine uptake would not have significantly affected the release of stored hormones. It is likely that the observed effect on the thyroid RAIU is physiological since a rebound increase in the RAIU was observed after perchlorate was discontinued, which may represent an increase in NIS. This rebound increase in the thyroid RAIU is almost identical to the increase reported by Stanbury and Wyngaarden in hyperthyroid patients receiving therapeutic doses of perchlorate (17). In our previous study of workers in the plant producing perchlorate, exposure to much higher levels of perchlorate for months and years did not affect thyroid function tests or cause clinical thyroid disease (15). However, thyroid RAIUs could not be measured in these workers.

Serum perchlorate levels were consistently elevated and varied only slightly among the 9 volunteers. The serum levels were essentially equal at the end of the first and second week of ingestion. There was considerable variation in urinary perchlorate values between individuals and between the 2 collections from each subject. This is most likely due to incomplete 24 hour urine collections and different patterns of perchlorate ingestion in relation to the urine collections. Since serum perchlorate values were consistent in all subjects, as noted above, incomplete urine collections is a more plausible explanation than incomplete perchlorate ingestion.

Perchlorate readily crosses the placenta and could pose a potential hazard to the fetus by decreasing fetal thyroid iodine stores and subsequent thyroid function. However, this possibility is unlikely since a recent report from regions of perchlorate-contaminated ground water, with levels as high as 16 μg/l, found no evidence of an increased incidence of congenital hypothyroidism (18).

Further studies will be carried out to determine a NOAEL for the effects of perchlorate on the thyroid RAIU, using lower daily doses of perchlorate in our iodine sufficient population. It seems unlikely, however, that the low levels of perchlorate detected in surface and ground waters pose a risk to the general population, since the daily dose of 10 mg perchlorate, which is at least 300 times greater than the dose ingested based on the highest amount found in public water supplies, did not affect serum thyroid hormone or TSH concentrations. Since no effect on thyroid function was observed in perchlorate plant workers exposed for months and years to as much as 34 mg perchlorate daily (15), it seems less likely that this low dose of perchlorate given over a prolonged period of time would eventually perturb thyroid function. However, a longer study period of 6 months using low doses of perchlorate is currently being undertaken to address this concern.

References

1. Office of Ground water and Drinking water. Perchlorate. Washington, D.C: Environmental Protection Agency; December 15, 1998.

2. Dai G, Levy O, Carrasco N. Cloning and characterization of the thyroid iodide transporter. Nature 1996 1;379:458–60.
3. Smanik PA, Liu Q, Furminger TL, Ryu K, Xing S, Mazzaferri EL, Jhiang SM. Cloning of the human sodium iodide symporter. Biochem Biophys Res Commun 1996; 13;226:339–45.
4. Wolff J 1998. Perchlorate and the Thyroid Gland. Pharmacological Reviews 1961; 50: 89–105.
5. Hobson QJ. Aplastic Anaemia Due to Treatment with Potassium Perchlorate. BMJ 1961;1: 1368–9.
6. Johnson SR, Moore WG. Fatal Aplastic Anaemia after Treatment of Thyrotoxicosis with Potassium Perchlorate. BMJ 1961;1: 1369–71.
7. Fawcett JW, Clarke CW. Aplastic Anaemia due to Potassium Perchlorate. BMJ. 1961;1: 1537.
8. Krevans JR, Asper SP, Rienhoff WF. Fatal Aplastic Anemia Following Use of Potassium Perchlorate in Thyrotoxicosis. JAMA 1962; 181:162–4.
9. Barzilai D and Sheinfeld M. Fatal complications following use of potassium perchlorate in thyrotoxicosis: report of two cases and a review of the literature. Israel J Med Sci 1966; 2,4: 453–6.
10. Wenzel KW and Lente JR. Similar effects of thionamide drugs and perchlorate on thyroid-stimulating immunoglobulins in Graves' disease: evidence against an immunosuppressive action of thionamide drugs. J Clin Endocrinol Metab 1984; 58:62–9.
11. Martino E, Aghini-Lombardi F, Mariotti S et al. Treatment of amiodarone associated thyrotoxicosis by simultaneous administration of potassium perchlorate and methimazole. J Endocrinol Invest 1986; 9:201–7.
12. Nolte W, Muller R, Siggelkow H, Emrich D, Hufner M. Prophylactic application of thyrostatic drugs during excessive iodine exposure in euthyroid patients with thyroid autonomy: a randomized study. Eur J Endocrinol 1996; 134: 337–41.
13. Bürgi H, Benguerel M, Knopp J, Kohler H and Studer H. Influence of Perchlorate on the Secretion of Non-Thyroxine Iodine by the Normal Human Thyroid Gland. Europ. J Clin Invest. 1974 ; 4:65–9.
14. Brabant G, Bergmann P, Kirsch CM, Kohrle J, Hesch RD, von zur Muhlen A. Early adaptation of thyrotropin and thyroglobulin secretion to experimentally decreased iodine supply in man. Metabolism 1992; 41:1093–6
15. Lamm SH, Braverman LE, Li FX, Richman K, Pino S, and Howearth G. Thyroid health status of ammonium perchlorate workers: a cross-sectional occupational health study. JOEM 1999; 41:248–60.
16. Benotti J, Benotti N, Pino S, Gardyna H. Determination of total iodine in urine, stools, diets, and tissue. Clin Chem 1965; 11:932–6.
17. Stanbury JB and Wyngaarden JB. Effect of perchlorate on the human thyroid gland. Metabolism 1952;1:533–9.
18. Lamm SH, Doemland M. Has Perchlorate in Drinking Water Increased the Rate of Congenital Hypothyroidism? JOEM 1999; 41: 409–11.

Short communication:

Nitrates (N) and organochlorine pesticides (OCP) elimination in subjects with normal and marginal iodine uptake and OCP effects on thyroid parameters

M. Simescu, [1]C. Neagu, [1]D. Rusea, [2]I. Zosin, E. Nicolaescu, E. Gudovan, [3]E. Marinescu

Institute of Endocrinology, Bucharest; [1]Institute of Public Health, Bucharest; [2]IMF Timisoara, Timisoara; [3]District Hospital RM Valcea, Valcea, Romania

Reassessment of IDD prevalence in our country has revealed discordance between goiter incidence (G) and urinary iodine (UI) values in some plain areas. The main endemic goiter area was localized in the mountains and hall areas with a geochemical iodine deficiency. This finding suggested to us that goitrogenic factors in the environment and diet could play a critical role in the high incidence of goiter in plain area. Nitrogenous (N) fertilizers and organochlorine pesticides (OCP) used in agriculture and found in high concentration in many vegetables were assumed to be goitrogenic factors. We studied: 1) the percentage elimination of nitrate (N) and pesticides (P) metabolites in the urine of certain groups of population in 3 towns from plain area: town B – UI 10.18 mg/dl, G 23.04 %; town S – UI 8.54 mg/dl, G 22.31 %; town T – UI 10.4 mg/dl, G 1 %. 2) implications of thyroid parameters among workers manufacturing hexachlorocyclohexane (h). For the N estimation we used Boehringer Kits. For pesticides, gas chromatography of OCP in urine, blood. Urinary iodine assays were performed on spot samples. The WHO method was used to determine goiter in children, ultrasonography to measure goiter volume in adults.

The values of urine nitrate analysis in schoolchildren were: in town B, among 324 children, the results were positive in 29 (8.95 %) N range 0.02–18.9, mean 2.46; in town S among 204 children, results were positive in 72 (35.29 %) N range 0.004–4.2, mean 1.34, SD 1.36; in town T among 100 children, results were positive in 2 (2 %) N range 0.3 l-0.69 mg/l.

The values of N in 2 groups of women, aged 18–35 years living in town B: among 164 women with simple non-toxic goiter, 111 had positive results range 0.012–22.4

mg/l, mean 1.37, SD 3.20; in the group of working women, results were positive in 38 (32 %), range 0.012–22.4, mean 1.3586, SD 1.92).

The assays for urine pesticides in a group of 32 women living in B town were positive in all investigated females with goiter and without goiter, range 0.35–78 μg/l.

The second group investigated included 15 workers (male) manufacturing H (exposed to H for 8–30 years). The value of thyroid parameters were: thyroid volumetry range = 12.7–31.7, mean free T_4 13.21, range 12.81-18.3, SD 1.91, mean TSH 1.77.

Our data suggest that N itself may be an indicator of environmental pollution; it is also possible that N itself interacts with the unavailability of iodide to the thyroid. Its influence expresses especially in situation were the iodine supplementation is already marginal. H can influence the peripheral metabolism of T_4. Further studies are required, because of the intensive use of fertilizers and pesticides in agriculture.

Session II:

Environment and autoimmune thyroid disease

Chairpersons: A. Pinchera, V. Zamrasil

Genetic predisposition versus environmental factors in autoimmune thyroid disease

Th. H. Brix, **L. Hegedüs**

Department of Endocrinology M, Odense University Hospital, 5000 Odense C, Denmark

Abstract

The autoimmune thyroid diseases, comprising Graves' disease, Hashimoto's thyroiditis, and atrophic thyroiditis, are the commonest autoimmune diseases in humans. The etiology of these diseases is incompletely understood. It is generally believed that the development of autoimmune thyroid disease, whether Graves' disease or Hashimoto's /atrophic thyroiditis, depends on complex interactions between genetic, environmental and endogenous factors. The importance of genetic factors is evident from clustering of autoimmune thyroid disease within families and by a higher concordance rate for Graves' disease as well as Hashimoto's/atrophic thyroiditis in monozygotic than in dizygotic twins. Recently, studies assessing the role of specific candidate genes or genetic markers in the etiology of autoimmune thyroid disease, have given conflicting results in various populations. However, there may well be single genes playing a major role within certain families or populations e.g., the human leukocyte antigen region, the cytotoxic T lymphocyte antigen-4, and the markers AITD-1, GD-1,GD-2, GD-3, HT-1, and HT-2, but the genes will vary from family to family. In addition, the family and twin studies also indicate a role for environmental factors in the etiology of autoimmune thyroid disease. Clearly, iodine and cigarette smoking are the most important environmental risk factors associated with the genesis of autoimmune thyroid disease. Other suggested risk factors include emotional stress, low birth weight, and certain drugs and infections. Ongoing studies focus on whole genome screening in multiplex families in combination with linkage analysis, as well as family based linkage disequilibrium analysis. As more susceptibility genes and their allelic variants are identified, assessing the nature of the gene-environment interaction in Graves' disease, Hashimoto's thyroiditis and atrophic thyroiditis will become an important research priority. Thus, systematic evaluation of nature-nurture interactions will replace the old nature versus nurture controversy.

Introduction

Autoimmune thyroid disorders (AITD) are common, affecting around 2% of women and 0.2% of men, while subclinical disease, reflected by the presence of thyroid antibodies in euthyroid individuals, is approximately 10-fold higher (1–3). AITD comprises several clinical variants. Roughly, patients can be divided into those with hyperthyroidism (Graves' disease, GD) and those with hypothyroidism with (Hashimoto's thyroiditis, HT) or without goiter (atrophic thyroiditis, AT). Although, GD and HT/AT are phenotypically very different, it is generally believed that they share a number of common etiological factors. Clearly, GD and HT/AT frequently occur in the same family (4, 5) and some individuals progress from one form to another. Moreover, there are descriptions of young monozygotic (MZ) twin pairs in which one has GD whereas the other has HT/AT (6).

Although GD and HT/AT are among the most common thyroid disorders their etiology is still incompletely understood (7). It is generally accepted that high iodine intake is a major environmental factor contributing to both GD and HT/AT (7, 8). In epidemiological studies, it has been demonstrated that differences in the prevalence of GD and HT/AT in different parts of the world closely mimic the magnitude of iodine intake, with GD and HT/AT being more prevalent in areas with a high iodine intake (9–11). In addition, constitutional factors, such as sex hormones, have been implicated in the etiology of AITD. Thus, in the general population the female to male prevalence ratio of AITD ranges from 5:1 to 10:1, the highest ratio reported in iodine

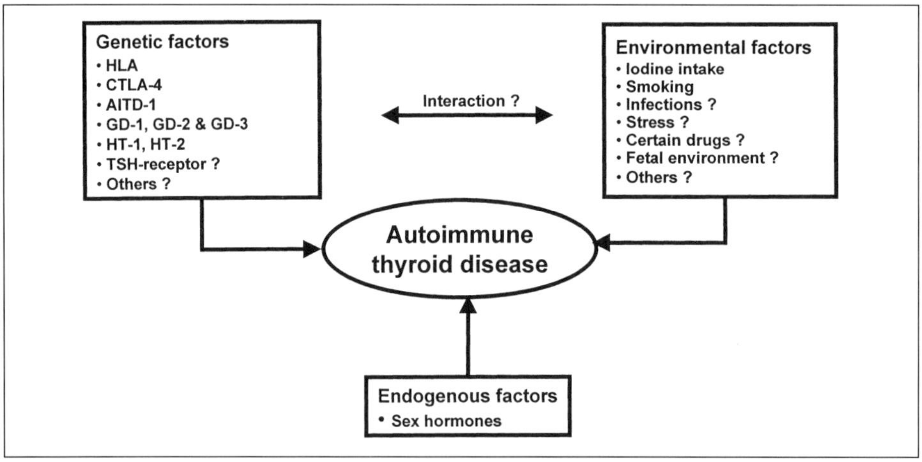

Fig. 1 Etiology of autoimmune Thyroid disease. The development of clinically overt AITD seems to involve complex interactions between environmental, genetic, and endogenous factors. However, at present it is not clear how and to what degree the candidate genes or genetic markers interact with the environmental risk factors.

deficient areas (1, 3, 11, 12). Other suggested risk factors include cigarette smoking (13, 14), emotional stress (15, 16), adverse fetal environment reflected by a low birth weight (17, 18), and certain infections (19). However, the majority of the background population is also exposed to one or more of these various environmental determinants and yet only a small fraction actually develop overt AITD. Consequently, it seems apparent that, if any of these environmental exposures do play an etiological role in the development of overt GD and/or HT/AT, none of them is sufficient or necessary to cause disease. This indicates that individual factors that predispose a part of the population to develop AITD must play a role in the etiology.

A role of genetic factors in the etiology of GD and HT/AT has long been suspected (20, 21). The strategies that have been applied in humans to estimate the magnitude of the genetic component in the etiology of AITD have been based on family and twin studies (22). With advances in genetic technology, recent studies have assessed the role of possible candidate genes or genetic markers in the etiology of AITD, with conflicting findings in various populations (7, 22). Consequently, it has become evident that both GD and HT/AT belong to the group of diseases referred to as "complex diseases", which include insulin dependent diabetes mellitus, rheumatoid arthritis, hypertension, and osteoporosis. These conditions are common, show no simple Mendelian mode of transmission, vary in their severity and are multifactorial, with the clinical phenotype representing the net effect of all the contributing genetic and environmental factors (Figure 1).

This chapter will review existing family and twin studies concerning AITD and focus on the influence of genetic factors in the etiology of AITD. Others contributions to this symposium will mainly highlight the importance of environmental factors in the etiology of AITD.

Family and twin studies in AITD

Family and twin studies are the classic methods of investigation in human genetics, the two methods being complementary to one another. Family studies examine whether there is evidence of aggregation of a disease within families, and sometimes this approach can provide information concerning the mode of inheritance (23). However, in complex conditions, such as AITD, classic family studies cannot determine whether the observed familial clustering is due to shared environment or a shared genetic predisposition (23). Twin studies, on the other hand, can provide evidence for both a genetic and an environmental contribution to disease development (24). Moreover, even in the absence of genotypic information, twin studies can shed light on the relative importance of genetic and environmental factors in the causation of disease (24). The basic premise of the classic twin study is that MZ twins carry identical genes, whereas dizygotic (DZ) twins are genetically as similar as ordinary siblings. Based on the assumption that the intrapair difference in environment is the same for MZ and DZ twins, a higher degree of similarity with respect to the presence of a disease, in this case AITD, among MZ pairs than among DZ pairs can be taken as evidence of a genetic contribution to its etiology. Similar concordance rates in MZ and DZ pairs indicate that the disease is mainly due to environmental factors.

Family studies

A family history of thyroid disease can be obtained in up to 40–50 % of patients with GD (20, 25), and, during the last century, family studies have repeatedly demonstrated a familial aggregation of GD (20, 25–28). Similarly, it is well recognized that HT/AT also has a high degree of familial aggregation (4, 29). The magnitude of familial clustering of a given disease can be estimated by the use of lambda statistic, K_R/K, where K_R equals the risk among relatives and K equals the cumulative lifetime risk in the background population (30). By assuming that the population prevalence at large equals the cumulative lifetime risk, it is possible to make a rough estimate of λ, which can be interpreted as the increased risk of disease for a relative given the presence of disease in the proband. Studies where proband ascertainment has been based on sampling of hospital patients indicate that the prevalence of GD among first degree relatives of patients is approximately 5–10 times higher than the prevalence of GD in the background population (Table 1). The λ_{Sister} for GD is around 8, which implies that the risk for a sister of developing GD, when a sister or brother already has GD, is approximately 8-fold compared with the risk in the general population. In HT/AT, several studies have suggested familial clustering of disease (4, 29, 31). However, because of a lack of prevalence data from the background population and

Table 1 Prevalence and magnitude of familial clustering (λ) of Graves' disease among the first degree relatives of probands.

Study	**Background population**	**Mothers**	**Fathers**	**Sisters**	**Brothers**	**Daughters**
Bartels (20)	0.4 %	3 % $\lambda_M = 7.5$	0 %	5 % $\lambda_S = 12.6$	0.9 % $\lambda_B = 2.1$	1.5 % $\lambda_D = 3.7$
Martin & Fisher (25)	1.1 % [a]	1.1 % $\lambda_M = 1$	0 %	10.1 % $\lambda_S = 9.2$	7.4 % $\lambda_B = 6.7$	–
Howel-Evans et al. (27)	1.1 % [a]	10.5 % $\lambda_M = 9.6$	0 %	5.9 % $\lambda_S = 5.4$	1.3 % $\lambda_B = 1.2$	–
Stenszky et al. (28)	0.65 %	4.3 % $\lambda_M = 6.6$	1.9 % $_F = 2.9$	5.3 % $\lambda_S = 8.1$	0 %	5.3 % $\lambda_D = 8.2$

– = No information available; [a] Estimated from the Whickham survey (1), since no prevalence data were given in the original article).

very small data sets involving only single families, it has not been possible to estimate the magnitude of this clustering.

Mode of inheritance

Despite the obvious familial clustering of GD, no clear pattern of inheritance has been defined. An autosomal dominant pattern of inheritance with diminished penetrance in males has been described in early reports (reviewed in 20). However, according to the author, most of these studies are based on inadequate clinical characterization of the subjects, hampering the interpretation of the data. An autosomal recessive pattern of inheritance has been described in two large well performed hospital-based studies from the 1940s (20, 25). Bartels (20) concluded that inheritance of GD was controlled by a single recessive gene with variable expression and a relative sex-limitation to women. Martin & Fisher (25) found evidence for the inheritance of a single recessive predisposing factor favorable to GD and perhaps necessary for its development. In contrast, the familial clustering of GD, observed in subsequent studies with a more well defined phenotype, does not seem to follow any simple Mendelian pattern of inheritance (26–28). A multifactorial mode of inheritance of GD has therefore been suggested (28). In contrast, only one study has evaluated the pattern of inheritance of HT/AT. In this study (29), the observed familial clustering of HT/AT was compatible with a simple sex-influenced recessive pattern of inheritance. Moreover, the findings pointed towards the presence of a genetic relationship between HT/AT, hyperthyroidism, and simple goiter.

Twin studies

Romberg was the first to report, in 1851, concordance for GD (20). Since then several case reports of twin pairs concordant for GD (22) as well as HT/AT (31) have been published. However, it is important to bear in mind that these isolated cases of concordant twin pairs do not give any etiologic information. To derive a valid assessment of the magnitude of genetic and environmental influences on disease development from twin data requires that a number of crucial issues are taken into account (32). Briefly, population-based rather than volunteer-based ascertainment methods should be used to avoid bias. It is crucial to establish zygosity and to ensure that the diagnoses/phenotypes are well defined. Finally, analysis of concordance should be by the probandwise instead of the pairwise method, since the former includes a correction for dual ascertainment of concordant pairs under incomplete sampling which makes it much more reliable.

Population based twin studies

There are only a few studies concerning the occurrence of clinically overt GD and HT/AT in unselected twin populations (Table 2). The two early studies (33, 34) dealt with self-reported hyperthyroidism, and one study (33) even included patients with self-reported simple nontoxic goiter, hampering if not invalidating any conclusions. In the study by Verschuer (34), the concordance rate for hyperthyroidism was found to be as high as 64 % in MZ compared with 6 % in DZ twins. Unfortunately, no effort was made to verify the self-reported diagnoses or to distinguish between autoimmune and nonautoimmune hyperthyroidism, making the interpretation of this study very difficult. In our two recent population-based twin studies (35, 36), all the probands had well-defined phenotypes. The concordance rates for GD were found to be much lower than previously reported by Verschuer (34) (pairwise; 22 % vs. 0 %, probandwise; 36 % vs. 0 % in MZ and DZ pairs, respectively), but still significantly higher for MZ than DZ pairs. Similarly, the probandwise concordance rates for HT/AT were significantly higher for MZ (55 %, 95 % CI 23%-83 %) compared with DZ twins (0 %, 95 % CI 0%-25 %). Our findings are supported by preliminary results

Table 2 Population based twin studies concerning hyperthyroidism, Graves' disease and Hashimoto's thyroiditis.

Phenotype	Study		Probandwise concordance rate in % (95 % CI)		MZ/DZ concordance ratio
			MZ	DZ	
Hyperthyroidism	Harvald & Hauge (33)		86 (71–95)	40 (19–64)	2.2
	Verschuer (34)		64 (52–75)	6 (2–15)	10.7
GD	Brix et al. (35)	self-reported GD	27 (15–42)	3 (0–10)	9
		confirmed GD	36 (17–60)	0 (0–11)	9[a]
	Ringold et al (37)		17[b]	1.9[b]	8.9[b]
HT/AT	Ringold et al. (37)		17.2[b]	2.1[b]	8.2[b]
	Brix et al. (36)		55 (23–83)	0 (0–25)	13.8[a]

[a] Based on a DZ probandwise concordance rate of 4 %. The finding of a probandwise concordance rate of 0.0 among the DZ twin pairs reflects the small number of affected twins and not the lack of aggregation or concordance for GD or HT/AT in DZ twins. In fact, according to the 95 % confidence interval, the concordance rate for the DZ twins could lie anywhere between 0 and 11 % and 0 and 25 % in GD and HT/AT, respectively. Assuming that the degree of aggregation of AITD in DZ twins is the same as reported for siblings (Table 1), one would expect a probandwise concordance rate of around 4 % in DZ twins which is clearly within the 95 % confidence interval.

[b] Only the pairwise concordance rates were reported.

from a very recent population-based twin study from California, USA (37). In this study, the pairwise concordance rate for GD was estimated to be approximately 17 % in MZ twins and 1.9 % in DZ twins, whereas the pairwise concordance rates for HT/AT were found to be 17.2 % in MZ and 2.1 % in DZ twins (37). Thus, in all three population-based studies (35–37) the concordance rate for GD as well as HT/AT was found to be significantly higher for MZ than DZ twins, confirming the presence of genetic factors in the etiology of these disorders. On the other hand, the fact that the concordance rate for both GD and HT/AT among MZ twins was well below 100 %, even with more than 25 years of follow-up, clearly demonstrates that environmental factors are also of etiological importance in GD as well as in HT/AT (Figure 1).

Magnitude of the genetic component in AITD

Accepting that there is a genetic component in the etiology of GD and HT/AT, how large is its effect? The finding of lower overall concordance rates for GD in the population based twin studies has led the authors of recent reviews to imply that the genetic contribution to disease etiology might not be as strong as previously believed (22, 38, 39). However, such simple calculations give an erroneous assessment of the genetic contribution to disease development. In complex diseases, the concordance rates are a function of both the prevalence of the disease in the general population, in this case GD and HT/AT, and the heritability (40). Thus, it follows that if the prevalence is low the concordance rate in MZ twins will also be low even though there is a high degree of heritability. In addition, one of the basic assumptions for the classical twin study, that MZ twins carry identical genes, may not be fulfilled in twin studies of immune-mediated diseases, such as AITD (22, 41). Clearly, the generation of immunoglobulins and T-cell receptors by somatic mutations of germline genes and rearrangements that take place during the differentiation of the immune system are a potential source of difference between the two twin individuals in a given MZ pair (22, 42). There is now evidence for a bias in the use of T-cell receptor V genes by T cells involved in autoimmune diseases including AITD (41). Therefore, the classic twin study will tend to underestimate the magnitude of the genetic component in AITD as well as in other autoimmune diseases. More sophisticated analyses of twin data (path analysis or structural equation modeling) give more precise and usually higher estimates for the genetic component of disease susceptibility. In rheumatoid arthritis, for example, the heritability has been estimated to be approximately 60 % despite a concordance rate of only 12 % in MZ twins (42).

One way to estimate the magnitude of the genetic contribution to disease etiology in complex traits using twin data is to calculate the ratio of concordance in MZ and DZ twin pairs (32). A concordance ratio of 1 implies no genetic contribution to disease. The fact that the concordance ratio between MZ and DZ twins is around 9 in both GD and HT/AT indicates a substantial genetic effect (Table 2). In comparison, the MZ/DZ concordance ratio in insulin dependent diabetes mellitus is approximately 4.9 (24). Another measure of the genetic contribution to disease development can be derived from the probandwise concordance rate in MZ and DZ twins divided by the prevalence of the disease in the background population (32). It follows that this measure of genetic risk is equivalent to the $\lambda_{sibling}$ (also named sibling recurrence risk) obtained in family-studies (30). Using this approach, the λ_{MZ} and λ_{DZ} for GD in Danish twins, can be estimated to be around 90 (95% CI, 43 to150) and 10 (95% CI, 0 to 30), respectively. This implies that the risk for a twin of developing GD when the co-twin already has GD is approximately 90 and 10 times greater than the risk in the general population in MZ and DZ twins, respectively. Moreover, the fact that the estimated λ_{DZ} is in close agreement with the λ_{sister} indicates that familial clustering of GD is, to a high degree, due to genetic effects and not the result of a shared environment.

These findings not only confirm the presence of a genetic component in the etiology of AITD, but also suggest that the magnitude of the genetic contribution in AITD may be of the same order as seen in other common autoimmune diseases such as rheumatoid arthritis and insulin dependent diabetes mellitus. However, it should be remembered that all the above estimates of the genetic contribution are functions of the heritability and the prevalence of the disease in the general population. Heritability, which is theoretically independent of the disease prevalence, may therefore be a much more useful indicator of the magnitude of the genetic influence. Unfortunately, it requires a very large population based twin study within a genetically homogeneous population to obtain a reliable estimate of the heritability of GD and HT/AT, and this is at present not available.

Candidate genes

Accepting that genes do play a substantial role in the etiology of AITD, can they be identified? During the last decade, much effort has been put into characterization of the genetic background of AITD, especially GD. Advances in genetic technology, such as restriction fragment length polymorphism (RFLP) and the polymerase chain reaction (PCR) have facilitated this search. By using these techniques in combination with association studies, family based linkage analysis, and family based linkage disequilibrium analysis, recent studies have assessed the role of specific candidate genes or genetic markers in the etiology of AITD (Table 3).

Since GD and HT/AT are immune mediated diseases, numerous studies have focused on genes involved in the immune response, with conflicting findings in various populations (Table 3, reviewed in (7, 22)). These studies have included the human leukocyte antigen (HLA) class II genes, as well as the genes for tumor necrosis factor (TNF), the immunoglobulin heavy chain region (IgH), the T-cell receptor, the

Table 3 Studies concerning association or linkage between genetic markers and overt AITD (since 1990)

Phenotype	Candidate gene	Chromosome number	Association studies		Linkage and linkage disequilibrium studies	
			positive	negative	positive	negative
Graves' disease	HLA class II	6	(44–51)		(51, 52)	(53–55)
	TNF	6	(56)	(57)		(58)
	IgH	15				(53, 59)
	T-cell-R	7 & 14		(48)		(59)
	IL-1-R	2	(60)	(61–63)		
	CTLA-4	2	(64–70)	(71, 72)	(52, 73)	(58, 59, 71)
	TSH-R	14	(69, 74, 75)	(76–79)		(58, 76, 79)
	TPO			(48)		(67)
	Tg	10				(67)
Hashimoto's thyroiditis	HLA	6	(80–84)	(44, 48)		(53, 58)
	TNF	6				(58)
	IgH	15				(59)
	T-Cell-R	7 & 14		(48)		(59)
	IL-1-R	2		(60, 63)		
	CTLA-4	2	(64, 65, 70, 85)	(71, 86)		(58, 59, 71)
	TSH-R	14		(74, 77)		(58)
	TPO			(48)		(58)
	Tg	10				(58)

HLA = human leukocyte antigen, TNF = tumor necrosis factor, IgH = immunoglobulin gene complex, T-Cell-R = T-cell receptor gene complexes, IL-1-R = interleukin-1 receptor, CTLA-4 = the cytotoxic T lymphocyte antigen 4, TSH-R = TSH receptor, TPO = thyroid peroxidase, Tg = thyroglobulin.

interleukin-1 receptor antagonist, and the cytotoxic T lymphocyte antigen-4 (CTLA-4). Other genes that could be implicated in the genesis of AITD include the TSH-receptor gene and the genes for thyroid peroxidase (TPO), and thyroglobulin (Tg). Again, studies have yielded contradictory results (Table 3).

Using classic linkage analysis in combination with whole genome screening in 56 multi-generation AITD families, Tomer et al. (43) recently identified 6 loci that showed preliminary evidence of linkage to AITD. Only one locus, AITD-1 on chromosome 6, was linked with both GD and HT/AT. Interestingly, this locus is close to, but distinct from, the HLA region. Three loci showed evidence for linkage with GD, GD-1 on chromosome 14, GD-2 on chromosome 20, and GD-3 on the X chromosome. The findings in HT/AT were less convincing, probably due to heterogeneity of their HT/AT phenotype. Nevertheless, two loci pointed towards linkage with HT/AT, HT-1 on chromosome 13 and HT-2 on chromosome 12. Until replication in another population, these data should be viewed with caution. However, if these genetic markers are major susceptibility loci they should not be difficult to replicate by others.

Thus, it follows that although a number of candidate genes have been investigated (Table 3), no single gene or genetic marker has been shown to be either necessary or sufficient for the development of clinically overt GD or HT/AT. This implies that GD and HT/AT are under the influence of multiple genes probably with variable penetrance.

Conclusion

The etiology of GD and HT/AT is incompletely understood. It is generally believed that the development of AITD, whether GD or HT/AT depends on complex interactions between genetic, environmental and endogenous factors. The importance of genetic factors is evident from clustering of AITD within families and by a higher concordance rate for both GD and HT/AT in MZ than in DZ twins. Recent studies assessing the role of specific candidate genes or genetic markers in the etiology of AITD have given conflicting results in various populations. However, there may well be single genes playing a major role within certain families or populations e.g. the HLA region, the CTLA-4, and the markers AITD-1, GD-1, GD-2, GD-3, HT-1 and HT-2, but the genes will vary from family to family. In addition, the family and twin studies also indicate a role for environmental factors in the etiology of AITD. Clearly, iodine and cigarette smoking are the most important environmental risk factors associated with the genesis of AITD. Other suggested risk factors include emotional stress, low birth weight, and certain drugs and infections.

However, despite several large investigations, no single gene or environmental risk factor has been shown to be either necessary or sufficient for the development of clinically overt GD or HT/AT. Furthermore, it is at present unknown how much of the etiology of AITD can be explained by allelic variation in these genes and how much is due to environmental variation. Neither is it clear how these susceptibility genes interact with environmental risk factors for AITD, such as iodine and cigarette smoking. Indeed, as more susceptibility genes and their numerous allelic variants are discovered, it is crucial to assess how modifiable risk factors such as iodine intake or smoking interact with these susceptibility genes to influence disease risk. Clearly, environmental risk factors in AITD, as in most chronic diseases, have poor predictive value for disease occurrence. Therefore, stratifying according to genetic susceptibility at one or more loci will improve the predictive value for disease occurrence among biologically susceptible individuals and may thus help target preventive and therapeutic interventions. In other words, the old nature versus nurture controversy is being replaced by a systematic investigation of nature-nurture interactions.

References

1. Tunbridge WMG, Evered DC, Hall R, Appleton D, Brewis M, Clark F et al. The spectrum of thyroid disease in a community: The Whickham survey. Clin Endocrinol 1977; 7:481–493.
2. Vanderpump MPJ, Tunbridge WMG, French JM, Appleton D, Bates D, Clark F et al. The incidence of thyroid disorders in the community: a twenty-year follow-up of the Whickham survey. Clin Endocrinol 1995; 43:55–68.
3. Knudsen N, Jørgensen T, Rasmussen S, Christiansen E, Perrild H. The prevalence of thyroid dysfunction in a population with borderline iodine deficiency. Clin Endocrinol 1999; 51:361–367.
4. Doniach D, Roitt IM, Taylor KB. Autoimmunity in pernicious anemia and thyroiditis: A family study. Ann N Y Acad Sci 1965; 124:605–625.
5. Tomer Y, Barbesino G, Greenberg DA, Concepcion E, Davies TF. Linkage analysis of candidate genes in autoimmune thyroid disease. III. Detailed analysis of chromosome 14 localizes Graves' disease-1 (GD-1) close to multinodular goiter-1 (MNG-1). J Clin Endocrinol Metab 1999; 83:4321–4327.
6. Ilicki A, Marcus C, Karlsson FA. Hyperthyroidism and hypothyroidism in monozygotic twins: Detection of stimulating and blocking TSH receptor antibodies using the FRTL5-cell line. J Clin Invest 1990; 13:327–331.
7. Weetman AP, McGregor AM. Autoimmune thyroid disease: Further developments in our understanding. Endocr Rev 1994; 15:788–830.
8. McGregor AM, Weetman AP, Ratanachaiyavong S, Owen GM, Ibbertson HK, Hall R. Iodine: an influence on the development of autoimmune thyroid disease? In: Hall R, Köbberling J, editors. Thyroid disorders associated with iodine deficiency and excess. New York: Raven Press, 1985: 209–216.
9. Laurberg P, Pedersen KM, Vestergaard H, Sigurdsson G. High incidence of multinodular toxic goitre in the elderly population in a low iodine intake area vs. high incidence of Graves' disease in the young in a high iodine intake area: Comparative surveys of thyrotoxicosis epidemiology in East-Jutland Denmark and Iceland. J Int Med 1991; 229:415–420.
10. Laurberg P, Pedersen KM, Hreidarsson A, Sigfusson N, Iversen E, Knudsen PR. Iodine intake and the pattern of thyroid disorders: A comparative epidemiological study of thyroid abnormalities in the elderly in Iceland and in Jutland, Denmark. J Clin Endocrinol Metab 1998; 83:765–769.
11. Vanderpump MPJ, Tunbridge WMG. The epidemiology of thyroid diseases. In: Braverman LE, Utiger RD, editors. Werner and Ingbar's The Thyroid. Philadelphia: Lippincott-Raven, 1996: 474–482.
12. Furszyfer J, Kurland LT, McConahey WM, Woolner LB, Elveback LR. Epidemiologic aspects of Hashimoto's thyroiditis and Graves' disease in Rochester, Minnesota (1935–1967), with special reference to temporal trends. Metabolism 1972; 21:197–204.
13. Bertelsen JB, Hegedüs L. Cigarette smoking and the thyroid. Thyroid 1994; 4:327–331.
14. Brix TH, Hansen PS, Kyvik KO, Hegedüs L. Cigarette smoking and risk of clinically overt thyroid disease – a population based twin case-control study. Arch Intern Med [In press].

15. Winsa B, Adami H-O, Bergström R, Gamstedt A, Dahlberg PA, Adamson U et al. Stressful life events and Graves' disease. Lancet 1991; 338:1475–1479.
16. Chiovato L, Pinchera A. Stressful life events and Graves' disease. Eur J Endocrinol 1996; 134:680–682.
17. Phillips DIW, Cooper C, Fall C, Prentice L, Osmond C, Barker DJP et al. Fetal growth and autoimmune thyroid disease. QJM 1993; 86:247–253.
18. Brix TH, Kyvik KO, Hegedus L. Low birth weight is not associated with clinically overt thyroid disease – a population based twin case-control study. Clin Endocrinol [In press].
19. Tomer Y, Davies T. Infection, thyroid disease, and autoimmunity. Endocr Rev 1993; 14:107–121.
20. Bartels ED. Heredity in Graves' disease. With remarks on heredity in toxic adenoma in the thyroid, non-toxic goitre, and myxoedema [Thesis]. 1941. Copenhagen, Einar Munksgaard.
21. Craig PE, Spann JL, Lowbeer L. Hashimoto's disease (struma lymphomatosa): a familial incidence of three cases. Am J Surg 1952; 84:286–292.
22. Brix TH, Kyvik KO, Hegedüs L. What is the evidence of genetic factors in the etiology of Graves' disease? – a brief review. Thyroid 1998; 8:627–634.
23. Khoury MJ, Beaty TH, Cohen BH. Epidemiologic approaches to familial aggregation. In: Kelsey JL, Marmot MG, Stolley PD, Vessey MP, editors. Fundamentals of genetic epidemiology. Oxford: Oxford University Press, 1993: 164–199.
24. Hawkes CH. Twin studies in medicine – what do they tell us ? QJM 1997; 90:311–321.
25. Martin L, Fisher RA. The hereditary and familial aspects of exophthalmic goitre and nodular goitre. QJM 1945; 14:207–219.
26. Farid NR, Barnard JM, Marshall WH, Woolfrey I, O'Driscoll RF. Thyroid autoimmune disease in a large Newfoundland family: The influence of HLA. J Clin Endocrinol Metab 1977; 45:1165–1172.
27. Howel-Evans AW, Woodrow JC, McDougall CDM, Chew AR, Evans RW. Antibodies in the families of thyrotoxic patients. Lancet 1967;l:636–641.
28. Stenszky V, Kozma L, Balazs C, Rochlitz S, Bear JC, Farid NR. The genetics of Graves' disease: HLA and disease susceptibility. J Clin Endocrinol Metab 1985; 61:735–740.
29. Hall PF. Familial occurrence of myxoedema. J Med Genet 1965; 2:173–180.
30. Risch N. Assessing the role of HLA-linked and unlinked determinants of disease. Am J Hum Genet 1987; 40:1–14.
31. McGregor AM, Roberts DF, Hall R. A study of triplets with Hashimoto's thyroiditis. Postgrad Med J 1979; 55:894–896.
32. MacGregor AJ. Practical approaches to account for bias and confounding in twin data. In: Spector TD, Snieder H, MacGregor AJ, editors. Advances in twin and sib-pair analysis. London: Greenwhich Medical Media Ltd., 1999: 35–52.
33. Harvald B, Hauge M. A catamnestic investigation of Danish twins – a preliminary report. Dan Med Bull 1956; 3:150–158.
34. Verschuer OV. Die zwillingsforschung im dienste der inneren medizin. Verh Dtsch Ges inn Med 1958; 64:262–273.
35. Brix TH, Christensen K, Holm NV, Harvald B, Hegedüs L. A population based study of Graves' disease in Danish twins. Clin Endocrinol 1998; 48:397–400.
36. Brix TH, Kyvik KO, Hegedüs L. A population-based study of chronic autoimmune hypothyroidism in Danish twins. J Clin Endocrinol Metab 2000; 85:536–540.
37. Ringold DA, Nicoloff JT, Kesler H, Davis H, Mack T. Graves' disease, genetics and environment: revised estimates of the concordance rates in monozygotic and dizygotic twin populations. The proceedings of the 72nd Annual Meeting of the American Thyroid Association. 1999. [Abstract 13].
38. Philippou G, McGregor AM. The aetiology of Graves' disease: What is the genetic contribution ? Clin Endocrinol 1998; 48:393–395.
39. Allahabadia A, Gough SCL. The different approaches to the genetic analysis of autoimmune thyroid disease. J Endocr 1999; 163:7–13.
40. Smith C. Concordance in twins: Methods and interpretation. Am J Hum Genet 1974; 26:454–466.
41. Davies TF. Autoimmune thyroid disease genes come in many styles and colors. J Clin Endocrinol Metab 1998; 83:3391–3393.
42. Worthington J, Silman AJ. Genetic control of autoimmunity, lessons from twin studies. Clin Exp Immunol 1995; 101:390–392.

43. Tomer Y, Barbesino G, Greenberg DA, Concepcion E, Davies TF. Mapping the major susceptibility loci for familial Graves' and Hashimoto's diseases: evidence for genetic heterogeneity and gene interactions. J Clin Endocrinol Metab 1999; 84:4656–4664.
44. Badenhoop K, Walfish PG, Rau H, Fischer S, Nicolay A, Bogner U et al. Susceptibility and resistance alleles of human leukocyte antigen (HLA) DQA1 and HLA DQB1 are shared in endocrine autoimmune disease. J Clin Endocrinol Metab 1995; 80:2112–2117.
45. Chen Q, Huang W, She JX, Baxter F, Volpe R, Maclaren NK. HLA-DRB1*08, DRB1*03/DRB3*0101, and DRB3*0202 are susceptibility genes for Graves' disease in North American Caucasians, whereas DRB1*07 is protective. J Clin Endocrinol Metab 1999; 84:3182–3186.
46. Yanagawa T, Mangklabruks A, Chang Y-B, Okamoto Y, Fisfalen M-E, Curran PG et al. Human histocompatibility leukocyte antigen-DQA1*0501 allele associated with genetic susceptibility to Graves' disease in a Caucasian population. J Clin Endocrinol Metab 1993; 76:1569–1574.
47. Yanagawa T, Mangklabruks A, DeGroot LJ. Strong association between HLA-DQA1*0501 and Graves' disease in a male Caucasian population. J Clin Endocrinol Metab 1994; 79:227–229.
48. Mangklabruks A, Cox N, DeGroot LJ. Genetic factors in autoimmune thyroid disease analyzed by restriction fragment length polymorphisms of candidate genes. J Clin Endocrinol Metab 1991; 73:236–244.
49. Barlow ABT, Wheatcroft N, Watson P, Weetman AP. Association of HLA-DQA1*0501 with Graves' disease in English Caucasian men and women. Clin Endocrinol 1996; 44:73–77.
50. Lavard L, Madsen HO, Perrild H, Jacobsen BB, Svejgaard A. HLA class II associations in juvenile Graves' disease: indication of a strong protective role of the DRB1*0701, DQA1*0201 haplotype. Tissue Antigens 1997; 50:639–641.
51. Heward JM, Allahabadia A, Daykin J, Carr-Smith J, Daly A, Armitage M et al. Linkage disequilibrium between the human leukocyte antigen class II region of the major histocompatibility complex and Graves' disease: replication using a population case control and family-based study. J Clin Endocrinol Metab 1998; 83:3394–3397.
52. Vaidya B, Imrie H, Perros P, Young ET, Kelly WF, Carr D et al. The cytotoxic T lymphocyte antigen-4 is a major Graves' disease locus. Hum Mol Genet 1999; 8:1195–1199.
53. Roman SH, Greenberg D, Rubinstein P, Wallenstein S, Davies TF. Genetics of autoimmune thyroid disease: lack of evidence for linkage to HLA within families. J Clin Endocrinol Metab 1992; 74:496–503.
54. O'Connor G, Neufeld DS, Greenberg DA, Concepcion ES, Roman SH, Davies TF. Lack of disease associated HLA-DQ restriction fragment length polymorphisms in families with autoimmune thyroid disease. Autoimmunity 1993; 14:237–241.
55. Shields DC, Ratanachaiyavong S, McGregor AM, Collins A, Morton NE. Combined segregation and linkage analysis of Graves disease with a thyroid autoantibody diathesis. Am J Hum Genet 1994; 55:540–554.
56. Badenhoop K, Schwarz G, Schleusener H, Weetman AP, Recks S, Peters H et al. Tumor necrosis factor gene polymorphisms in Graves' disease. J Clin Endocrinol Metab 1992; 74:287–291.
57. Rau H, Donner H, Usadel KH, Badenhoop K. Polymorphisms of tumor necrosis factor receptor 2 are not associated with insulin-dependent diabetes mellitus or Graves' disease. Tissue Antigens 1997; 49:535–536.
58. Tomer Y, Barbesino G, Keddache M, Greenberg DA, Davies TF. Mapping of a major susceptibility locus for Graves' disease (GD-1) to chromosome 14q31. J Clin Endocrinol Metab 1997; 82:1645–1648.
59. Barbesino G, Tomer Y, Concepcion E, Davies TF, Greenberg D. Linkage analysis of candidate genes in autoimmune thyroid disease: 1. selected immunoregulatory genes. J Clin Endocrinol Metab 1998; 83:1580–1584.
60. Blakemore AIF, Watson PF, Weetman AP, Duff GW. Association of Graves' disease with an allele of the interleukin-1 receptor antagonist gene. J Clin Endocrinol Metab 1995; 80:111–115.
61. Mühlberg T, Kirchberger M, Spitzweg C, Herrmann F, Herberling H-J, Heufelder AE. Lack of association of Graves' disease with the A2 allele of the interleukin-1 receptor antagonist gene in a white European population. Eur J Endocrinol 1998; 138:686–690.

62. Cuddihy RM, Bahn RS. Lack of an association between alleles of interleukin-1a and interleukin-1 receptor antagonist genes and Graves' disease in a North American Caucasian population. J Clin Endocrinol Metab 1996; 81:4476–4478.
63. Heward J, Allahabadia A, Gordon C, Sheppard MC, Barnett AH, Franklyn JA et al. The interleukin-1 receptor antagonist gene shows no allelic association with three autoimmune diseases. Thyroid 1999; 9:627–628.
64. Kotsa K, Watson PF, Weetman AP. A CTLA-4 gene polymorphism is associated with both Graves' disease and autoimmune hypothyroidism. Clin Endocrinol 1997; 46:551–554.
65. Awata T, Kurihara S, Iitaka M, Takei S, Inoue I, Ishii C et al. Association of CTLA-4 gene A-G polymorphism (IDDM12 locus) with acute-onset and insulin-depleted IDDM as well as autoimmune thyroid disease (Graves' disease and Hashimoto's thyroiditis) in the Japanese population. Diabetes 1998; 47:128–129.
66. Yanagawa T, Hidaka Y, Guimaraes V, Soliman M, DeGroot LJ. CTLA-4 gene polymorphism associated with Graves' disease in a Caucasian population. J Clin Endocrinol Metab 1995; 80:41–45.
67. Donner H, Rau H, Walfish PG, Braun J, Siegmund T, Finke R et al. CTLA4 alanine-17 confers genetic susceptibility to Graves' disease and to type 1 diabetes mellitus. J Clin Endocrinol Metab 1997; 82:143–146.
68. Yanagawa T, Taniyama M, Enomoto S, Gomi K, Maruyama H, Ban Y et al. CTLA4 gene polymorphism confers susceptibility to Graves' disease in Japanese. Thyroid 1997; 7:843–846.
69. Sale MM, Akamizu T, Howard TD, Yokota T, Nakao K, Mori T et al. Association of autoimmune thyroid disease with a microsatellite marker for the thyrotropin receptor gene and CTLA-4 in a Japanese population. Proceedings of the Association of American Physicians 1997; 109:453–461.
70. Braun J, Donner H, Siegmund T, Walfish PG, Usadel KH, Badenhoop K. CTLA-4 promotor variants in patients with Graves' disease and Hashimoto's thyroiditis. Tissue Antigens 1998; 51:563–566.
71. Heward JM, Allahabadia A, Carr-Smith J, Daykin J, Cockram C, Gordon C et al. No evidence of allelic association of a human CTLA-4 promotor polymorphism with autoimmune thyroid disease in either population-based case-control or family-based studies. Clin Endocrinol 1998; 49:331–334.
72. Djilali-Saiah I, Larger E, Harfouch-Hammoud E, Timsit J, Clerc J, Bertin E et al. No major role for the CTLA-4 gene in the association of autoimmune thyroid disease with IDDM. Diabetes 1998; 47:125–127.
73. Heward JM, Allahabadia A, Armitage M, Hattersley A, Dodson PM, Macleod K et al. The development of Graves' disease and the CTLA-4 gene on chromosome 2q33. J Clin Endocrinol Metab 1999; 84:2398–2401.
74. Cuddihy RM, Dutton CM, Bahn RS. A polymorphism in the extracellular domain of the thyrotropin receptor is highly associated with autoimmune thyroid disease in females. Thyroid 1995; 5:89–95.
75. Cuddihy RM, Schaid DS, Bahn RS. Multivariate analysis of HLA loci in conjunction with a thyrotropin receptor codon 52 polymorphism in conferring risk of Graves' disease. Thyroid 1996; 6:261–265.
76. de Roux N, Shields DC, Misrahi M, Ratanachaiyavong S, McGregor AM, Milgrom E. Analysis of the thyrotropin receptor as a candidate gene in familial Graves' disease. J Clin Endocrinol Metab 1996; 81:3483–3486.
77. Watson PF, French A, Pickerill AP, McIntosh RS, Weetman AP. Lack of association between a polymorphism in the coding region of the thyrotropin receptor gene and Graves' disease. J Clin Endocrinol Metab 1995; 80:1032–1035.
78. Kotsa KD, Watson PF, Weetman AP. No association between a thyrotropin receptor gene polymorphism and Graves' disease in the female population. Thyroid 1997; 7:31–33.
79. Allahabadia A, Heward JM, Mijovic C, Carr-Smith J, Daykin J, Cockram C et al. Lack of association between polymorphism of the thyrotropin receptor gene and Graves' disease in United Kingdom and Hong Kong Chinese patients: Case control and family-based studies. Thyroid 1998; 8:777–780.
80. Jenkins D, Penny MA, Fletcher JA, Jacobs KH, Mijovic CH, Franklyn JA et al. HLA class II gene polymorphism contributes little to Hashimoto's thyroiditis. Clin Endocrinol 1992; 37:141–145.
81. Bogner U, Badenhoop K, Peters H, Schmieg D, Mayr WR, Usadel KH et al. HLA-DR/DQ gene variation in nongoitrous autoimmune thyroiditis at the serological and molecular level. Autoimmunity 1992; 14:155–158.

82. Shi Y, Zou M, Robb D, Farid NR. Typing for major histocompatibility complex class II antigens in thyroid tissue blocks: Association of Hashimoto's thyroiditis with HLA-DQ0301 and DQB0201 alleles. J Clin Endocrinol Metab 1991; 75:943–946.
83. Badenhoop K, Schwarz G, Walfish PG, Drummond V, Usadel KH, Bottazzo GF. Susceptibility to thyroid autoimmune disease: Molecular analysis of HLA-D region genes identifies new markers for goitrous Hashimoto's thyroiditis. J Clin Endocrinol Metab 1990; 71:1131–1137.
84. Tandon N, Zhang L, Weetman AP. HLA associations with Hashimoto's thyroiditis. Clin Endocrinol 1991; 34:383–386.
85. Donner H, Braun J, Seidl C, Rau H, Finke R, Ventz M et al. Codon 17 polymorphism of the cytotoxic T lymphocyte antigen 4 gene in Hashimoto's thyroiditis and Addison's disease. J Clin Endocrinol Metab 1997; 82:4130–4132.
86. Waterman EA, Watson PF, Lazarus JH, Parkes AB, Darke C, Weetman AP. A study of the association between a polymorphism in the CTLA-4 gene and postpartum thyroiditis. Clin Endocrinol 1998; 49:251–255.

Autoimmune thyroid disorders, maternal hypothyroxinemia, and its potential repercussions for the progeny

D. Glinoer

Université Libre de Bruxelles, University Hospital Saint-Pierre, Department of Internal Medicine, Thyroid Investigation Clinic, 322 Rue HAUTE, 1000 Brussels, Belgium

Abstract

An interesting study was recently published (NEJM, 1999) concerning maternal thyroid deficiency during pregnancy and its possible consequences on fetal and child development. The authors investigated the children of 62 women, who had had an elevated TSH with hypothyroxinemia (hypo-T_4) during pregnancy (15–17th wk) and had given birth to healthy infants, 7–9 years before the study. Among children born to hypo-T_4 mothers, the overall full-scale IQ score was 4 points lower (103 vs. 107, $p = 0.06$), than in controls. Moreover, mean IQ was 7 points lower among children born to mothers with undiagnosed (and, hence, untreated) hypo-T_4, while IQ was normal among the progeny of mothers treated for hypothyroidism during gestation. Finally, IQ was 85 (or lower) among 19 % of children of women with early gestational hypo-T_4, compared with 5 % among controls. Other studies on the potential neuropsychological developmental consequences of maternal hypo-T_4 during pregnancy were also critically examined. The author presents an overview of this important public health and medical topic and proposals for the systematic screening, as well as the diagnosis and management of thyroid dysfunction during pregnancy.

Introduction

The recent article by *Haddow and colleagues* and the accompanying Editorial by *Bob Utiger*, published in August 1999 in the New England Journal of Medicine, have focused the attention of the press and the medical community on the complex relations that exist between maternal thyroid deficiency during pregnancy and their possible consequences for the neuropsychomotor development of the fetus and child (1, 2).

Haddow's study dealt primarily with thyroid deficiency related to autoimmune thyroid disorders (AITD) during pregnancy. Because of the wide public health interest in this topic, the strong public reactions by scientific societies and medical associations, and finally because only a limited number of studies have investigated this topic, it was felt that a critical discussion of the available data could be useful to help our understanding and perhaps delineate bases for future action.

Critical analysis of available data

1. The "Klein-Mitchell-Haddow" studies in the United States

In 1991, *Klein and colleagues* reported the results of a retrospective population-based survey of serum TSH concentrations in 2,000 sera from consecutive pregnancies (in Maine) obtained at 15–18 weeks gestation (3). The study was organized within the scope of the "New England Newborn Screening Program in Boston". Sera assayed for TSH were obtained (by random selection?) from a group of 25,216 consecutive pregnancies. Forty-nine women were identified with serum TSH values above 6 mU/L, a prevalence of 2.5 %. Among them, 6 women not only had elevated serum TSH (7–54 mU/L) but also markedly lowered thyroid hormone concentrations (with a mean free T_4 of 6.1 pmol/L, compared with 13.4 pmol/L in control pregnancies), thus yielding a 0.3 % prevalence of overt thyroid deficiency in this unselected population. The other 43 women were considered to have compensated thyroid disease, although the authors could not exclude that some women may have been hypothyroid at some stage during pregnancy. Finally, 58 % of these 49 women had positive thyroperoxidase antibodies (TPO-Ab), compared with 11 % positive TPO-Ab among controls. Because the study was retrospective, the authors admitted that the inherent constraints of their investigation precluded any identification of the causes of hypothyroidism (which may, for instance, have resulted from the treatment of Graves' disease with PTU, as well as from insufficient l-T_4 administration to women with known hypothyroidism). Also, the obstetric outcomes of the pregnancies as well as the status of the offspring were not available at the time of the publication. Given the concerns about the relation between maternal hypothyroidism and potential alterations of fetal brain development, the authors concluded that "*a sufficient number of women have gestational thyroid dysfunction to warrant further investigation of the subject*".

The recent work by *Haddow and colleagues* is a prospective follow up investigation (carried out in 1996–97) of the neuropsychological development of the children (now 7–9 years of age) born to the mothers previously identified as having variable degrees of thyroid deficiency during the pregnancy that had taken place 8–10 years previously (1). Given this clinical setting, the investigators recruited 75 women with serum TSH above the 99.7th percentile of controls (TSH: 〉9 mU/L). They contacted 55/75 women, and 47/55 women agreed to participate. At the "*urging of a grant review panel*", they recruited 18 additional women to represent a range of milder cases, with serum TSH levels between the 98th-99.6th percentiles (TSH: 4.5–8 mU/L), and total T_4 below 7.75 µg/dl (< 99.7 nmol/L): 15/18 women agreed to participate. It is of interest that 15 of these women had a diagnosis of hypothyroidism before pregnancy and 14 of them were actually taking l-T_4 during pregnancy. Mothers participating in the study during pregnancy (17th wk) had a mean (geometric) serum TSH of 13.2 (vs. 1.4 for controls) mU/L, total T_4 7.4 (vs. 10.6) µg/dl, and free T_4 0.7 (vs. 1.0) ng/dl, with significant differences between hypo-T_4 and control mothers. Hence, the final study group comprised the 62 children born to these mothers. The investigators also established a suitable control group of 124 healthy mothers and children born to mothers with normal TSH during pregnancy, matched for mother's age at delivery, number of years of education of the mother, gestational age at sampling time, duration of frozen serum storage, sex of the child, and "Hollingshead scores" to account for possible socioeconomic differences among the families. Neuropsychological testing of the children included the evaluation of performances for 15 tests relating to intelligence, attention, language, reading abilities, school performance, and visual-motor performance.

The case children performed less well on all the tests, although only 2/15 differences in test performance reached statistical significance. The mean full-scale IQ score was 4 points lower in study children compared with controls, and the overall difference (103 vs. 107) was at the limit of significance ($P = 0.06$). More striking differences in performance were found in children from the untreated hypothyroid mothers, with worse scores for all items tested and 9/15 tests significantly different, when compared with controls: mean full-scale IQ score was 7 points lower (100 vs. 107; $p = 0.005$). By contrast, IQ was similar among children born to thyroxine-treated hypothyroid mothers and control children (111 vs. 107). Another important finding was that 9/48 children (19 %) of untreated hypothyroid mothers had an IQ below 86, compared with only 6/124 children (5 %) whose mothers were normal controls. Finally, 77 % of hypothyroid women had positive thyroid antibodies, indicating that, as expected, chronic "asymptomatic" AITD was the most frequent underlying cause. A majority of women (64 %) with previously undisclosed hypo-T_4 during pregnancy had confirmed definitive hypothyroidism at the time of follow up about eleven years later, with a median five-year interval between the pregnancy and clinical diagnosis.

In another article discussing the same study, published also in 1999 (4), the investigators insisted that the hypo-T_4 women whose children were investigated for IQ performances had similar thyroid function parameters, irrespectively of having received ($N = 14$) or not ($N = 48$) thyroxine during pregnancy: elevated TSH (17.8 vs. 12.1 mU/L), low serum total T_4 (98 vs. 98 nmol/L) and free T_4 (9 vs. 9 pmol/L). They proposed therefore as an hypothesis to explain the better performance scores in children of thyroxine-treated mothers, that in the latter cases thyroid function may have been normal during early pregnancy at a critical earlier time for fetal brain development.

From their studies, the authors concluded that:
1. Decreased intellectual and school performances in the offspring may occur even if a pregnant woman has mild and presumably asymptomatic hypothyroidism;
2. Chronic AITD is the most frequent underlying cause of thyroid insufficiency, and a large percentage of such women subsequently develop clinically apparent hypothyroidism, with a median time to diagnosis of 5 years;
3. IQ and school attainment of the offspring are not affected when hypothyroid mothers receive thyroxine during pregnancy (even though l-T_4 dosage was not adequately adjusted), and
4. Systematic screening for hypothyroidism early in pregnancy may be worthwhile, preferably at the first prenatal visit.

In an Editorial accompanying Haddow's article in the NEJM, *Bob Utiger* rightly insisted that *"it is likely that both chronic AITD and iodine deficiency contribute to the occurrence of hypothyroidism in pregnant women in many countries"* (2). Even in the United States, iodine intake has declined substantially in the past 15 years, with 15 % of women in the childbearing age and 7 % of pregnant women having urinary iodine concentrations lower than 50 µg/L (5).

In the late 1960s and early 1970s, pioneering studies by *Evelyn Man and colleagues* reported that 3 % of women had "*thyroid underfunction*" during pregnancy, and that the offspring of inadequately treated hypothyroid pregnant women had significantly lower mental scores compared with controls, when tested at 8 months and 4 years of age. At 4 and 7 years of age, 33–35 % of the children born to such mothers had IQs under 1 SD below the mean IQ of the offspring of euthyroid mothers, that is low IQ was 2.3-fold more prevalent than among controls. In a summary report of their earlier studies, published in 1991, the authors "*encouraged prenatal and/or early gestational screening for maternal hypo-T_4 and urged prescription of adequate thyroid replacement therapy for hypothyroxinemic women*" (6).

Despite the intrinsic, historical, and scientific merits of these early studies, the interpretation of Man's data has remained somewhat difficult. One was not prepared in the seventies to recognize that pregnancy constituted a challenge for the maternal thyroid gland, and precise laboratory means for such assessments were not yet available: measurements of thyroid volume by ultrasonography, free thyroid hormones determinations, measurements of serum thyroglobulin, etc., which we now know all constitute good indicators of early stimulatory thyroidal events. The thyroidal challenge, i.e. the requirement for increased hormone production during gestation, can only be met if iodine intake levels are adequate (150–200 µg/day) and if the functional capacity of the glandular machinery is intact (which has subsequently been shown not to be the case, when AITD is present) (7–9). Also, our understanding of the complex thyroidal pathophysiology in the pregnant state, both for the woman, the fetus, and the fetoplacental unit was only beginning (10). For instance, the notion that thyroid hormones originating from the pregnant woman through placental transfer might be important for fetal brain development in early gestational stages was non-existent (11). Man's early studies also lacked appropriate controls for confounding variables. To cite just a few examples: no information was available concerning iodine intake levels in the population studied; the causes of maternal hypothyroidism were not systematically identified; there was little information on the adequacy of treatment with thyroid extracts or thyroxine; no precise thyroid function tests were carried out, as most data were based on maternal BEI (butanol extractable iodine) determinations.

2. The "Pop" studies in the Netherlands

In 1993, *Victor Pop and colleagues* reported their first study, carried out in 1988–89, on 293 women during and after pregnancy (12). The presence of thyroid autoantibodies was evaluated at 32 weeks gestation and women were followed after parturition, until 34 weeks postpartum. Among the 38 women identified with positive thyroid antibodies (13 %), 27 were positive at 32 weeks gestation and 11 only showed a rise in antibody titer in the postpartum period. Altogether, 40 % of these women had thyroid dysfunction during postpartum (unfortunately, no results were given for thyroid function during pregnancy). The investigators also assessed mental depression during pregnancy and postpartum, using the Research Diagnostic Criteria. According to these criteria, women with AITD had a slightly increased risk (1.7-fold) of developing postpartum depression (unfortunately, no results were given for depression during pregnancy).

In 1995, the same investigators published their second study on the same cohort (230/293 women reevaluated 5 years after delivery), in which they also investigated the children's development (at 5 years of age) using the "MSCA" (McCarthy Scales of Children's Abilities) (13). Two interesting features were observed. Among the mothers, there was a high percentage of depression (23 %) five years after delivery, although the prevalence of depression among antibody-positive and antibody-negative women during the pregnancy period did not differ. The results also showed that at least half of the women with postpartum depression suffered from another episode of depression (some women may perhaps have remained chronically depressed?) within several years of the delivery. It was noteworthy that 56 % of the women diagnosed with AITD in the pregnancy period still had positive thyroid antibodies five years later. Among the offspring, the "MSCA" scores at preschool age were significantly lower in the children of women with postpartum depression and among the children of women with AITD, when compared with children of women without postpartum depression and without AITD, respectively. After correction for possible confounding variables, maternal TPO-Ab positivity during gestation was found to be the most important factor associated with lower scores on the general cognitive scale (odds ratios: 10.5; $P = 0.003$). The authors concluded that children born to mothers with AITD are at risk for impaired cognitive development and asked the crucial question whether "*development in children of AITD mothers might be positively influenced by low dose l-T_4 substitution during early pregnancy*".

In their most recent study reported in 1999, the same investigators assessed, in early infancy, the neuropsychological development of children born to mothers with low-normal free T_4 concentrations in early pregnancy (14). The study was conducted in 1994 in an iodine-sufficient area in the Netherlands. A cohort of 448 consecutive women was initially tested for thyroid function during early pregnancy: 310 women consented to participate, with 291 women completing the study. After excluding 71 women for various methodological reasons, a final group of 220 women, and their infants born full-term, constituted the study groups. Two cut-off points were used to define low-normal free T_4 concentrations at 12 weeks gestation: the lowest 1–5th percentiles ($N = 11$; free $T_4 < 9.8$ pmol/L) and 1–10th percentiles ($N = 11$; free $T_4 < 10.4$ pmol/L). The infants' development was evaluated at 10 months of age using the Bailey Psychomotor Developmental Index (PDI). The children born to mothers in the 1–5th percentiles group had a significant 14.1 % negative difference on PDI score, and those born to mothers in the 1–10th percentiles group a 7.4 % negative difference on PDI score, compared with control infants from the same cohort. The results also showed a linear correlation between maternal serum free T_4 at 12 weeks of gestation (but not at 32 weeks) and the infants' PDI score.

Scrutinizing the results from the data at hand, it is worth mentioning that although significant ($r = 0.46$; $p = 0.03$), the correlation was relatively weak with $r^2 = 0.21$. This suggests that the PDIs of 4–5/22 infants, at most, were truly concerned by a statistical correlation with maternal low-normal early free T_4 values during pregnancy. Moreover, even though there was no correlation between infants' performance and maternal thyroid function during late gestation, the authors mentioned that a few women were probably hypothyroid (with moderately elevated serum TSH and low free T_4) at 32 weeks' gestation. Another important feature was that 23 % of the women were depressed during pregnancy, and as many as 37 % had depression in the postpartum period (while only 3–7 % of the women had AITD during pregnancy and 6 % postpartum thyroid dysfunction). Notwithstanding, after appropriate corrections for confounding variables, the authors concluded that early maternal hypo-T_4 represented a 5.8 relative risk factor for impaired development during the first year of age.

3. The "Matsuura & Konishi" nationwide study in Japan

In 1990, *Matsuura and Konishi* reported the results of a retrospective study carried out in Japan (15). The investigators identified 31 children, born to 16 mothers with chronic thyroiditis. Of these children, 24/31 were born after their mother had developed hypothyroidism; 23/24 infants had a diagnosis of "transient" hypothyroidism in the perinatal period, and 18/23 children received thyroxine treatment for 5–117 months. Thus, the clinical situation in this study was different from that of the other studies analyzed above, both because mothers and children presented hypothyroidism, with variable degrees of severity and because there was wide variation in the interval between the diagnosis and initiation of treatment. For instance, at the time of diagnosis of hypothyroidism in the offspring – that is after parturition – maternal serum TSH concentrations showed that the majority of mothers (75 %) were severely hypothyroid, with serum TSH values as high as 105–480 mU/L. During pregnancy (or at delivery), 50 % of the women were hypothyroid, with serum TSH values of 13–170 mU/L.

Concerning the progeny, 5 (of the 23) children were clearly mentally retarded when tested at 2–9 years of age (IQ 54–76) and presented evidence of abnormal physical development. One child remained untreated and the other 4 children in this group received thyroxine treatment, started on average more than 3 weeks after birth. Furthermore, in the majority of mothers, the diagnosis of hypothyroidism was not made during (or rapidly after) pregnancy, and hence the mothers remained untreated for several months (or years). The other subgroup consisted of 18 (of the 23) children, tested between 0.5–7 years. This group had normal IQ (range 86–122, mean IQ 104) and normal physical development. The major differences between this subgroup and the other subgroup of children were:

- that the majority of these 18 children had received thyroxine treatment soon after birth (on average at 2 weeks of age),
- that most of their mothers were treated for hypothyroidism during pregnancy, and,
- that only two women had mild TSH elevations during gestation.

The authors concluded *"that impaired thyroid function during pregnancy may represent an important factor in the final prognosis of infants born to mothers with chronic thyroiditis"*.

Comments

The complex fetal-maternal unit's interrelations, when the mother has hypothyroidism, are schematically illustrated in Figure 1. Maternal hypothyroidism results usually from autoimmune thyroiditis and also (at least in our experience) from glan-

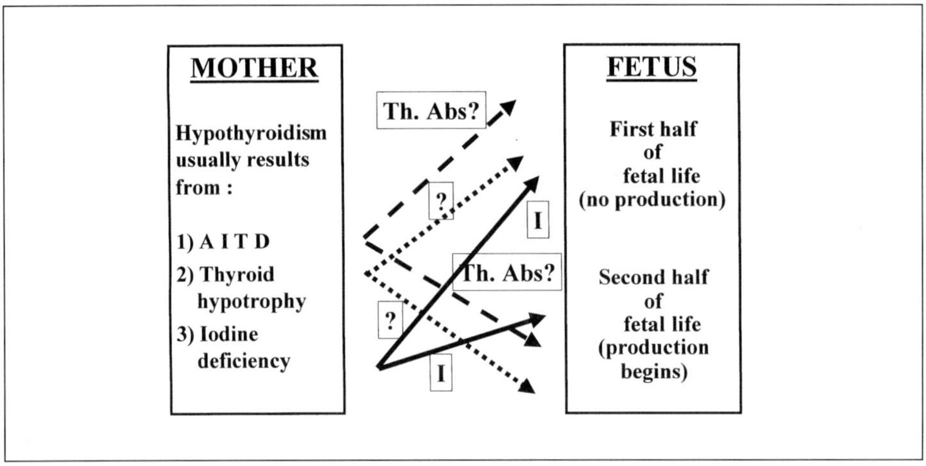

Fig. 1 Maternal hypothyroidism is mainly caused by autoimmune thyroiditis (AITD), glandular hypotrophy (thyroid volumes below 7 milliliters, without detectable thyroid antibodies in serum), and iodine deficiency in many areas in Europe and elsewhere. In AITD, thyroid antibodies have only rarely been implicated in abnormal development of the fetal thyroid gland. No factor has been delineated, so far, that would directly link maternal thyroid hypotrophy with abnormal fetal thyroid gland development or function. When iodine deficiency is present, it is the lack of iodine that constitutes the direct link to explain defective thyroid function in both the mother and fetus.

dular hypotrophy, in conditions with an adequate iodine nutrition status. Hypothyroidism, when present already in the first half of gestation, may lead to impairment of fetal development, since at this early stage the fetal thyroid gland is not yet productive, and thyroid hormones are probably critical for maturation of several thyroid hormone responsive tissues in the fetus (16, 17). In conditions with iodine deficiency disorders (IDD), the lack of iodine affects thyroid function both in the pregnant woman (already in early gestation) and her developing fetus (later in gestation), and the subsequent impairment of fetal development is directly dependent upon the severity and duration of iodine restriction (18). That thyroid hormones play an essential part in normal brain development and that maternal hypothyroidism in areas with overt IDD is associated with neurodevelopmental alterations in the offspring have been known for years. What has been learned from the recently published studies of Haddow (1) and Pop (14) is that neuropsychological developmental alterations may occur in the progeny even in the absence of detectable abnormalities of thyroid function in the child at birth.

Brain development is a complex process involving neuronal differentiation, organization, maturation, and myelinogenesis. It starts during the first weeks of fetal life, and continues throughout gestation and after birth (17). Thyroid hormones have an

Major developmental event	*T.H.*	*Peak time of occurrence*
• **primary neurulation**	??	**3-4 weeks gestation**
• **prosencephalic development**	??	**2-3 months gestation**
• **neuronal proliferation**	+++	**3-4 months gestation**
• **neuronal migration**	+++	**3-5 months gestation**
• **organization**	+++	**5 months gest. ---> years postnatal**
• **myelination**	+++	**birth ---> years postnatal**
• **environmental factors necessary to reach the optimal final human intelligence & learning abilities**	+++	**all life ?**

Fig. 2 Major events in human brain development, with their peak time of occurrence during fetal, neonatal, and perinatal life, and the role of thyroid hormones in these processes (adapted from Rovet (24).

important role in neuronal proliferation, migration, and organization. Thus, maternal hypothyroxinemia, even when restricted to the first trimester (i.e. before the fetal thyroid gland becomes productive), represents a real concern. Delicately timed neuronal processes may be irreversibly impaired because of a lack, at a crucial period, of adequate amounts of thyroid hormones of maternal origin (Figure 2).

In most clinical circumstances where a woman's has thyroid dysfunction, maternal hypothyroxinemia is not restricted to the first trimester of gestation. For instance, in hypothyroidism due to AITD, thyroid hormone deprivation tends to worsen as gestation progresses, especially if undiagnosed and untreated. Therefore, the fetus may be deprived of adequate amounts of thyroid hormones (through placental transfer) in the early stages of brain development, and also during the neurological development later on, thereby reinforcing the potential deleterious effects of early hypothyroxinemia. We have attempted to show, by critically reviewing the available data, that there are reasons to suspect that a combination of both early and late events may indeed have occurred in several patients investigated, since chronic autoimmune thyroiditis was the underlying cause for impaired thyroid function in the majority.

Concerning the causal relationship between maternal thyroid deficiency and the risk of altered neuropsychological development, it was recently proposed that "*the coin may have two faces*". The "hardware" part of the relationship may be related to missed or impaired neuronal connections during brain development, because of the inadequate availability of thyroid hormones transferred from the maternal circulation, both early and also later during gestation, leading to irreversible damage. Furthermore, as indicated by the studies discussed above, maternal and fetal-neonatal hypothyroidism may have been present before birth and around birth, and may have persisted after birth. This combination of factors may potentially have important repercussions in the final achievement of the intelligence quotient in the offspring. This is what we referred to as the "software" part of the problem, namely that maternal hypothyroidism (with fatigue, gestational depression, postpartum thyroiditis, postpartum depression, etc.) may affect the mother's ability to raise a child in the most psycho-stimulating manner. Thus, any delay in diagnosing and treating maternal hypothyroxinemia may ultimately cost "IQ" points in the offspring, with the educational socioeconomic, and public health consequences that may be foreseen. In a world of strong individual competition, the best chance of personal achievement should be given to every child, and no child should be deprived of remediable intellectual capacity (19).

Hypothyroidism is not a rare occurrence in women in the childbearing age and, as shown in several studies, is far from systematically diagnosed during pregnancy. In unselected female populations with an adequate iodine intake, undiagnosed hypothyroidism probably has a prevalence of 2–3 % in all pregnancies (7, 20). Even when hypothyroidism is correctly diagnosed before a woman becomes pregnant, the condition is not always adequately treated, because of inadequate monitoring of thyroid function or late and inadequate adjustment of thyroid hormone replacement doses during gestation (21). One of the striking features in Haddow's study was the fact that both the treated and non-treated hypothyroid pregnant women had similar elevations of serum TSH values, clearly indicating insufficient thyroxine replacement. The present consensus is that women already diagnosed with hypothyroidism before they become pregnant require increments of thyroxine dosage of the order of 30–50 % above preconception daily thyroxine doses. Because thyroxine dosage increments are highly variable among hypothyroid pregnant patients, women need to be monitored closely (by measuring serum TSH and free T_4) from early gestation. For women diagnosed with asymptomatic AITD and who maintain normal thyroid function parameters in the early stages of gestation, it has been proposed that the decision as to whether to administer thyroxine treatment should be based on both serum TSH values (below versus above 2 mU/L) and TPO-Ab titers (below versus above 750 U/ml) in the first half of gestation (9, 20).

Screening pregnant women for hypothyroidism is probably worthwhile, and can in principle easily be achieved with simple blood tests (by measuring thyroid antibodies and serum TSH), either before or as soon as pregnancy is confirmed, and particularly when there is a family history of AITD. Whether systematic screening of thyroid immunity and/or dysfunction should be instituted nationwide is a political, more than a medical issue. In our opinion, the systematic screening of chronic autoimmune thyroiditis and the detection of inadequate levels of iodine nutrition, followed by their correction and treatment, will be beneficial both for the neurointellectual potential of the offspring and also the health of the mothers. Many hospital centers in Europe have embarked on such detection, monitoring, and patient management procedures, without waiting for institutional or governmental bodies to propose consensus guidelines. Such medical decisions appear particularly pertinent for Europe, because of the persistence of iodine deficiency in many European regions. To date, only one large voluntary program of systematic screening of thyroid dysfunction during pregnancy has briefly been reported, carried out in the Sapporo area of Japan (22). Over 70,000 pregnancies have been screened, and the overall rate of reexamination because of abnormal results was 2 %, with half being referred for further medical evaluation. Hyperthyroidism was diagnosed more often than hypothyroidism (an unexpected finding), but the unusual pattern of thyroid dysfunction may be related to a bias in the voluntary acceptance of the women who were screened, and also to the peculiarities of high iodine intake, which is frequent in many Japanese regions.

In Europe, because iodine deficiency is still prevalent in many regions and is also a subject of concern to several important groups of thyroidologists, pediatricians, epidemiologists, etc., maternal hypothyroxinemia and its potential repercussions on the mother and her progeny have been and remain today a major topic of scientific and public health interest. Since the introduction of the systematic screening for congenital hypothyroidism (in the mid-1970s), using serum TSH determinations in the first days of life, it has been well established that neonatal transient hyperthyrotropinemia (elevated TSH) is frequent and is mainly due to maternal iodine deficiency (when no other cause is present). Studies in experimental animals have also indicated that hypothyroxinemia is present in several fetal tissues when the pregnant animals are deprived of an adequate supply of iodine. Over the last decade, several investigators have clearly shown that mild iodine deficiency during pregnancy was associated with hypothyroxinemia and excessive thyroidal stimulation, resulting in frequent goiter formation in the mother and her newborn, among other features. European investigators have therefore proposed, for several years, that iodine prophylaxis be introduced systematically for pregnant women in order to provide mothers with an adequate iodine supply throughout pregnancy. Finally, European scientists have recently proposed screening pregnant populations systematically for the presence of thyroid autoimmunity and hypothyroidism and precise algorithms to this effect have been published (20). Finally, more studies are needed to evaluate alterations of thyroid function during pregnancy more completely in the mother and the fetal-placental unit, with the aim of assessing potentially detrimental neurodevelopmental repercussions in the offspring, of thyroid disorders occurring during gestation (23).

Conclusions and perspectives

The recent article by Haddow et al. has generated commentaries, controversies, letters to Editors, and questions in the U.S. press and the American public, as well as rapid reactions, statements and proposals by several medical associations, including the American Endocrine Society, and the American and European Thyroid Associations. Many questions remain that will require more studies and future work, as well as also rational debates. The recent articles by Haddow and Pop, when placed in the context of the accumulated knowledge in this field during the last two decades, have the merit of having drawn public attention to a potentially important and remediable cause of reduced well being for the children in the future.

References

1. Haddow JE, Palomaki GE, Allan WC, Williams JR, Knight GJ, Gagnon J, O'Heir CE, Mitchell ML, Hermos RJ, Waisbren SE, Faix JD, Klein RZ. Maternal thyroid deficiency during pregnancy and subsequent neuropsychological development of the child. N Engl J Med 1999; 341; 549–55.
2. Utiger RD. Maternal hypothyroidism and fetal development (Editorial). N Engl J Med 1999; 341; 601–2.
3. Klein RZ, Haddow JE, Faix JD, Brown RS, Hermos RJ, Pulkkinen A, Mitchell ML. Prevalence of thyroid deficiency in pregnant women. Clin Endocrinol 1991; 35; 41–6.
4. Klein RZ, Mitchell ML. Maternal hypothyroidism and child development. Horm Res 1999; 52; 55–9.
5. Hollowell JG, Staehling NW, Hannon WH, Flanders DW, Gunter EW, Maberly GF, Braverman LE, Pino S, Miller DT, Garbe PL, DeLozier DM, Jackson RJ. Iodine nutrition in the United States. Trends and public health implications: iodine excretion data from national health and nutrition examination surveys I and III (1971–1974 and 1988–1994). J Clin Endocrinol Metab 1998; 83; 3401–8.
6. Man EB, Brown JF, Serunian SA. Maternal hypothyroxinemia: psychoneurological deficits of progeny. Annals Clin Lab Sci 1991; 21; 227–39.
7. Glinoer D. The regulation of thyroid function in pregnancy: pathways of endocrine adaptation from physiology to pathology. Endocr Rev 1997; 18; 404–33.
8. Glinoer D. Maternal and fetal impact of chronic iodine deficiency. Clin Obstet Gynecol 1997; 40; 102–16.
9. Glinoer D, Rihai M, Grün JP, Kinthaert J. Risk of subclinical hypothyroidism in pregnant women with asymptomatic autoimmune thyroid disorders. J Clin Endocrinol Metab 1994; 79; 197–207.
10. Burrow GN, Fisher DA, Larsen PR. Maternal and fetal thyroid function. N Engl J Med 1994; 331; 1072–8.
11. Vulsma T, Gons MH, de Vijlder JJ. Maternal-fetal transfer of thyroxine in congenital hypothyroidism. N Engl J Med 1989; 321; 13–6.
12. Pop VJ, de Rooy HA, Vader HL, ven der Heide D, van Son MM, Komproe IH. Microsomal antibodies during gestation in relation to postpartum thyroid dysfunction and depression. Acta Endocrinol 1993; 129; 26–30.
13. Pop VJ, de Vries E, van Baar AL, Waelkens JJ, de Rooy HA, Horsten M, Donkers MM, Komproe IH, van Son MM, Vader HL. Maternal thyroid peroxidase antibodies during pregnancy: a marker of impaired child development? J Clin Endocrinol Metab 1995; 80; 3561–6.
14. Pop VJ, Kuijpens JL, van Baar AL, Verkerk G, van Son MM, de Vijlder JJ, Vulsma T, Wiersinga WM, Drexhage HA, Vader HL. Low maternal free thyroxine concentrations during early pregnancy are as-

sociated with impaired psychomotor development in early infancy. Clin Endocrinol 1999; 50; 149–55.
15. Matsuura N, Konishi J, and the transient hypothyroidism study group in Japan. Transient hypothyroidism in infants born to mothers with chronic thyroiditis: a nationwide study of twenty-three cases. Endocr Japan 1990; 37; 369–79.
16. Fisher DA, Polk DH, Wu SY. Fetal thyroid metabolism: a pluralistic system. Thyroid 1994; 4; 367–71.
17. Porterfield SP, Hendrich CE. The role of thyroid hormones in prenatal and neonatal neurological development: current perspectives. Endocr Rev 1993; 14; 94–106.
18. Delange F. Endemic cretinism. An overview. In: Delong GR, Robbins J, Condliffe PG (Eds). Iodine and the Brain. Plenum Press (New York) 1989; 219–29.
19. Glinoer D. Potential repercussions for the progeny of maternal hypothyroxinemia during pregnancy. Thyroid 2000; 10; 59–62.
20. Glinoer D. The systematic screening and management of hypothyroidism and hyperthyroidism during pregnancy. Trends Endocrinol Metab 1998; 9:403–11.
21. Kaplan MM. Monitoring thyroxine treatment during pregnancy. Thyroid 1992; 2; 147–54.
22. Fukushi M, Honma K, Fujita K. Letter to the Editor (untitled). N Engl J Med 1999; 341; 2016.
23. Delange F. Perinatal thyroidology and brain development in iodine deficiency. Biology of the Neonate 2000 (in press).
24. Rovet J. Congenital hypothyroidism: long-term outcome. Thyroid 1999; 9; 741–8.

Fetal growth and autoimmune thyroid disease

D. I. W. Phillips, B. Rees-Smith

MRC Metabolic Programming Group, Southampton General Hospital, Tremona Road, Southampton SO16 6YD, United Kingdom

Abstract

To determine whether events in early life could influence susceptibility to autoimmune thyroid disease, the occurrence of thyroid autoantibodies was studied in 305 women born in Hertfordshire, UK, between 1924–30 for whom details of birthweight, infant growth and feeding were routinely recorded. Using highly sensitive assays, thyroglobulin antibodies were detected in 37 % of the women and thyroid peroxidase antibodies in 41 %. Overt autoimmune thyroid disease defined as the presence of autoantibodies together with hypothyroidism was present in 5.6 %. The proportion of women with thyroid antibodies fell with increasing birthweight but was not related to weight at one year or the method of infant feeding. The prevalence of both antibodies was also related to the current body habitus of the women, rising with increasing body mass index but falling as the waist to hip ratio increased. Overt autoimmune thyroid disease was not associated with fetal or infant weight.

These results suggest that the early environment may affect susceptibility to autoimmune thyroid disease. The contrasting effects of adult body mass index and waist to hip ratio on antibody prevalence could be explained by their associations with different hormonal environments.

Introduction

Autoimmune thyroid disease encompasses a range of disorders from Hashimoto's thyroiditis, the commonest cause of hypothyroidism, to Graves' disease, which in iodine sufficient areas are the commonest causes of hyperthyroidism. The link between these extremes is the presence of antibodies to various components within the thyroid gland. The most frequently found are antibodies to thyroid peroxidase and thyroglobulin, which occur in both patients with Hashimoto's thyroiditis and Graves' disease.

In the late 1980s we developed very sensitive assays for Tg and TPO antibodies

(1). These assays depend on the direct interaction between antibody and highly purified ^{125}I-labeled antigen. Using these assays as a marker for thyroid autoimmunity we carried out a series of investigations to attempt to define their etiological basis. We hypothesized that the mechanisms underlying spontaneous autoantibody production may be less complex than those of overt autoimmune thyroid disease. Initial studies in groups of patients with Hashimoto's thyroiditis and Graves' disease showed that almost all patients with Hashimoto's disease had detectable antibody to both antigens but that the prevalence of antibody in Graves' patients was lower. However, we were also able to detect antibody in a surprisingly high proportion of healthy subjects without a history of thyroid disease. Thus, in blood donors we found prevalences of 10–11 % in men and 18 % in women. As with other thyroid autoantibody assays we found that the prevalence of antibody increased with age. Among the women blood donors we studied that the prevalence of TPO antibody rose from 16 % in the youngest age group to 31 % at age 65. The prevalence of Tg antibody showed a similar pattern (2).

Because it has been known for a long time that Tg and TPO antibodies tend to cluster in families, we examined their distribution in a group of families with autoimmune thyroid disease. In the 16 pedigrees studied, the results showed that where one or other parent was affected equal numbers of daughters were found to be antibody positive and antibody negative. This finding suggested a dominant Mendelian characteristic. However, when we examined the male offspring in these families we found that most sons were unaffected. The ratio of antibody positive and antibody negative sons differed significantly from the expected 50/50 ratio for a dominant gene and suggested that if a dominant gene were involved in autoantibody production that this would have to show impaired penetrance in men (3). Because of the bias inherent in studying families known to have autoimmune thyroid disease, we carried out a segregation analysis in a series of families unselected for thyroid autoimmunity and obtained very similar results (4). These results accorded with studies of spontaneous autoimmunity in experimental animals which suggested that antibody production may be a dominant or co-dominant characteristic (5).

We proceeded to carry out a more elaborate segregation analysis with the computer program POINTER. The advantage of complex segregation analysis is that it enables various possible genetic models to be tested and compared. In the study, which was based on a large series of pedigrees with neuropsychiatric disorders, we were able to confirm the marked familial clustering of antibody, but we could not distinguish between a single gene and multifactorial inheritance. This analysis suggested the need to consider that other factors might be involved in the production of these autoantibodies (6).

Recent research has suggested that the processes of growth and development occurring during intrauterine life can have a profound influence on the pattern of disease in adult life up to 7 decades later. This work has come from a series of studies originally carried out in the country of Hertfordshire where birthweight and the weight at one year, together with the method of infant feeding, were routinely recorded for all infants born in the county. Using these records, we were able to trace adults still resident in Hertfordshire and from studies of these adults a remarkably strong series of correlations have emerged between fetal growth and common disorders in adult life including coronary heart disease, hypertension and non-insulin-dependent diabetes (7).

Results

Using the birth records in Hertfordshire we traced 514 women aged 60–71 who are still resident in the area. Of these, 388 agreed to be interviewed and blood samples were obtained from 305 (303 for thyroglobulin antibody) of them. Using the sensitive assays, Tg antibody was detected in 37 % and TPO antibody in 41 %. Autoimmune thyroiditis, defined as hypothyroidism (low FT4 and/or a raised TSH) in association with TPO or Tg antibody occurred in 5.6 %. The mean birthweight of the women positive for antibody against thyroglobulin, 7.37 lb, was significantly lower than that of the 159 women who were negative for both antibodies, 7.71 lb (difference 0.34lb, p = 0.026). A similar difference was observed in women with thyroid peroxidase antibody (0.28lb, p = 0.06) (8). Table 1 shows the relationship between birthweight and the prevalence of antibody in these late middle aged women. The relative risk or odds ratio of having Tg or TPO antibody is shown for each birthweight

Table 1 Proportions of women aged 60–71 with thyroglobulin or thyroid peroxidase antibody according to birthweight

Birth-weight (lb)	Thyroglobulin antibody				Thyroid peroxidase antibody			
	No of women	No (%) of women with antibody	Odds ratio* (95 % C.I.)	*p* value for trend	No of women	No (%) of women with antibody	Odds ratio* (95 % C.I.)	*p* value for trend
≤ 5.5	14	9 (64)	5.5 (1.0–30.1)		14	6 (43)	2.3 (0.4–12.4)	
– 6.5	57	24 (42)	2.3 (0.6–9.7)		57	28 (49)	3.1 (0.7–12.8)	
– 7.5	112	45 (40)	2.1 (0.5–8.2)		113	50 (44)	2.5 (0.6–9.7)	
– 8.5	74	18 (24)	1.0 (0.2–4.0)		74	24 (32)	1.5 (0.4–6.0)	
– 9.5	34	14 (41)	2.1 (0.5–9.5)		35	13 (37)	1.8 (0.4–8.0)	
> 9.5	12	3 (25)	1.0 –	0.019	12	3 (25)	1.0 –	0.037

* Odds ratio adjusted for BMI and age

Table 2 Multiple regression analysis of the effects of birthweight, body mass index, waist to hip ratio and age on the prevalence of thyroglobulin and thyroid peroxidase antibody

	Thyroglobulin antibody		Thyroid peroxidase antibody	
	Odds ratio (95% C.I.)	*p* value for trend	Odds ratio (95% C.I.)	*p* value for trend
Birthweight (lb)				
≤ 5.5	5.4 (0.9–31.3)		2.4 (0.4–13.3)	
– 6.5	2.5 (0.6–10.8)		3.2 (0.8–13.7)	
– 7.5	2.1 (0.5–8.6)		2.5 (0.6–9.9)	
– 8.5	0.9 (0.2–3.7)		1.4 (0.3–5.7)	
– 9.5	2.0 (0.4–9.2)		1.7 (0.4–7.7)	
> 9.5	1.0 –	0.014	1.0 –	0.04
Body mass index (kg/m²)				
≤ 24.0	1.0 –		1.0 –	
– 26.0	1.2 (0.6–2.6)		1.9 (0.9–3.9)	
– 29.0	1.2 (0.6–2.5)		1.4 (0.7–2.8)	
> 29.0	2.1 (1.1–4.4)	0.025	2.3 (1.1–4.6)	0.04
Waist to hip ratio				
≤ 0.76	3.0 (1.4–6.6)		2.4 (1.1–4.9)	
– 0.80	1.9 (0.9–4.1)		1.6 (0.8–3.2)	
– 0.84	1.6 (0.7–3.4)		1.1 (0.5–2.3)	
> 0.84	1.0 –	0.005	1.0 –	0.05
Age (years)				
≤ 62	1.0 –		1.0 –	
– 65	1.6 (0.9–2.8)		1.3 (0.7–2.2)	
> 65	1.4 (0.7–2.5)	0.024	1.4 (0.7–2.5)	0.16

group. There is a remarkable correlation between birthweight and the prevalence of both Tg and TPO antibody. Compared with the highest birthweight group, the odds ratio of developing thyroglobulin antibody is increased 5-fold and the odds ratio of developing TPO antibody increased 2.5-fold in women who had a birthweight less than 5.5 pounds. There was a gradient of falling prevalence with increasing birthweight, which was statistically significant for both Tg and TPO antibody. We carried out a further analysis looking at the relationships with age at one year. Although birthweight is correlated with weight at one year, we found no correlation between antibody prevalence and the weight at one year. There was also no relationship between the method of infant feeding and antibody prevalence.

We carried out a further analysis using multiple logistic regression to look at other variables that could influence the occurrence of Tg and TPO antibody (Table 2). Apart from birthweight, the prevalence of Tg and TPO antibody was also influenced by obesity (expressed as body mass index, wt/height^2) as well as by the waist to hip ratio – a measure of the centrality of obesity. As expected we found that age influenced antibody prevalence. However, the other variables we examined, including smoking and social class, did not show any correlation. Table 2 shows the effect of obesity on antibody prevalence. The prevalence of Tg antibody, expressed as the odds ratio or relative risk, increased with increasing body mass but fell as the waist to hip ratio increased. This is a surprising finding as a high waist to hip ratio is strongly correlated with a tendency to obesity and one would therefore have expected factors associating with one variable to associate with the other. We obtained similar findings with TPO antibody, again showing contrasting effects of obesity and central obesity on antibody prevalence. Table 3 shows how the waist to hip ratio and body mass index simultaneously affect the percentage of women with antibody. Waist to hip ratio and body mass index have been divided into approximate thirds. Antibody prevalence increased with body mass but at each level of body mass the prevalence of antibody fell with increasing waist to hip ratio. The lowest prevalence of 18 % was in the thin women with the greatest waist to hip ratio; the highest of 69 % in the most

Table 3 Percentage of women aged 60–71 with thyroglobulin or thyroid peroxidase antibody according to waist to hip ratio and body mass index (numbers of women are in parentheses)

Waist to hip ratio	Body mass index (kg/m^2)			
	< 24.5	– 28.0	> 28.0	All
Thyroglobulin antibody				
≤ 0.775	41 (44)	34 (38)	69 (16)	43 (98)
– 0.822	36 (33)	39 (36)	38 (34)	38 (103)
> 0.822	18 (22)	33 (30)	36 (50)	31 (102)
All	34 (99)	36 (104)	42 (100)	37 (303)
Thyroid peroxidase antibody				
≤ 0.775	45 (44)	41 (39)	69 (16)	48 (99)
– 0.822	33 (33)	39 (36)	38 (34)	37 (103)
> 0.822	23 (22)	43 (30)	41 (51)	38 (103)
All	36 (99)	41 (105)	45 (101)	41 (305)

obese women with the lowest waist to hip ratios. Similar trends were observed with TPO antibody.

Only 17 women had overt thyroiditis defined as clinical or biochemical hypothyroidism in association with thyroid antibody. The birth and infant weights of these women did not differ significantly from those of the women without autoimmune thyroid disease. Neither was autoimmune thyroid disease associated with the pattern of infant feeding.

Conclusion

This study suggests that adults who go on to develop thyroid antibodies have a lower prenatal weight gain. Weight at one makes no additional contribution suggesting that the processes leading to antibody production are the outcome of reduced prenatal rather than postnatal growth. The associations we have observed are limited to the development of thyroid antibodies. Patients with overt autoimmune thyroid disease as evidenced by the development of hypothyroidism did not have a lower birthweight although the failure to detect an association in this group may be due to the much smaller of subjects.

The mechanisms linking reduced fetal growth with increased autoantibody production must be speculative. One possibility may lie in the effects of reduced fetal growth on the development and maturation of the thymus. The thymus plays a central role in the maintenance of immunological tolerance via the production of suppressor/cytotoxic T-cells. The thymus reaches its maximum size in relation to body weight at birth. After birth there is a progressive decline in thymic weight, and it has been suggested that the emergence of autoimmunity with increasing age is due to thymic involution and the associated decline in suppressor T-cells (9). There is evidence from animal studies that prenatal influences that reduce fetal growth reduce the relative size of the thymus at birth. Babies born small for their gestational age also have a reduced thymic weight (10,11). It is possible therefore that babies born small at birth would show more rapid thymic involution with age which in turn would permit the earlier emergence of autoreactive, antibody-producing B-cell cones.

Our second finding was that Tg and TPO antibody prevalence rose with increasing body mass index but fell as the waist to hip ratio increased. A possible explanation of this effect is that they reflect the different hormonal environments associated with the different forms of obesity. In postmenopausal women the degree of obesity correlates with the blood levels of estrone and estradiol (12). In contrast, central fat predominance is associated with a decrease in sex hormone binding globulin and a corresponding increase in free testosterone levels (13). Evidence from several animal models suggests that gonadal steroids are important in the pathogenesis of autoimmune disease. In rat and chicken models of thyroiditis, estrogens appear to exacerbate while testosterone ameliorates the disease (14).

The associations reported in this study suggest that thyroid autoimmunity may have its origins during early life. Future research directed towards the causes of autoimmunity should address the development of the immune system and the nutritional or other influences that regulate it.

References

1. Beever K, Bradbury J, Phillips D, et al., 1989. Highly sensitive assays of autoantibodies to thyroglobulin and to thyroid peroxidase. Clin Chem. 35: 1949–1954.
2. Prentice LM, Phillips D.I.W., Sarsero D, Beever K, McLachlan SM, Rees Smith B., 1990 Geographical distribution of subclinical autoimmune thyroid disease in Britain: a study using highly sensitive direct assays for autoantibodies to thyroglobulin and thyroid peroxidase. Acta Endocrinol (Copenh). 123: 493–498.
3. Phillips D, McLachlan SM, Stephenson A, et al., 1990. Autosomal dominant transmission of autoantibodies to thyroglobulin and thyroid peroxidase. J Clin Endocrinol Metab. 70: 742–746.
4. Phillips D, Prentice L, Upadhyaya M, et al., 1991. Autosomal dominant inheritance of autoantibodies to thyroid peroxidase and thyroglobulin – studies in families not selected for autoimmune thyroid disease. J Clin Endocrinol Metab. 72: 973–975.
5. Knight JG, Adams DD, 1981. Genes determining autoimmune disease in New Zealand mice. J Clin Lab Immunol. 5: 165–170.
6. Phillips D.I.W., Shields DC, Dugoujon JM, Prentice L, McGuffin P, Rees-Smith B, 1993. Complex segregation analysis of thyroid autoantibodies: are they inherited as an autosomal dominant trait? Human Hered. 43: 141–146.
7. Barker DJP. Mothers, babies and health in later life. Edinburgh: Churchill Livingstone, 1998
8. Phillips DIW, Cooper C, Fall C, et al. 1993. Fetal growth and autoimmune thyroid disease. Quart J Med. 86: 247–253.
9. Talor E, Rose NR 1991. The ageing paradox and autoimmune disease. Autoimmunity. 8: 245–249.
10. Winick M, Noble A 1966. Cellular Response in Rats during Malnutrition at Various Ages. J Nutrition. 89: 300–306.
11. Chandra RK. Interaction between early nutrition and the immune system. In: Barker DJP, Ed. The Childhood Environment and Adult Disease. Chichester: John Wiley, 1992 77–89.
12. Vermeulen A, Verdonck L, 1978. Sex hormone concentrations in post-menopausal women. Clin Endocrinology. 9: 59–66.
13. Evans DJ, Hoffman RG, Kalkhoff RK, Kissebah AH, 1983. Relationship of androgenic activity to body fat topography, fat cell morphology, and metabolic aberrations in premenopausal women. J Clin Endocrinol Metab. 57: 304–310.
14. Gause WC, March JA. 1986 Effect of testosterone treatment for varying periods on autoimmune development and on specific infiltrating leukocyte populations in the thyroid gland of obese strain chickens. Clin Immunol Immunopathol. 39: 464–478.

Short communication:

Low birth weight is not associated with clinically overt thyroid disease – a twin study

T.H. Brix, K.O. Kyvik, L. Hegedüs

Dept. of Endocrinology, Odense University Hospital, Odense, Denmark

Objective. In recent years low birth weight has been proposed as a risk factor for the development of several chronic diseases in adult life, including diabetes and autoimmune thyroid disease. The association could, however, also be due to genetic or environmental factors affecting both birth weight and adverse health outcomes in adult life. These confounders can to some extent be controlled for through studies of disease discordant twin pairs. The aim of the present study was to investigate the impact of birth weight and several other birth characteristics on the development of clinically overt thyroid disease.

Design. A matched twin case-control study of same sex twin pairs.

Patients. 131 same sex twin pairs (262 individuals) discordant for clinically overt thyroid disease, ascertained from a population based nation-wide twin register.

Measurements. Information about birth weight, birth length, birth order and prematurity was obtained from the original midwife records.

Results. Forty-nine twin pairs were discordant for clinically overt autoimmune thyroid disease (Graves' disease = 35 and Hashimoto's thyroiditis = 14) and 82 pairs were discordant for overt non-autoimmune thyroid disease (simple goiter = 79 and toxic nodular goiter = 3). Overall, there was no difference in birth weights between probands and the healthy co-twins in monozygotic (MZ, n = 39) or in dizygotic (DZ, n = 92) pairs (MZ: mean ± SE: 2619 ± 93 g vs 2553 ± 89 g, p = 0.40; DZ: 2576 ± 45 g vs 2585 ± 49, p = 0.86). By means of logistic regression, the impact of other birth characteristics such as birth length, birth order (first or second born), and prematurity was tested. None of the variables reached statistical significance. Subdividing the twin pairs into those discordant for clinically overt Graves' disease, Hashimoto's thyroiditis, and non-autoimmune thyroid disease did not alter the results.

Conclusion. This is the first study of the effect of birth weight and other birth characteristics on the subsequent development of clinically overt thyroid disease in which maternal, socioeconomic, and genetic factors have been controlled for. Our study did not show any effect of birth weight or any of the other birth characteristics on the risk of developing clinically overt autoimmune or non-autoimmune thyroid disease.

Cigarette smoking and thyroid autoimmunity

E. Martino, F. Bogazzi, A. Pinchera, L. Bartalena

Dipartimento di Endocrinologia e Metabolismo, University of Pisa, Via Paradisa 2, 56124 Pisa, Italy

Abstract

Cigarette smoking has been associated with minor and probably physiologically not important variations in serum thyroid hormone and thyrotropin concentrations. More relevant appears to be the goitrogenic effect of smoking, probably due to thiocyanate (or other smoke products), which is more evident in iodine deficient areas. Smoking has several immunological effects, although it is not clear whether they play an important role in the pathogenesis of smoking-related disorders or are irrelevant epiphenomena. As far as thyroid autoimmune disorders are concerned, an increased prevalence of smokers has been reported in many studies among patients with Graves' disease, and smoking has been associated with an increased risk of developing Graves' disease. It is, however, unclear whether this association is pathogenetically important. The prevalence of smokers is even higher among patients with Graves' ophthalmopathy. The degree of smoking may be somehow related to the severity of eye disease. This relation between cigarette smoking and Graves' ophthalmopathy might have, at least in part, an immunological basis, because smoke-induced hypoxia in the retrobulbar space might stimulate synthesis and secretion of cytokines that are involved in the ongoing immune reactions in the orbit. Cigarette smoking increases the likelihood of progression of non-severe Graves' ophthalmopathy following radioiodine therapy for hyperthyroidism. In addition, cigarette smoking appears to reduce the effectiveness of orbital radiotherapy and high-dose systemic glucocorticoids for severe eye disease. It is presently unknown whether smoking withdrawal may be beneficial for the ophthalmopathy. In contrast with Graves' disease, no relation between smoking and the other thyroid autoimmune disease, Hashimoto's thyroiditis, has been reported, although studies in vitro showed that anthracene products can induce experimental autoimmune thyroiditis. Likewise, no relation has been observed (with the exception of one study) between cigarette smoking and post-partum thyroid dysfunction. The reason for this difference between Graves' disease and Hashimoto's thyroiditis is unknown.

Introduction

Cigarette smoking can influence thyroid function (for a review, see 11; 2). Minor and not unequivocal changes in thyroid function tests, such as an increase or a slight decrease in serum triiodothyronine (T_3) concentration (12; 38), an increase or a decrease in serum thyroxine (T_4) concentration (18; 38), a decrease in serum thyrotropin (TSH) levels (25; 38) were reported. In addition, a relation between serum thyroid hormone and TSH variations and the degree of smoking (and plasma thiocyanate levels) was observed in one study (44), suggesting a possible causative role of thiocyanate in these changes. However, many other studies have failed to find relevant changes in thyroid function tests (11; 2). Interestingly, among women with subclinical hypothyroidism, smokers had higher serum TSH levels than nonsmokers; likewise, smokers had a greater degree of hypothyroidism than nonsmokers with comparable serum TSH concentrations (34). These results do not indicate that smoking causes hypothyroidism, but that it may increase the severity and peripheral effects of hypothyroidism (48).

It has been proposed that smoking might play a significant role in the development of goiter; this action might be related to the goitrogenic effect of thiocyanate (and other smoke products), well established in the presence of iodine deficiency (20). In iodine-sufficient area, smoking may not be a very important goitrogenic cofactor (10). In general, however, an increased prevalence of goiter among smokers was observed in most studies (12; 25; 19; see also 11; 2 for review). In addition, smoking in pregnancy may be associated with transient thyroid enlargement in the newborn (14).

This paper will focus on the relation between cigarette smoking and thyroid autoimmune disorders, with particular regard to Graves' disease and ophthalmopathy.

Cigarette smoking and immunity

Numerous studies have evaluated the immunological actions of cigarette smoking, based on the assumption that immune function abnormalities might contribute to inflammatory and neoplastic complications of smoke. A detailed description of the effects of tobacco smoke is beyond the scope of this article and can be found in recent reviews (22; 31). In experimental animals, during the course of tobacco smoking exposure, T cell dependent humoral and cell-mediated immune responses showed a biphasic pattern, with enhancement during the first months of exposure, followed by suppression during prolonged exposure (see 28, for review). Other findings in experimental animals included profound depression of T cell function in the respiratory tract, as well as the development of expanded and functionally abnormal population of alveolar macrophages (see 28, for review). Marked depression of natural kill (NK) cell activity, which plays a central role in the immune surveillance against tumors and infections, was found in heavy smokers, while it was normal in light-to-moderate smokers (40). Smoking interacts with major depression to decrease NK activity (30). Abnormalities in the number and function of circulating T lymphocytes, including an increase in both CD4+ (helper/inducer) and CD8+ (suppressor/cytotoxic) T cells, was reported in light-to-moderate smokers (29). In heavy smokers a decrease in CD4+ and an increase in CD8+ T cells (with a decrease in the CD4+/CD8+ ratio) was observed, these changes being reversible after smoking withdrawal (33). Studies in twins showed that smoking was associated with an enhancement of humoral immune responses and a decrease of cell-mediated immune responses (51). A decreased CD4+/CD8+ cell ratio, together with reduced cytokine production, was observed in the bronchoalveolar lavage fluid of HIV patients, suggesting that smoking may have a negative impact on lung defenses in these patients (52). Serum immunoglobulin (Ig) G, IgM and IgA levels were found to be decreased by 10–20% (40), whereas IgE levels were increased in light-to-moderate smokers and decreased in heavy smokers (1).

The smoking-associated immunological changes might have some importance in human pathophysiology. For example, a decrease in the concentration of Langerhans cells, the most prominent type of antigen-presenting cell in the normal cervical epithelium, was found in smokers (9): this might facilitate persistence of local viral infection and predispose to the development of virally induced neoplastic transformation. In addition, it has been shown that smoking is strongly associated with Crohn's disease, while ulcerative colitis is strongly associated with not smoking (13). Finally, an association between rheumatoid arthritis and cigarette smoking has been reported (50), together with an increased prevalence of anti-nuclear antibody among smokers (43).

In summary, as briefly outlined above, cigarette smoking is associated with numerous abnormalities of the immune system, although it remains unclear whether these play an important role in the pathogenesis of smoking-related disorders or are irrelevant epiphenomena.

Smoking and thyroid autoimmune disorders

Graves' disease

Graves' disease is an autoimune disease to the pathogenesis of which genetic and environmental factors contribute. The latter seem to include stressful life events (53; 15) and infections (47). Smoking may represent an additional environmental factor (2). An increased prevalence of smokers has been observed among patients with Graves' disease (2). In a large survey of the smoking habits of 1730 women with thyroid disorders or normal controls, the prevalence of smokers was about 30% among

Table 1 Prevalence of smokers among patients with Graves' disease without relevant ophthalmopathy.

Author	Year	Number of Patients	Prevalence of Smokers
Hagg (23)	1987	24	46%
Bartalena (7)	1989	167	48%
Shine (45)	1990	62	27%
Balazs	1990	45	22%
Tellez	1992	103	28%
Winsa (54)	1993	208	41%
Prummel (41)	1993	100	56%
Total		709	41%

Compiled from Bartalena et al. (1995), with some modifications (2).

patients with nontoxic goiter, toxic nodular goiter, Hashimoto's thyroiditis or in normal controls, but as high as 48 % among Graves' patients without ophthalmopathy and 62 % among those with ophthalmopathy (5, 6, 7) (Table 1). Subsequent studies have confirmed this finding. A consecutive entry case-control study documented a higher prevalence of smokers in Graves' patients (56 %) than in controls (41 %), with an odd ratio of 1.9 (41). Similar results were obtained in a case-control study of 208 patients with newly diagnosed Graves' disease, 41 % of whom smoked, compared to 30 % of controls (odds ratio, 1.4) (54). A 52 % prevalence of smokers was observed among 171 patients randomly assigned to different forms of treatment for hyperthyroidism (46). At variance with the above studies, an English study failed to find any difference in the prevalence of smokers between Graves' patients (without ophthalmopathy) and controls (45).

Why should cigarette smoking confer an increased risk for the development of Graves' disease? Smoking might simply be an innocent bystander, and Graves' patients might smoke more because they are nervous and stressed. Stress is indeed associated with an increased desire to smoke (37). It should be mentioned that, in most cases, Graves' patients smoked prior to the development of hyperthyroidism. Alternatively, smoking might enhance other activities (e.g., drinking alcohol or coffee) or other factors which bear the true responsibility for the occurrence of the disease (17). However, it cannot presently be excluded that smoking is effectively involved in the pathogenesis of the disease. This might happen through different smoke-related mechanisms, such as alteration in TSH receptor structure, enhancement of responsiveness to factor(s) responsible for the initiation of the disease, and impairment of restoration of tolerance to thyroid autoantigens (49). The demonstration that these hypothetical mechanisms participate in the development of Graves' ophthalmopathy is presently lacking. In this regard, it should be mentioned that one preliminary study reported no differences in the prevalence and levels of TSH receptor antibodies in smoker and nonsmoker Graves' patients (24). These data still await confirmation.

Graves' ophthalmopathy

Graves' ophthalmopathy is the most frequent extrathyroidal manifestation of Graves' disease and represents a complex therapeutic problem (8). A possible relation between cigarette smoking and Graves' ophthalmopathy was initially suggested in a small series of patients (23) and subsequently confirmed in a large number of patients in different series (see 2, for review) (Table 2). In our own series we found a 64% prevalence of smokers among 307 patients with Graves' ophthalmopathy, a figure much higher than that of Graves' patients without ophthalmopathy (6, 7). In a consecutive entry case-control study, smoking was found to increase greatly the risk for Graves' ophthalmopathy (odds ratio, 7.7) (41). Both the above studies also reported a relation between smoking and the severity of the disease. Recently, 253 patients with Graves' disease of recent onset were followed prospectively (39). Cigarette smoking was associated with a 1.3-fold increased incidence of clinically relevant Graves' ophthalmopathy, and 2.6-fold and 3.1-fold increases in the incidence of proptosis and diplopia, respectively (39). In this study, the current number of daily cigarettes, but not lifetime tobacco consumption, was an independent risk factor, and former smokers had a lower risk of developing severe Graves' ophthalmopathy than current smokers with a comparable lifetime tobacco consumption (39).

This association of cigarette smoking with Graves' ophthalmopathy is unexplained. In addition to direct irritative effects, cigarette smoking might influence ongoing immune reactions in the orbit. It is well accepted that cytokines play an important role in the pathogenesis of Graves' ophthalmopathy (26). Cigarette smoking

Table 2 Prevalence of smokers among patients with Graves' disease and ophthalmopathy.

Author	Year	Number of Patients	Prevalence of Smokers
Hagg (23)	1987	12	83%
Bartalena (7)	1989	307	64%
Shine (45)	1990	85	62%
Balazs	1990	38	95%
Tellez	1992	52	44%
Winsa (54)	1993	62	48%
Prummel (41)	1993	100	81%
Total		656	66%

Compiled from Bartalena et al. (1995), with some modifications (2).

Table 3 Smoking behavior and outcome of treatment of severe Graves' ophthalmopathy with orbital radiotherapy and high-dose systemic glucocorticoids.

Outcome	Smokers		Nonsmokers	
	N	%	N	%
Responders	58	68	61	94
Nonresponders	27	32	4	6

Compiled from Bartalena et al. (1998b) (6).

may affect the process, because smoking-induced hypoxia in the retrobulbar tissue has been shown to increase the release of cytokines from orbital fibroblasts (32). In this regard, it has been reported that, compared to nonsmokers, smokers have lower circulating levels of soluble IL-1 receptor antagonist levels, an anti-cytokine antagonizing the effects of IL-1 (27). It should be mentioned that we were unable to reproduce these data in a different series of patients with Graves' ophthalmopathy (3).

Cigarette smoking may also affect treatment outcomes of Graves' ophthalmopathy. It has recently been reported that in patients submitted to orbital radiotherapy and high-dose systemic glucocorticoid treatment for severe Graves' ophthalmopathy, a favorable response to treatment was observed in 61 of 65 nonsmokers (94 %) and only in 58 of 85 smokers (68 %) (6) (Table 3). Among patients with non-severe Graves' ophthalmopathy, radioiodine treatment may cause a progression of eye disease in about 15 % of cases (4). This progression can be prevented by concomitant short-term course of oral glucocorticoid treatment (5). In a randomized, single-blind study, progression of ophthalmopathy occurred only in about 6 % of nonsmokers and in 23 % of smokers ($p = 0.007$); improvement of preexisting Graves' ophthalmopathy with the concomitant glucocorticoid treatment occurred in 64 % of nonsmokers and 15 % of smokers ($p < 0.001$) (6).

In summary, although the mechanisms whereby cigarette smoking operates remain to be defined, the relation between smoking and eye disease is well established, in terms of both the epidemiology of the disease and its influence on the severity of the disease and the efficacy of its management. Accordingly, Graves' ophthalmopathy patients should be vigorously encouraged to undertake any effort to refrain from smoking, even though it remains to be proven that smoking withdrawal beneficially affects the course of the disease.

Hashimoto's thyroiditis

In a 12-year follow-up study of randomly selected samples of women, a strong association between smoking at the time of initial screening and the subsequent development of autoimmune hypothyroidism was reported, the relative risk for a female smoker becoming hypothyroid being 3.9 (35). However, this association has not been confirmed in other studies. In our own study carried out in a large series of patients, the prevalence of smokers in women with Hashimoto's thyroiditis did not differ from that observed in patients with nontoxic goiter, toxic nodular goiter and in control subjects, and was significantly lower than that in Graves' patients (7). Similar negative results were obtained in a consecutive entry case-control study (prevalence of smokers among Hashimoto's patients and controls, 43 % and 35 %, respectively) (41). Likewise, no relation between smoking and autoimmune thyroiditis was reported in a Swedish study (19).

It is intriguing that two related thyroid autoimmune diseases (Graves' disease and Hashimoto's thyroiditis) show such diversity in their relation with cigarette smoking. An obvious explanation might be that the effects of cigarette smoking on the development of Graves' disease are unrelated to a direct action on the immune system. However, in addition to the immune effects of cigarette smoking described above, it should be mentioned that anthracene derivatives have been reported to cause experimental autoimmune thyroiditis in susceptible rats (16). Therefore, the observed differences in the prevalence of smokers between Graves' and Hashimoto's patients remain unexplained.

Post-partum thyroid dysfunction

In a study of post-partum thyroid function in a series of 220 women, thyroid dysfunction occurred in 49 subjects (22 %) and was significantly related to smoking more than 20 cigarettes/day and to the presence of thyroid microsomal antibodies (21). This relationship (in particular with the development of long-term post-partum thyroid dysfunction) has not been confirmed in subsequent studies from the same (Othman et al., 1990) or other (42) groups. Although patient selection and the small number of patients may, at least in part, have influenced this discrepancy, it is apparent that cigarette smoking does not play a relevant role in the occurrence of post-partum thyroid dysfunction.

Concluding remarks

The relationship between cigarette smoking and the thyroid is multifaceted and far from being fully clarified. Smoking causes marginal (and not unequivocal) changes in thyroid function of uncertain (and probably marginal) pathophysiologic importance. Smoking has a more established goitrogenic effect, possibly related to the action of thiocyanate (and other smoke products).

The most interesting information to have emerged in the past few years is the association of cigarette smoking with Graves' hyperthyroidism and, even more, with Graves' ophthalmopathy. The reason and the mechanisms for this association remain to be elucidated, but smoking appears to influence negatively the course and the treatment outcome of Graves' ophthalmopathy. While autoimmune reactions are likely to play an as yet undefined role in these effects of smoking, this remains to be definitely proven in view of the observation that the other closely related thyroid autoimmune diseases, Hashimoto's thyroiditis and post-partum thyroiditis, do not show the same association with cigarette smoking.

Acknowledgements

This work was supported in part by grants from the University of Pisa (Fondi d'Ateneo) to Professor Enio Martino.

References

1. Bahna SL, Heiner DC, Myhre BA. Immunoglobulin E pattern in cigarette smokers. Allergy 1983; 38: 57–64.
2. Bartalena L, Bogazzi F, Tanda ML, et al. Cigarette smoking and the thyroid. Eur J Endocrinol 1995; 133: 507–12.
3. Bartalena L, Manetti L, Tanda ML, et al. Soluble interleukin-1 receptor antagonist concentration in patients with Graves' ophthalmopathy is neither related to cigarette smoking nor predictive of subsequent response to glucocorticoids. Clin Endocrinol (Oxf) 2000a; 52, in press.
4. Bartalena L, Marcocci C, Bogazzi F, et al. Relation between therapy for hyperthyroidism and the course of Graves' ophthalmopathy. N Engl J Med 1998a; 338: 73–8.
5. Bartalena L, Marcocci C, Bogazzi F, et al. Use of corticosteroids to prevent progression of Graves' ophthalmopathy after radioiodine therapy for hyperthyroidism. N Engl J Med 1989a; 321: 1349–52.
6. Bartalena L, Marcocci C, Tanda ML, et al. Cigarette smoking and treatment outcomes in Graves ophthalmopathy. Ann Intern Med 1998b; 129: 632–5
7. Bartalena L, Martino E, Marcocci C, et al. More on smoking habits and Graves' ophthalmopathy. J Endocrinol Invest 1989b; 12: 733–7.
8. Bartalena L, Pinchera A, Marcocci C. Management of Graves' ophthalmopathy: reality and perspectives. Endocr Rev 2000b; 21: 138–69.
9. Barton SE, Maddox PH, Jenkins D, et al. Effect of cigarette smoking on cervical epithelial immunity: a mechanism for neoplastic change? Lancet 1988; 2: 652–4.
10. Berghout A, Wiersinga WM, Smits NJ, et al. Determinants of thyroid volume as measured by ultrasonography in healthy adults in a non-iodine deficient area. Clin Endocrinol (Oxf) 1987; 26: 273–80.
11. Bertelsen JB, Hegedus L. Cigarette smoking and the thyroid. Thyroid 1994;4: 327–31.
12. Borup Christensen S, Ericsson U-B, Janzon L, et al. Influence of cigarette smoking on goiter formation, thyroglobulin, and thyroid hormone levels in women. J Clin Endocrinol Metab 1984; 58: 615–8.
13. Calkins BM. A meta-analysis of the role of smoking in inflammatory bowel disease. Dig Dis Sci 1989; 34: 1841–54.
14. Chanoine JP, Toppet V, Bourdoux P, et al. Smoking during pregnancy: a significant cause of neonatal thyroid enlargement. Br J Obstet Gynaecol 1991; 98: 65–8.

15. Chiovato L, Pinchera A. Stressful life events and Graves' disease. Eur J Endocrinol 1996; 134: 680–2.
16. Cohen SB, Weetman AP. Characterization of different types of experimental autoimmune thyroiditis in the Buffalo strain rat. Clin Exp Immunol 1987; 69: 25–32.
17. Cooper DS. Tobacco and Graves' disease. Smoking gun or smoke and mirrors? JAMA 1993; 269: 518–9.
18. Edèn S, Jagenburg R, Lindstedt G, et al. Thyroregulatory changes associated with smoking in 70-year-old men. Clin Endocrinol (Oxf) 1984; 21: 605–10.
19. Ericsson U-B, Lindgarde F. Effects of cigarette smoking on thyroid function and the prevalence of goitre, thyrotoxicosis and autoimmune thyroiditis. J Intern Med 1991; 229: 67–71.
20. Ermans AM, Mbulamoko NM, Delange F, et al. Role of cassava in the etiology of endemic goitre and cretinism. International Development Research Centre, Ottawa, 1980.
21. Fung HYM, Kologlu M, Collison K, et al. Postpartum thyroid dysfunction in Mid Glamorgan. Br Med J 1988; 296: 241–4.
22. George J, Levy Y, Shoenfeld Y. Smoking and immunity: an additional player in the mosaic of autoimmunity. Scand J Immunol 1997; 45: 1–6.
23. Hagg E, Asplund K. Is endocrine ophthalmopathy related to smoking? Br Med J 1987; 295: 634–5.
24. Hegedus L, Bliddal H, Karstrup S, et al. Thyroid stimulating immunoglobulins are not influenced by smoking in healthy subjects. Thyroidol Clin Exp 1992; 4: 91–2.
25. Hegedus L, Karlstrup S, Veiergang D, et al. High frequency of goitre in cigarette smokers. Clin Endocrinol (Oxf) 1985; 22: 287–92.
26. Heufelder AE. Pathogenesis of Graves' ophthalmopathy: recent controversies and progress. Eur J Endocrinol 1995; 132: 532–41.
27. Hofbauer LC, Muhlberg T, Konig A, et al. Soluble interleukin-1 receptor antagonist serum levels in smokers and nonsmokers with Graves' ophthalmopathy undergoing orbital radiotherapy. J Clin Endocrinol Metab 1997; 82: 2244–7.
28. Holt PG. Immune and inflammatory function in cigarette smokers. Thorax 1987; 42: 241–9.
29. Hughes DA, Haslam PA, Townsend PJ, et al. Numerical and functional alterations in circulatory lymphocytes in cigarette smokers. Clin Exp Immunol 1985; 61: 459–66.
30. Jung W, Irwin M. Reduction of natural killer cytotoxic activity in major depression: interaction between depression and cigarette smoking. Psychosom Med 1999; 61: 263–70.
31. McAllister-Sistilli CG, Caggiula AR, Knopf S, et al. The effects of nicotine on the immune system. Psychoneuroendocrinology 1998; 23: 175–87.
32. Metcalfe RA, Weetman AP. Stimulation of extraocular muscle fibroblasts by cytokines and hypoxia: possible role in thyroid-associated ophthalmopathy. Clin Endocrinol (Oxf) 1994; 40: 67–72.
33. Miller LG, Goldstein G, Murphy M, et al. Reversible alterations in immunoregulatory T cells in smoking. Chest 1982; 82: 526–9.
34. Muller B, Zulewski H, Huber P, et al. Impaired action of thyroid hormone associated with smoking in women with hypothyroidism. N Engl J Med 1995; 333: 964–69.
35. Nystrom E, Bengtsson C, Lapidus L, et al. Smoking – A risk factor for hypothyroidism. J Endocrinol Invest 1993; 16: 129–31.
36. Ohtman S, Phillips DIW, Parkes AB, et al. A long-term follow-up of postpartum thyroiditis. Clin Endocrinol (Oxf) 1990; 32: 559–64.
37. Perkins KA, Grobe JE. Increased desire to smoke during acute stress. Br J Addict 1992; 87: 1037–40.
38. Petersen K, Lindstedt G, Lundberg P A, et al. Thyroid disease in middle-aged and elderly Swedish women: thyroid-related hormones, thyroid dysfunction and goitre in relation to age and smoking. J Intern Med 1991; 229: 407–14.
39. Pfeilschifter J, Ziegler R. Smoking and endocrine ophthalmopathy: impact of smoking severity and current vs. lifetime cigarette consumption. Clin Endocrinol (Oxf) 1996; 45: 477–81.
40. Phillips B, Marshall ME, Brown S, et al. Effect of smoking on human natural killer cell activity. Cancer 1985; 56: 2789–92.
41. Prummel MF, Wiersinga WM. Smoking and risk of Graves' disease. JAMA 1993; 269: 479–82.
42. Rasmussen N, Hornnes PJ, Feldt-Rasmussen U, et al. Thyroid size and function in healthy pregnant

women with thyroid autoantibodies. Relation to development of postpartum thyroiditis. Acta Endocrinol (Copenh) 1990; 123: 395–401.
43. Regius O, Lengyel E, Borzsonnyi L, et al. The effect of smoking on the presence of antinuclear antibodies and the morphology of lymphocytes in aged subjects. Z Gerontol 1988; 21: 161–3.
44. Sepkovic DW, Haley NJ, Wynder EL. Thyroid activity in cigarette smokers. Arch Intern Med 1984; 144: 501–3.
45. Shine B, Fells P, Edwards OM, et al. Association between Graves' ophthalmopathy and smoking. Lancet 1990; 335: 1261–3.
46. Tallstedt L, Lundell G, Taube A. Graves' ophthalmopathy and tobacco smoking. Acta Endocrinol (Copenh) 1993; 129: 147–50.
47. Tomer Y, Davies TF. Infection, thyroid disease and autoimmunity. Endocr Rev 1993; 14: 107–20.
48. Utiger RD. Cigarette smoking and the thyroid. N Engl J Med 1995; 333: 1001–2.
49. Utiger RD. Effects of smoking on thyroid function. Eur J Endocrinol 1998; 138: 368–9.
50. Vessey MP, Villard-Macintosh L, Yeates D. Oral contraceptives, cigarette smoking and other factors in relation to arthritis. Contraception 1987; 35: 457–64.
51. Von Hertzen L, Surcel HM, Kaprio J, et al. Immune responses to Chlamydia pneumoniae in twins in relation to gender and smoking. J Med Microbiol 1998; 47: 441–6.
52. Wewers MD, Diaz PT, Wewers ME, et al. Cigarette smoking in HIV infection induces a suppressive inflammatory environment in the lung. Am J Respir Crit Care Med 1998; 158: 1543–9.
53. Winsa B, Adami H-O, Bergstrom R, et al. Stressful life events and Graves' disease. Lancet 1991; 338: 1475–9.
54. Winsa B, Mandahl A, Karlsson FA. Graves' disease, endocrine ophthalmopathy and smoking. Acta Endocrinol (Copenh) 1993; 128: 156–60.

Stress and autoimmune thyroid disease

J. F. Leclère

Clinique Médicale et Endocrinologique, Centre Hospitalier Universitaire de Nancy, Hôpital de Brabois, 54511 Nancy-Vandœuvre-Cédex, France

Abstract

The triggering role of stress in some thyroid diseases has been suggested since the early description of Graves' thyrotoxicosis. Thanks to specific methodology for identification and scoring stressful life events, this hypothesis is now supported by prospective studies. Based on these studies, one can conclude that patients genetically predisposed to autoimmunity may develop thyroid autoimmune disease when exposed to stress. The nature of stress is not different from the control population but the number of events is greater and they are more distressing. Recent knowledge concerning neuroendocrine-immune relations accounts for the onset of thyroid autoimmunity, with the hypothalamic-pituitary-adrenal axis playing a key role.

Introduction

Autoimmune diseases are influenced by multiple factors of genetic, endogenous and environmental origin. For the clinician, certain stressful life events seem to precede the onset of thyroid pathology, at least in Graves' disease. *Parry* and *Von Basedow* suggested that psychological factors had an influence in their descriptions of the disease. The relationships between stress and other autoimmune thyroid diseases are difficult to ascertain because of their insidious development. In a recent review on the pathogenesis of chronic autoimmune disease, stress is not taken into consideration among environmental factors (9). There have been several studies concerning the possible influence of stress in the pathogenesis of Graves' disease.

Clinical studies

Two groups of studies are available, retrospective (sometimes anecdotal) and prospective studies.

Retrospectives studies

Parry, Graves, and *von Basedow* suggested stressful life events as inducers of hyperthyroidism in their early descriptions. We should also mention the publications of *Conrad* (8), *Katzenlbogen* (21), and *Lidz* (26), who identified a number of stressful life events in the recent history of hyperthyroid patients. However, the most convincing series were reported by *Bram* (4) and *Forteza* (11) who detected stress life events in 85 % of 3343 and 75 % of 116 patients, respectively, suffering from Graves' disease.

Civil and international wars also represent particular circumstances relating to the onset of autoimmune diseases influenced by stress. *Meulengracht* (28) found an increase of thyrotoxicosis in the Danish population during the Second World War compared with the 1945 – 1948 period. *Grelland* came to the same conclusion in Norway (13). More recently, *Paunkovic* (30) found an increase of Graves' disease in Serbia during and immediately after the Yugoslavian civil war. Nevertheless, some other studies, such as those of *Bastenie* (2) during the Second World War and *Hadden* (14) in Ireland, come to different conclusions.

However, all these studies come in for sharp criticism because of their methodologies and the technical limitations in the diagnosis of Graves' disease for the oldest reports. These remarks cannot be directed against the recent paper of *Paunkovic* (30).

Prospective studies

The term "prospective" is not appropriate because these studies are based on recall, which may be biased by failure of memory as well as by emotional hypersensitivity due to thyrotoxicosis (7).

There are also some concerns about the methods used to quantify the role of stress:

- Over what period can events influence the onset of the disease? It is usually considered that a 1 to 2 year period is adequate
- How does one quantify the impact of stress on the patient? The most frequently used methods are the life events scales of *Holmes* (18), *Paykel* (31), and *Sarason* (34). These scales have been widely validated, but they do not consider coping. However important an event may be, its impact differs according to whether the

subject copes or not. This aspect can be quantified by the Ways of Coping Checklist of *Folkman* and *Lazarus* (10).

In 1991, *B. Winsa and colleagues* (39) published an important study of 208 Graves' disease patients who completed a mailed questionnaire based on the Sarason life survey. Each patient's answers were compared with those of 2 controls. The thyroid status of the controls is not stated in the paper. Apart from this last criticism, careful analysis allowed the authors to conclude that the patients experienced more negative events during the 12 months before diagnosis. The scores for events were higher among patients than controls. On the other hand, there were no differences for positive events between the two groups. Moreover, by means of the Jenkins' activity survey (19), which measures the degree of mastery, patients exhibited type "A" behavior. This psychological profile predisposes individuals to be more dissatisfied and to recall negative events more readily than positive events. Although the methodology used in this work may be criticized (3, 32) it represents the first substantial study concerning the connection between stress and thyroid autoimmunity.

At the same time (24), we presented the results of a prospective study based on 27 unselected consecutive Graves' disease patients. The diagnosis was based on classical signs, high levels of free T_3 and T_4, low TSH, presence of TSH receptor antibodies, and diffuse thyroid scintiscan. The clinical signs had been present for less than 3 months. At the same time, each case was matched with one euthyroid control recruited from the Worker Health Care Service at our Institution where they attended for routine annual check. Matching criteria included similar age (± 2 years) and socioeconomic status according to the 9 categories of the national system of classification (National Institute of Statistics and Economic Studies – INSEE). Cases and controls data were obtained at the same time during interviews conducted by a single psychologist. Life events were recorded using the Holmes rating (43 items distributed over 5 domains, scored on a scale of intensity from 0 to 100) and the French adaptation of Paykel's method, including 53 items scored 0 to 100. This second scale was used in order to corroborate the first scale and to avoid any bias due to French culture. The records were divided into 2 periods: 0 to 1 year and 1 to 2 years before the diagnosis of Graves' disease. The statistical analysis used the two-sided paired Student test for each one-year period and the overall. Comparison of the score within each one-year period in each group was used to detect any effect of time on the number and intensity of reported life events. Our results (Table 1) led to the conclusion that the impact of some but not all life events was slightly different between patients and controls. However, the difference was highly significant when considering the number of negative events ($p < 0.0001$).

The greater number of life events among patients with Graves' disease was confirmed by the study of *Harris* (15) in 1992 (odds ratio 6.3, 95 % confidence interval 2.7–14.7).

Table 1 Statistical analysis of the number and scoring of life stress events in 27 patients and 27 matched controls

		Death	Illness	Economic	Relations	Positive	Total
Paykel (modified)	< 1 y	0.054	0.207	0.204	0.191	0.147	0.0001
Scale	> 1 y	0.556	0.009	0.036	0.148	0.879	0.0001
Holmes	< 1 y	0.020	0.031	0.092	0.189	0.135	0.0001
Scale	> 1 y	0.541	0.085	0.021	0.161	0.777	0.008

Later prospective studies are in agreement with earlier series:

- *N. Sonino* (36) interviewed 70 consecutive Graves' disease patients and 70 controlled carefully matched using the Paykel's Interview for Recent Life Events and found a greater number of life events among patients than among controls. In contrast to other studies, the number of positive events was also statistically significant.
- Using very careful methodology employing 3 different questionnaires measuring retrospective life events (18), coping (10) and daily stresses (20), *A. Kung* (22) did not find any influence of positive or neutral events on Graves' disease in her 95 patients. The patients experienced more negative events ($p < 0.0001$) with more severe rating ($p < 0.0001$) than controls. There was no difference in the coping ability between the two groups.
- *Radoslavjevic* (33) also found more life events in the 12 months before diagnosis among 100 Graves' disease patients than among 100 controls ($p < 0.0001$).
- In contrast to these results, *Gray and Hoffenberg* (12) found no differences between toxic and non-toxic goiters. However, this study did not indicate the type of thyrotoxic goiters and has to be considered with circumspection.

In spite of eventual bias due to recalls, all these studies come to broadly the same conclusions: stressful life events are more frequent among Graves' disease patients than among healthy subjects. The nature of these events is not different but they are perceived more severely. These conclusions might be biased by increased sensitivity due to hyperthyroidism (7). This seems to be not the case in a recent presentation of *A. Matos Santos and colleagues* (27), who compared stress life events among controls and patients suffering from Graves' disease and thyrotoxic non-autoimmune goiters. The impact of stress life events was more pronounced in Graves' disease than in hyperfunctioning goiters ($p < 0.004$).

Pathogenesis

A genetic predisposition is now well established for thyroid autoimmunity. A 6-fold increased risk has been found among patients with HLA DR3 or DR5. Among Graves' disease families, specific HLA-DR and -Gm haplotype associations are found in nearly all thyrotoxic patients. More precisely, a strong statistical linkage disequilibrium ($p < 0.00001$) can be seen between the haplotype DRB1*0304 – DQB1*02 – DQA1*0501 and Graves' disease (16). CTLA-4 and CD 28 have an opposite role in the regulation of T cell responses to antigen presentation. Linkage disequilibrium has been recently described between CTLA – 4 and Graves' disease using the Transmission Disequilibrium Test among 179 families (17). This last method is a more powerful tool than the usual studies based on linkage analysis. In summary, genetic susceptibility to thyroid autoimmunity seems to be definitely established and is probably not restricted to the above genes.

It is difficult to determine the importance of genetic factors in autoimmune diseases, but their onset requires some other factors, including environmental influences. Infections and iodide excess are recognized as factors able to induce thyroid damage followed by release of antigens. Normal subjects are able to modulate and finally end the immune response to environmental injuries, but in predisposed patients the immune response is amplified and autoimmunity develops. This may be due to a failure of immunoregulation, leading to inability to maintain self-tolerance. This maintenance is dependent on the different steps of development of the immune system and any circumstances tending to disturb the immune equilibrium may lead to the development of autoimmunity in a predisposed patient.

The mechanisms by which stress could be one of these factors depend on interactions between neuroendocrine and immune systems. The endocrine reactions to stress have been extensively studied since the historical concept proposed by Selye, in which took into account participation of the immune system. Besides the metabolic and endocrine reactions to stress, *Selye* (35) described involution of the thymus and lymphatic organs, a reduction in circulating lymphocytes, an increase in plasma gamma globulins and the presence of antibodies, as well as the occurrence of inflammatory diseases (periarteritis nodosa and polyarthritis).

Stress acts on different areas of the brain and induces a series of responses leading to stimulation of the autonomic nervous system (ANS) and consequently to release of noradrenaline (NA), adrenaline (A, from the adrenal medulla) and acetylcholine (AC) and later to the stimulation of hypothalamic-pituitary-adrenal axis (HPA).

The ANS is regulated by integrating neurons located in the hypothalamus, which receive a large amount information from various origins including the environment. The ANS innervates numerous organs, including endocrine glands and lymphoid tissues.

The impact of acute stress on hypothalamic neurons also influences other endocrine secretions like prolactin, GH, gonadal steroids, and thyroid hormones.

Autonomic and endocrine impact on immune function

HPA stimulation occurs later and is under the influence of various pathways, including the ventral and dorsal ascending noradrenergic bundles, hippocampus, amygdala, and limbic system. Many neuromediators originate from these structures: NA, AC, GABA, neuropeptide Y, VIP, and serotonin. Most of these – except GABA which inhibits – stimulate release of corticotrophin releasing hormones CRH and arginine vasopressin (AVP) and consequently the secretion of POMC and its derivatives ACTH and β-endorphin, as well as cortisol (5). This cascade of reactions is observed in acute stress but – apart from HPA axis there is little information concerning the magnitude of reactions consequent on chronic or repeated stress. In these cases, the response is ubiquitous, but is sometimes attenuated due to a kind of "tolerance", and sometimes amplified. Sustained hyperstimulation of HPA axis has been clearly demonstrated during chronic stress. Interestingly, the HPA reaction is more pronounced in female (38) and in the elderly (6). The impact of acute stress on hypothalamic neurons also influences other endocrine secretions like PRL, GH, gonadal steroids, and thyroid hormones. The influence of autonomic and endocrine reactions on the immune system is suggested by the presence of receptors for NA and AC on immune cells. Receptors have also been demonstrated for corticosteroids, PRL, GH, ACTH, endorphins, and VIP.

It is likely that all these hormones modify the equilibrium of immunoregulation through their receptors. Concerning the thyroid axis, it is interesting to note that, during chronic stress, secretion of TSH is normal or decreased, excluding the participation of hypothalamic-pituitary-thyroid axis in the onset of thyroid hyperfunction (1).

It appears that the most important consequence of stress on the endocrine system concerns HPA and it could be paradoxical if this axis induces autoimmunity since corticosteroids are strong immunodepressors. In fact, the effects of corticosteroids are dose-dependent: they have opposite effects on immune cells at low (which approximate the endogenous levels obtained after stress) and high concentrations. In addition, the number of receptors is not equal on different types of cells. In decreasing order, the expression of b adrenergic receptors is higher in B than in T helper (CD4+) and T suppressor (CD8+) lymphocytes (23). One of the most convincing argument for a link between stress-endocrine system and autoimmunity is the selective suppressor effect of corticoids on Th1 cells, whereas Th2 are somewhat unaffected (37). This selection could favor humoral immunity.

In turn, immune cells may influence the neuroendocrine system by production of cytokines. In experimental studies, it has been demonstrated that IL-1, IL-6, IL-8 and TNF α stimulate CRH / AVP neurones and secretion of ACTH (29).

The complexity of the neuroendocrine-immune system is compounded by the expression of CRH, AVP, and POMC in immune tissues.

Conclusions

In conclusion, we can conceive the pathogenesis of thyroid autoimmune disorders induced by stress as follows:

- Genetically predisposed patients maintain a self tolerance until they are exposed to any factor leading to immune disequilibrium.
- This disequilibrium may be due to thyroid lesions (secondary to viral or other thyroid injury) or to sustained stimulation of endocrine system by powerful and/or successive stresses.
- Autoimmunity is then triggered and may be maintained by the thyroid lesions induced by cytotoxic antibodies.

Thus, the causes of thyroid autoimmunity are obviously multiple. There are convincing clinical reports indicating that stress may be one of them. The role of stress is explained by the tight relations between the central nervous system, hypothalamic endocrine regulation, and the immune system.

References

1. Armario A, Lopez-Calderon A, Jolin T, Balasch T. Response of anterior pituitary hormones to chronic stress. The specificity of adaptation. Neurosci Behav Rev 1986; 10: 245–250.
2. Bastenie P A. Disease of the thyroid gland in occupied Belgium. Lancet 1947; i: 789 – 792.
3. Ben-Shlomo Y, Chaturvedi N. Stress and Graves' disease. Lancet 1992; 339: 427.
4. Bram I. Psychic trauma in the pathogenesis of exophthalmic goiter. Endocrinology 1927; 11: 106-116.
5. Buckingham J C, Cowell A M, Gillies G E, et al. The neuroendocrine system: anatomy, physiology and responses to stress. In: Stress, stress hormones and the immune system. Buckingham J C, Gillies G E, Cowell A M, eds. London: Wiley 1997: 9 – 47.
6. Buckingham J C, Loxley H D, Christian H C, Philip J G. Activation of the HPA axis by immune insults: roles and interactions of cytokines, eicosanoids and glucocorticoids. Pharmacol Biochem Behav 1996; 51: 285 – 296.
7. Chiovato L, Pinchera A. Stressful life events and Graves' disease. Eur J Endocrinol 1996; 134: 680 – 682.
8. Conrad A. The psychiatric study of hyperthyroid patients. J Nerv Ment Dis 1934; 79: 505–529.
9. Dayan C M, Daniels G H. Chronic autoimmune thyroiditis. N Engl J Med 1996; 335: 99 – 107.
10. Folkman S, Lazarus R S. An analysis of coping in a middle-aged community sample. J Health Soc Behav 1980; 21: 219 – 239.
11. Forteza M E. Precipitating factors in hyperthyroidism. Geriatrics 1973; 28: 123 126.
12. Gray J, Hoffenberg R. Thyrotoxicosis and stress. Q J Med 1985; 54: 153–160.
13. Grelland R. Thyrotoxicosis at Ulleval hospital in the years 1934–44 with a special view to frequency of the disease. Psychosom Med 1955; 125: 420–427.
14. Hadden D R, McDevitt D G. Environmental stress and thyrotoxicosis. Lancet 1974; ii: 577–578.
15. Harris T, Creed F, Brugha T S. Stressful life events and Graves' disease. Br J Psychiatry 1992; 161: 535–541.
16. Heward J M, Allahabadia A, Daykin J, et al. Linkage disequilibrium between the human leukocyte antigen class II region of the major histocompatibility complex and Graves' disease: replication us-

ing a population case control and family-based study. J Clin Endocrinol Metab 1998; 83: 3394–3397.
17. Heward J M, Allahabadia A, Armitage M, et al. The development of Graves' disease and the CTLA-4 gene on chromosome 2q33. J Clin Endocrinol Metab 1999; 84: 2398–1401.
18. Holmes T H, Rahe R H. The social readjustment rating scale. J Psychosom Res 1967; 11: 213–218.
19. Jenkins C, Rosenman R H, Zyzanski S J. The Jenkins Activity Survey for health prediction. Jenkins A C, ed. Chapel Hill 1965.
20. Kanner A D, Coyne J C, Schaefer C, Lazarus R S. Comparison of two modes of stress measurement: daily hassles and uplifts versus major life events. J Behav Med 1981; 4: 1–39.
21. Katzenlbogen S, Luton F H. Hyperthyroidism and psychobiological reactions. Am Psychiatry 1935; 91: 969–981
22. Kung A W C. Life events, daily stresses and coping in patients with Graves' disease. Clin Endocrinol (Oxf) 1995; 42: 303–308.
23. Landmann R M A, Wesp M, Box R, et al. Distribution and function of b-adrenergic receptors in human blood lymphocytes. Interactions among CNS, neuroendocrine and immune systems. Hadden J W, Masek K, Nistico G, eds. Rome: Pythagora Press 1989: 251–264.
24. Leclere J, Germain M, Weryha G, et al. Role of stressful life-events in the onset of Graves' disease. Ann Endocrinol (Paris) 1991; 52: 100.
25. Leclere J, Weryha G. Stress and auto-immune endocrine diseases. Horm Res 1989; 31: 90–93.
26. Lidz T, Whitehorn J C. Life situations, emotions and Graves' disease. Psychosom Med 1950; 12: 184–186
27. Matos Santos A, Lacerda Nobre E, Garcia E Costa J, et al. Stressful life events, Graves' disease and toxic goitre. Presented at the 26th Annual Meeting of the European Thyroid Association, Milan, Italy, August 28 – September 1, 1999. Abstr. J Endocrinol Invest 1999; 22: 81.
28. Meulengracht E. Epidemiological aspects of thyrotoxicosis. Arch Intern Med 1949; 83: 119–134.
29. Navarra P, Schettini G, Grossman A B. Responses of the stress axis to immunological challenge: the role of eicosanoids and cytokines. In: Stress, stress hormones and the immune system. Buckingham J C, Gillies G E, Cowell A M, eds. London: Wiley 1997: 283–298.
30. Paunkovic N, Paunkovic J, Pavlovic O, et al. The significant increase in incidence of Graves' disease in eastern Serbia during the civil war in the former Yugoslavia. Thyroid 1998; 8: 37–41.
31. Paykel E S. Methodology of life events research. In: Research paradigms in psychosomatic medicine. Fava G A, Wise T N, eds. Basel: Karger 1987: 13–29.
32. Petticrew M. Stress and Graves' disease. Lancet 1992; 339: 427.
33. Radoslavjevic V R, Jankovic S M, Marinkovic J M. Stressful life events in the pathogenesis of Graves' disease. Eur J Endocrinol 1996; 134: 699–701.
34. Sarason I G, Johnson J H, Seigel J M. Assessing the impact of life changes: development of the Life Experience Survey. J Consulting Clin Psychol 1978; 46: 932–946.
35. Selye H. The general adaptation syndrome and the diseases of adaptation. J Clin Endocrinol Metab 1946; 6: 117- 230.
36. Sonino N, Girelli M E, Boscaro M, et al. Life events in the pathogenesis of Graves' disease. A controlled study. Acta Endocrinol (Kbh) 1993; 128: 293–296.
37. Stam W B, Van Oosterhout A J, Nijkamp F P. Pharmacological modulation of Th1 and Th2 – associated lymphokine production. Life Sci 1993; 53: 1921–1934.
38. Vamvakopoulos N C, Chrousos G P. Hormonal regulation of human corticotrophin releasing hormone gene expression: implications for the sexual dimorphism of the stress response and immune/inflammatory reaction. Endocrine Rev 1994; 15: 409–420.
39. Winsa B, Adami H-O, Berström R, et al. Stressful life events and Graves' disease. Lancet 1991; 338: 1475–1479.

Iodine and thyroid autoimmune disease

H. A. Drexhage, H. J. de Wit, P. Mooij

Dept. of Immunology, Erasmus University Rotterdam, Dr. Molewaterplein 50; 3000 DR Rotterdam, The Netherlands

Abstract

Thyroid autoimmune diseases are complex, polygenic afflictions the penetrance of which is heavily dependent on various environmental influences. In their pathogenesis, an afferent stage (enhanced autoantigen presentation), a central stage (excessive expansion and maturation of autoreactive T and B cells), and an efferent stage (effects of autoreactive T cells and B cells on their targets) can be discerned. At each stage, a plethora of inborn, endogenous or exogenous factors is able to elicit the abnormalities characteristic of that stage, thus opening the gateway to thyroid autoimmunity.

Iodine is an important exogenous modulating factor of the process. In general, iodine deficiency attenuates, while iodine excess accelerates autoimmune thyroiditis in autoimmune prone individuals. In non-autoimmune prone individuals, the effects of iodine are different. Here iodine deficiency precipitates a mild (physiological?) form of thyroid autoimmune reactivity. Iodine excess stimulates thymus development. Iodine exerts these effects via interference in the various stages of the autoimmune process. In the afferent and efferent stage iodine-induced alteration in thyrocyte metabolism and even necrosis most likely play a role. By contrast, in the central phase iodine has direct effects on thymus development, the development and function of various immune cells (T cells, B cells, macrophages and dendritic cells) and the antigenicity of thyroglobulin.

Introduction

One of the important functions of the immune system is the discrimination between "self" and "nonself", or perhaps better between "danger" and "non-danger". Currently, such distinctions are thought to be made through a series of complicated and multistep interactions between various cells and components of the immune system. Immune cells sometimes erroneously establish an immune reaction towards self anti-

Table 1 Overview of major organ-specific autoimmune diseases

Disease	Major autoantigens	Effector mechanisms Result autoantibodies/ T cells	Clinical symptoms	Animal models		
				Sponteaneous	Experimental (allergic)	
					Antigen/procedure	Animal
Hashimoto's thyroiditis	Thyroperoxidase (TPO) Thyroglobulin (Tg)	ADCC and Th1 mediated thyrocyte destruction	Goiter, followed by thyroid failure	BB rat NOD mouse OS chicken	Tg in FCA	Normal rats and rabbits
Primary hypo-thyroidism	TSH-receptor (TSH-R)	Antibodies blocking the TSH-R	Hypothyroidism and thyroid atrophy		TSH-R ECD	NOD mouse
Graves' disease	TSH-R	Antibodies stimulating the TSH-R	Goiter and hyper-thyroidism		$TSH-R^+$, MHC class II^+ fibroblasts TSH-R ECD	AKR/N mouse Balb-C mouse
Type 1 diabetes mellitus	Insulin GAD IA-2 ICA-69	Th1 mediated destruction of β cells	Hyperglycemia	BB rat NOD mouse	Streptozotocin	Normal rats and mice
Pernicious anemia	Na^+/H^+ ATP-ase Intrinsic Factor	Th1 mediated destruction of gastric parietal cells and neutralization of intrinsic factor by antibodies	Atrophic gastritis Anemia		Tx (3 day)	Balb/C mouse A/J mouse
Addison's disease	21-hydroxylase 17 α-hydroxylase	Th1 mediated destruction of steroid-producing cells	Adrenalitis and Oöphoritis		Tx (3 day)	Balb/C mouse A/J mouse

Vitiligo	Tyrosinase	Disappearence of melanocytes	Depigmentation	Smyth-line chicken	Melanosomal proteins + IL-2/DC	Melanoma therapy man
Sjögren syndrome	Phodrin M3-muscarinic receptor	Destruction/blockade salivary/lacrimal glands (sialoadenitis)	Dry eyes Dry mouth	NOD	Tx (3 day)	NFS/sld mouse
Multiple sclerosis	Myelin Basic Protein (MBP) Proteolipid Protein (PLP) Myelin Oligodendrocyte Glycoprotein (MOG)	Th1 mediated destruction of myelin sheaths	Diverse neurological symptoms	None	MBP, PLP or MOG in FCA	Lewis/DA rat SJL mouse Marmoset monkey

GAD, glutamic acid decarboxylase; IA-2, tyrosine phosphatase; Tx, 3 day thymectomy model (see text); FCA, Freund complete adjuvants; ADCC, antibody dependent cell mediated cytotoxicity, ECD = extracellular domain, DC=dendritic cells.

gens during conditions of apparent "non-danger". When such immune reactions are so aberrantly and vigorously self-directed, they inflict pathological damage on tissues. So-called "autoimmune diseases" are the consequence.

Autoimmune diseases can be divided into two main categories: "organ-specific" and "systemic" autoimmune diseases. In organ-specific autoimmune diseases, the immune attack is confined to one organ or organ system. In the majority of organ-specific autoimmune diseases, target tissues are neuroendocrine in character. One of these target tissues is the thyroid. The most extensively studied and well characterized organ-specific autoimmune diseases are listed in Table 1, and include thyroid disorders such as Hashimoto's thyroiditis, primary hypothyroidism and Graves' disease.

Multifactorial nature of organ-specific autoimmune disease

There are logical restrictions to the study of the etiology and the pathogenesis of the various organ-specific autoimmune diseases in humans. These autoimmune diseases often have long non-clinical prodromal phases, which are difficult to study since clinical signs and symptoms are (still) absent. Over the past 30 years, various inbred animal models of spontaneously occurring variants of the human organ-specific autoimmune diseases have become available (Table 1). These models have greatly contributed to the knowledge concerning the etiology and the pathogenesis of various organ-specific autoimmune diseases, most notably the events occurring in the very early prodromal phases.

Collectively, studies over the past 20 years have culminated in an awareness that organ-specific autoimmune diseases must be regarded as polygenic diseases, in which penetrance is strongly influenced by environmental factors. Multiple genes, e.g., more than 15 in the Nonobese Diabetic (NOD) mouse model of type 1 diabetes, determine part of the aberrant immune response towards self. The most important genes are those in the MHC region. However, other genes are also involved, including those with a role in regulation of the metabolism of the target tissue, e.g., the insulin gene in type 1 diabetes, and genes involved in general regulation of the immune system, e.g., the CTLA-4 gene (24). However, genetic polymorphisms are not the whole story. Monozygotic twin studies in type 1 diabetes, for example, have shown a concordance rate of, at best, 40–50 percent between twins. This demonstrates the important roles of environmental eliciting factors, e.g., environmental agents altering the target tissue and/or the immune system.

The development of organ-specific autoimmune diseases

Afferent, central and efferent phase (Figure 1)

The pathogenesis of autoimmune thyroiditis, autoimmune diabetes, autoimmune sialoadenitis, and autoimmune vitiligo have been studied in detail in animals that spontaneously develop forms of these autoimmune diseases, such as the Obese Strain of chicken (OS chicken) (25), the Bio Breeding (BB) rat (4), the NOD mouse (1), and the Smyth line chicken (21) (Table 1). A synopsis of the outcomes of these studies is given here. A word of caution is necessary when trying to extrapolate data obtained in these animal models to the human situation. The animal models clearly show caricatural, homogenous and extreme forms of the various diseases, which differ between the various models for a single disease (let alone from patients). Hence, general conclusions drawn from studies in one of the animal models should always be verified in other animal models and in humans.

The studies of the animal models have shown that the pathogenesis of the autoimmune failure of a gland or tissue is a multistep process, requiring several genetic and environmental abnormalities (or variants) to converge before full-blown autoimmune disease develops. Hence, organ-specific autoimmune diseases are the outcome of an unfortunate combination of various genetic traits and environmental circumstances that by themselves may not be harmful, and may even be advantageous.

In short, the following stages in the pathologic immune process can be distinguished:

1. An initial, *afferent phase* of an accumulation of antigen presenting cells (APC), particularly of dendritic cells (DCs) and subclasses of macrophages (Mϕ) in the target-tissue-to-be (Figure 1).
2. A later, *central phase* of an apparently uncontrolled production of autoreactive $CD4^+$ T cells, $CD8^+$ T cells and of autoantibodies of the IgG class (Figure 1). Initially this production of specific cells and antibodies takes place in the draining lymph nodes. Later, however, often a lymphoid tissue develops locally in the diseased tissue itself, e.g., in the thyroid gland of the BB rat. These local lymphoid tissues have a high degree of histological organization, with clearly distinguishable T-cell areas, B-cell follicles with germinal centers, and areas and cords of plasma cells in the periphery of the lymphoid tissue. These latter cells produce anti-thyroglobulin (α-Tg) antibodies. Often these lymphoid tissue areas are non-destructive and show a peaceful coexistence with adjacent thyrocytes. In fact, the adjacent thyrocytes often show signs of metabolic and proliferative stimulation.
3. A final, *efferent phase* in which the target tissue becomes excessively susceptible to the autoimmune influence exerted by the autoreactive T cells and autoantibodies now accumulated in large numbers in the target tissue. This commonly results

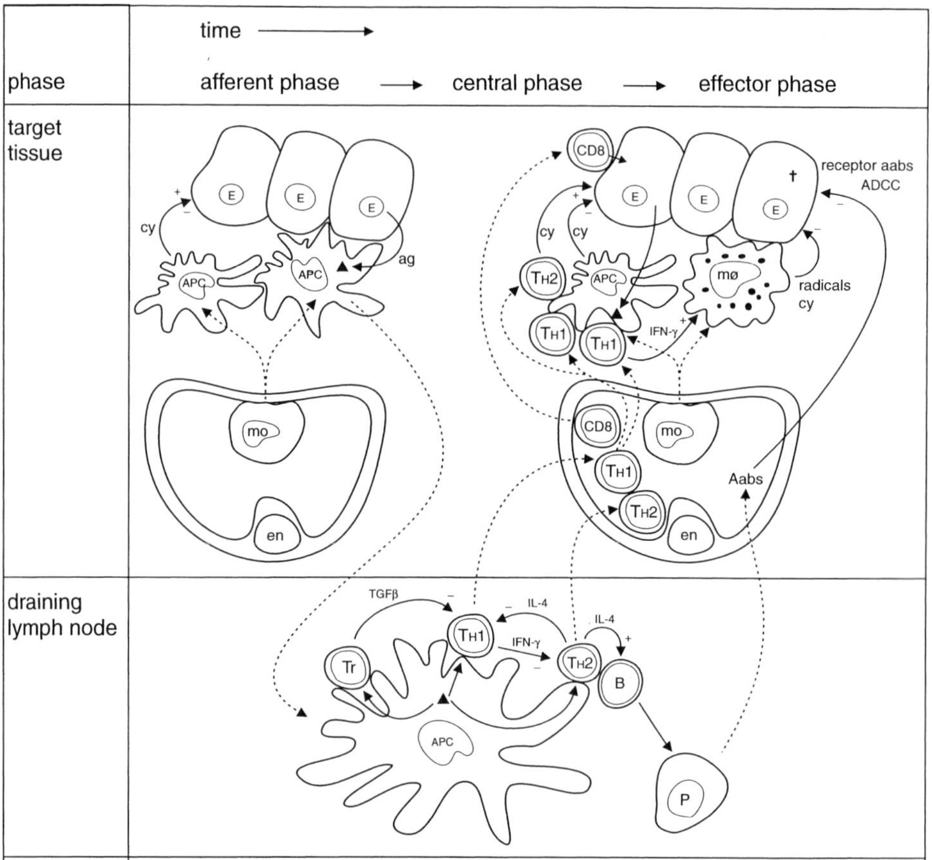

combination of conditions generating autoimmune disease	APC influx induced by:	aberrant regulation of immune response:	pathological reaction of target cells
	1. aspecific necrosis of target cells (virus, toxins) 2. altered metabolism or growth of target cells	1. defects in intrathymic generation of T cells 2. defects in T cell deletion (AICD) 3. TH1 : TH2 dysbalance 4. defects in Tr circuits due to altered APC function	1. excessive accumulation of lymphoid cells and their products. Effects of a. receptor abs b. ADCC c. blocking/toxic effects cytokines and mø derived radicals d. CD8 cytotoxicity 2. excessive susceptability of target cells

Fig. 1 A scheme of the immunopathogenic events that take place during the development of autoimmunity. These events ultimately lead to an autoimmune glandular failure. In the first, *afferent phase* APC – probably mostly monocyte derived – accumulate in the target-gland-to-be. The APC influx may be induced by nonspecific inflammatory stimuli, such as necrosis of

in destruction of the tissue or blockade of its function or growth, as is the case in Hashimoto's thyroiditis and primary hypothyroidism, respectively. Occasionally, it may also result in excessive stimulation of the target tissue, as is the case in Graves' disease.

Target abnormalities related to the afferent phase

Blood monocytes are able to mature into various subsets of Mϕ as well as into various subsets of DC (20). DC are the APC par excellence, and essential for stimulation of naive T cells, leading to clonal expansion of the latter. Mϕ have various functions, ranging from the phagocytosis and degradation of unwanted material, via the regulation of immune responses, to the production of factors for wound healing and remodeling of bone (12). Increased numbers of MHC class II-positive DC and specific subsets of Mϕ have been found both inside and outside lymphocytic accumulations in the thyroids of patients with Graves' disease or Hashimoto goiter, in the islets of diabetics, in the salivary glands of Sjögren patients, and in the thyroids, islets, and salivary glands of the animal models of these diseases (5). In the animal models, the first sign of a developing autoimmune reaction is in fact an increase in the number of DC and Mϕ in the future target-glands, as well as a local homotypic clustering of these cells. The potential APC accumulated in these tissues subsequently enter the lymphatics to travel to the draining lymph nodes while transporting self antigens.

What attracts these DC and Mϕ to the target glands? First, attraction signals may simply be inflammatory in nature. Early necrosis of future target-cells due to a viral or bacterial infection, or due to toxins (e.g., iodine, see later) and drugs, with the concomitant release of self antigens has been described as eliciting factors (Figure1).

target cells by viruses or toxins. Altered metabolism or growth of the target cells may also be an induction factor for APC accumulation (see text). The accumulated APC take up relevant autoantigens and leave the tissues to travel to the draining lymph nodes. In the second, *central phase* the APC seek contact with T cells and B cells in the draining lymph nodes. Apparently, an aberrant immune response results. Instead of reinforcing tolerance the APC generate an autoimmune reaction. The figure lists the various abnormalities found in animal models underlying this aberrant regulation of the autoimmune response. In the final, *afferent phase* the generated autoreactive T cells, B cells and antibodies have their effect on the target cells after having gained access to the target gland (see text for various mechanisms). mo = monocyte, EC = endothelial cell, APC = antigen presenting cell, Aag = ▲ = autoantigen, cy = cytokines, E = endocrine cell, Mϕ = macrophage, ADCC = antibody-dependent cell mediated cytotoxicity, P = plasma cell, Th1 = T helper 1 cell, Th2 = T helper 2 cell, Tr = T regulator cell, B = B cell, Aabs = autoantibodies.
+ = stimulation, – = suppression, → = traffic

This variety in eliciting factors indicates the heterogeneity of causal factors at the level of induction of organ-specific autoimmune disease.

Secondly, DC and Mϕ may accumulate not to exert an immune function, but to regulate growth and function of endocrine cells or to play a role in tissue homeostasis. It is relevant to note that DC and Mϕ are normal constituents of almost all tissues. In endocrine tissues, the cells regulate the growth and function (both in a positive and negative sense) of neighboring hormone producing cells (9). In other tissues, DC and Mϕ are involved in homeostasis during, e.g., regeneration processes such as wound healing. The recognition that monocyte-derived cells constitute a recruitable cell system that, on the one hand, is capable of regulating tissue homeostasis, but on the other hand is also capable of initiating immune responses, has implications for our understanding of the induction phase of an endocrine autoimmune reaction. Alterations in the structure, growth and function of tissues may necessitate an influx of DC and Mϕ to regulate tissue homeostasis. This 'non-inflammatory' influx may however be a first step on the way to autoimmunity. There are arguments for such a concept:

1. Very early (and even fetal) abnormalities in the proliferative capability and hormone production of thyrocytes and pancreatic islet cells have been described in the OS chicken (23), the BB rat (22), and the NOD mouse (10). In addition, the salivary glands of NOD mice and the melanocytes of the Smyth-line chicken show inborn errors of growth and metabolism.
2. The pre-autoimmune islet abnormalities in the NOD mouse can in part be corrected by prophylactic insulin treatment. Such early correction of the pre-autoimmune target cell abnormality leads to a lower influx of DC and attenuation of the subsequent autoimmune reaction (11).

The early DC and Mϕ influx does however not suffice for full development of an autoimmune endocrine disease. In addition, aberrations at the DC/Mϕ and lymphocyte level are required to initiate the inappropriate and pathological autoimmune response.

Dysregulation of the immune system in the central phase

In endocrine autoimmune diseases, the initial phase of the tissue accumulation of DC and Mϕ is followed by a phase of clonal expansion and maturation of autoreactive effector T and B cells in the draining lymph nodes. In the diabetes prone (DP) BB rat, the NOD mouse, and the OS-chicken, there are strong indications that genetically determined immunodysregulation leads to intolerance towards presented self-antigens, explaining the apparently uncontrolled clonal expansion of lymphocytes. These immunodysregulation mechanisms are partly associated with the presence of particular MHC class I and class II haplotypes, but other genes are also involved.

The exact mechanisms for maintaining tolerance in non-autoimmune individuals are far from clear. There exist mechanisms of central tolerance induction (e.g., T cell deletion in the thymus), mechanisms of peripheral tolerance induction (e.g., activation-induced T cell death (AICD) and the suppressor activity of regulatory T cells), mechanisms of anergy induction, and immunological ignorance. Various defects in these mechanisms have been described in the animal models.

The BB-DP rat lacks a particular regulator (suppressor) population of T cells in its peripheral immune system, so-called $RT6^{+}$ T cells. Interestingly, it is particularly this subset of T cells that is weakly stimulated by splenic DC of the BB-DP rat. In this and other aspects, this important splenic APC population also appears to be abnormal. Thymic abnormalities are also evident in the BB-DP rat, suggesting deviations at the level of central tolerance as well. Interestingly, the OS strain of chickens also has defects in its regulatory T cell system (25), as has the neonatally thymectomized Balb/C mouse (see Table 1). The NOD mouse has clear defects in T cell apoptosis, leading to decreased ability of the cells to undergo AICD, a major mechanism in both central and peripheral tolerance induction. Moreover, NOD mice are characterized by an abnormal thymic architecture.

Whether there are similar (inborn) defects in the lymphoid organs and in the immunoregulatory cells of patients needs to be investigated. There are, however, numerous reports of human studies showing both numerical and functional deficits in T cells with suppressive function. In addition, various DC and Mϕ defects have been described among patients with autoimmune thyroid disease and type 1 diabetes.

Enhanced susceptibility of the target cells for the excessive autoimmune response in the efferent phase

After the excessive generation of autoreactive T cells and IgG autoantibodies, another factor or factors, at least in the OS chicken and probably in the NOD mouse also, determine whether or not full blown autoimmune disease will develop (25). A prerequisite for clinical failure is susceptibility of the target tissue to autoimmune attack by the generated autoreactive T cells, the Mϕ, and IgG autoantibodies. Experiments have shown that in the OS-chicken, this susceptibility factor is genetically determined, and it has been speculated that this factor might be an abnormality induced by an endogenous retrovirus. Whether such susceptibility factors are also important in human autoimmune disease needs further investigation.

Dietary iodine changes and thyroid autoimmunity

Iodine deficiency

Besides goiter formation and hypothyroidism, iodine deficiency may lead to triggering of thyroid autoimmunity. We have previously described (16) accumulation of DC in the thyroids of female Wistar rats, followed by an intrathyroidal increase in T cells and a higher incidence of anti-colloid antibodies in the serum of the animals (see also Table 2). These observations in the Wistar rat are in agreement with observations made in human populations, in which low dietary iodine intake leads not only to goiter formation and hypothyroidism, but also to increased numbers of intrathyroidal aggregations of dendritic cells, epithelioid cells and giant cells (Wilders et al, 1989). There is also an increased incidence of anti-thyroglobulin (Tg) antibodies and of other thyroid reactive antibodies (7; 26).

We feel that the intrathyroidal accumulations of dendritic cells during iodine deficiency described above serve a physiological function, and are involved in the regulation and protection of the iodine-deprived stimulated thyrocytes. They therefore do not necessarily represent an autoaggressive infiltration (see earlier remarks on the endocrine regulatory role of DC and Mϕ earlier). Production of anti-colloid antibodies and the increased intrathyroidal infiltration with T cells following the DC infiltration in the iodine-deficient state may play also a physiological role. There are indications that these immune phenomena are also involved in regulation of hyperfunctioning thyroid tissue. A "physiological" role for Tg autoantibodies in the clearance of waste Tg in situations of overproduction of this thyroidal product was reported as early as 1959 by Grabar et al.(8) Furthermore, high titers of monoclonal anti-Tg antibodies have been reported to result in mice in the hypofunction of thyroid glands without inflammatory leukocyte inflammation (27). With regard to T cell infiltration, cytokines produced by thyroid infiltrating T cells (such as IFN-γ) are known to be capable of altering the hormone production and growth of stimulated thyrocytes (2).

Not every individual, however, shows such reactivity to iodine deficiency and the response is variable. Indeed, in our hands females of another rat strain, the autoimmune-prone BB rat, showed a different response to iodine deficiency in comparison with the normal Wistar rat:

1. Endocrinologically, the AI-prone BB rat is capable of compensating relatively mild low dietary iodine intake by a rapid and increased goiter formation. After 9 weeks on an iodine deficient diet full euthyroidism is restored (15; see also Table 2). On the one hand, it is possible that this rapid goiter formation reflects an intrinsic alteration in the growth rate of BB-DP thyrocytes (22, see also earlier). On the other hand, it may be due to the effects of the infiltrated lymphoid cells. During iodine deficiency, BB goiters show increased numbers of intrathyroidal DC

Table 2 The effects cf several iodine regiments on thyroid endocrine reactions, thyroid autoimmune reactions and the immune system

	Thyroid endocrine reactions		**Thyroid autoimmune reactions**		**Reaction of the immune system in general**	
	Wistar rat (normal)	**BB rat (AI-prone)**	**Wistar rat (normal)**	**BB rat (AI-prone)**	**Wistar rat (normal)**	**BB rat (AI-prone)**
Iodine deficiency						
Mild	goiter + hypothyroid +	goiter ++ euthyroid	DC ↑, T cells ↑ Abs ↑ (TGAb, colloid)	DC ↑↑, T cells ↑ Abs ↑	=	=
Severe	goiter ++ hypothyroid ++	goiter ++ hypothyroid ++	DC ↑, T cells ↑↑ Abs ↑↑ (TGAb, colloid)	Inflammation ↓ Abs ↓↓	↓↓	↓↓
Iodine excess						
Mild chronic	euthyroid	euthyroid, tendency to become hypothyroid	ectopic thymus Abs ↓↓ (colloid) DC ↓, T cells ↓	TALT> Abs ↑↑ (colloid) DC ↑↑, T cells ↑↑	=	=
Severe acute on hyperplastic goiter	hyperthyroidism followed by hypo-thyroidism (transient outburst of thyroiditis)	outburst of thyroiditis, followed by thyroid AID (hypothyroidism)	DC ↑↑, mϕ ↑↑ (transient)	DC ↑↑, mϕ ↑↑ (permanent) Induction of thyroid AID	ND	ND

Reference point nomal Wistar rat from our colony fed normal iodine diet (urinary iodine excretion 7 μg per day).
↑: increase, ↓: decrease, =: no difference, ND: not done, AI: autoimmunity, Abs: antibodies, TGAb: thyroid growth stimulating antibodies, DC: dendritic cells, AID: autoimmune disease, TALT: thyroid-associated lymphoid tissue.

and T cells compared with BB rats maintained on a normal iodine diet. It should also be noted that numbers of such intrathyroidal cells are higher anyway in BB rats than in Wistar rats (see Table 2). The observation that this rat strain with a clear genetically determined predisposition to thyroid autoimmunity is capable of coping with mild iodine deficiency may be helpful in explaining the heterogeneous response to iodine deficiency observed in random human populations. There might be individuals with a "BB likeness (autoimmune-proneness)" who remain euthyroid in conditions of moderately low dietary iodine intake. However, this is at the expense of rapid goiter formation with various signs and symptoms of an involvement of the local immune system.

2. Immunologically, under iodine deficient conditions, the autoimmune-prone BB-DP rat shows less severe thyroid lymphocytic infiltration and produces fewer anticolloid antibodies (Table 2). This is generally ascribed to a lower degree of Tg iodination, making the molecule less antigenic (see below). Severe iodine deficiency itself also leads to an immunodeficient state in general, hampering autoreactive T cell generation and autoantibody production normally seen in iodine-sufficient BB-DP rats.

Iodine excess

Iodine excess also results in complex modulation of thyroid autoimmune responsiveness in animal models. In the non-autoimmune-prone Wistar rat thyroid autoimmune reactivity is depressed. In the autoimmune-prone BB rat and NOD mouse, however, thyroid autoimmune reactivity is accelerated.

In the early phases of chronic iodine excess the Wistar rat develops thyroid-associated ectopic thymic tissue. We have previously speculated that this is related to tolerance induction since its development is associated with mild intrathyroidal infiltration by lymphoid cells and production of low levels of anti-colloid antibodies (18; Table 2). There are no disturbances in thyroid function. This relatively high dietary iodine intake therefore seems to be optimal for Wistar rats.

In the BB-DP rat, however, the same relatively high chronic dietary iodine intake results in an acceleration of the intrathyroidal development of the lymphoid tissue that normally occurs in 50 % of BB rats older than 18–22 weeks of age (17). This lymphoid tissue plays a prominent role in the production of autoantibodies and autoreactive T cells and therefore in the aggravation of thyroid autoimmunity.

When an acute large dose of iodine rather than chronic iodine excess is given to NOD mice with a hyperplastic goiter, this iodine administration is toxic to thyrocytes (see also below). The necrotic thyrocytes induce nonspecific inflammation, which also includes the infiltration of many APC, such as DC and macrophages. Against the NOD background (immunodysregulation) this nonspecific inflammation forms the impetus for the thyroid autoimmune reaction (14).

Our observations concerning the immunomodulatory effects of a high dietary iodine intake in rats and mice are in agreement with observations in human populations. In areas with relatively high iodine intake (for instance the United States and Japan), the incidence of classical Hashimoto's thyroiditis is higher compared with areas with a normal or relatively low iodine intake. The observations in the autoimmune-prone BB rat and NOD mice – in contrast to the normal Wistar rat – suggest that individuals already genetically prone to thyroid autoimmunity easily develop thyroid autoimmune disease under the influence of a high iodine diet, whereas those without such a tendency may even be protected by the high iodine intake (Table 2).

In the autoimmune-prone OS chicken, iodine is also a clear modulator of the spontaneously occurring thyroid autoimmune response. Again, a low iodine intake leads to a low incidence of thyroiditis, whereas a high iodine intake accelerates autoimmune thyroiditis (23). The iodine is, however, of minor importance in comparison with the two major factors playing a role in thyroid autoimmune development in this bird: a genetically determined target organ abnormality and genetically determined immune dysregulation.

Possible mechanisms by which dietary iodine modulates thyroid autoimmune reactivity

Toxicity for thyrocytes

One of the mechanisms by which iodine may precipitate thyroid autoimmune reactivity was demonstrated in experiments (14) in which a large dose of iodine was administered to iodine deficient mice and hamsters with hyperplastic goiter. Thyrocytes of such hyperplastic goiters are metabolically highly active, and they were damaged by the iodine. It was argued that excessive amounts of the iodide ion in the hyperplastic thyrocytes were rapidly oxidized by TPO thereby producing excessive amounts of either hypoiodous acid or oxygen radicals, reactive elements reported as intermediates in TPO catalyzed oxidation of iodine. These oxidative elements damage thyroid cell membranes by oxidation of membrane lipids or proteins. This mechanism probably plays a primary role in iodine supplementation in bolus form in iodine deficient individuals with a hyperplastic goiter.

There are also indications that chronic iodine excess has toxic effects on thyrocytes in autoimmune-prone individuals (13): iodide treated BB-DP rats exhibited marked signs of subcellular disruption: accumulation of secondary lysosomes and lipid droplets, swollen and disrupted mitochondria and extreme dilation of RER. There is also some indirect evidence that oxidative damage is an early event in the development of the spontaneous thyroiditis of the OS chicken, even under normal iodine conditions. Treating the OS chicken from the time of hatching with anti-oxidants reduced the intrathyroidal lymphocytic infiltration and anti-Tg antibody synthesis. The drugs were ineffective after disease initiation (23).

Immunogenicity of highly iodinated thyroglobulin

The creation of immunogenic epitopes in the Tg molecule by ingestion of excess iodide may also explain the acceleration of the above-described iodine-induced thyroid autoimmune phenomena. It has been demonstrated that highly iodinated Tg is a better immunogen than Tg with a low iodine content, both *in vivo* and *in vitro* (3; 23).

Although there is thus evidence emphasizing the importance of highly iodinated Tg as an immunogen, it must be noted that real autoimmune thyroiditis can only be elicited with this immunogen in genetically susceptible rats (6). Among OS chickens, BB-DP rats, and among patients suffering from Hashimoto's thyroiditis it is not clear whether highly iodinated Tg is a major causal factor for the development of autoimmune thyroid reactivity.

Direct stimulating effects of iodine on cells of the immune system, in particular on DC

Direct stimulating effects of iodine on immune cells, such as macrophages, T cells and B cells have been reported to play a role in the development of thyroid autoimmune reactivity. We have reported that iodinated Tg enhances the transition from monocyte to veiled/dendritic cells (19). This phenomenon may also play a role in the higher antigenicity of highly iodinated Tg.

References

1. Bach, J.F., Mathis, D. (1997) The NOD mouse. Res Immunol 148, 285–286.
2. Bendtzen, K. (1989) Immune hormones (cytokines); pathogenic role in autoimmune rheumatic and endocrine diseases. Autoimmunity 2, 177–189.
3. Champion, B., Rayner, D.C., Byfield, P.G.H., Page, K.R., Chan, C.T.J, Roitt, I.M. (1987) J Immunol 139, 3665–3670.
4. Delemarre, F.G.A., Simons, P.J., Drexhage, H.A. (1996) Histomorphological aspects of the development of thyroid autoimmune diseases: consequences for our understanding of endocrine ophthalmopathy. Thyroid 4, 367–375.
5. Drexhage, H.A., Delemarre, F.G.A., Radosevic, K, Leenen, P.J.M. (1999) Dendritic cells in autoimmunity. In: Dendritic cells. Biology and Clinical Applications. (Eds. Lotze, M.T., Thomson, A.W.) Academic Press.
6. Ebner, S.A., Lueprasitsakul, W., Alex, S., Fang, S.L., Appel, M.C., Braverman, L.E. (1992) Iodine content of rat thyroglobulin affects its antigenicity in inducing lymphocytic thyroiditis in the BB/Wor rat. Autoimmunity 13, 209–214.

7. Fenzi, G.F., Giani, C., Ceccarelli, P., Bartalena, L., Macchia, E., Aghini-Lombardi, F., Vitti, P., Lari, R., Ceccarelli, C., Baschieri, L., Pinchera, A. (1986) Role of autoimmune and familial factors in goiter prevalence. Studies performed in a moderately endemic area. J Endocrinol Invest 9, 161–164.
8. Grabar, P., Miescher, P., (eds). Immunopathology, 1st International Symposium 1959, Schnaabe, B., and Co, Verlag, Basel/Stuttgart.
9. Hoek, A., Allaerts, W., Leenen, P.J.M., Schoemaker, J., Drexhage, H.A. (1997) Dendritic cells and macrophages in the pituitary and the gonads. Evidence for their role in the fine regulation of the reproductive endocrine response. *Eur. J. Endocrinol.* 136, 8–24.
10. Homo-Delarche, F. (1997) Beta-cell behaviour during the prediabetic stage. Part II. Non-insulin-dependent and insulin-dependent diabetes. Diabetes Metab 23, 473–505.
11. Jansen, A., Rosmalen, J.G.M., Homo-Delarche, F., Dardenne, M., Lieter, E.H., Drexhage, H.A. (1996) Effect of prophylactic insulin treatment on the number of ER-MP23^{+} macrophages in the pancreas of NOD mice. Is the prevention of diabetes on ß-cell rest? J Autoimmunity 9, 341–348.
12. Leenen, P.J.M. and Campbell, P.A. (1993) Heterogeneity of mononuclear phagocytes. An interpretive review. In *Blood Cell Biochemistry* 5 (ed. M.H. Horton) pp. 29–84, Plenum Press, New York.
13. Li, M., Boyages, S.C. (1994) Iodine induced lymphocytic thyroiditis in the BB/W rat: evidence of direct toxic effects of iodine on thyroid subcellular structure. Autoimmunity 18, 31–40.
14. Many, M-C., Maniratunga, S., Varis, I., Dardenne, M., Drexhage, H.A., Denef, J-F. (1995) Two step development of a Hashimoto-like thyroiditis in genetically autoimmune prone non obese diabetic (NOD) mice. Effects of iodine-induced cell necrosis. J Endocrinol 147, 311–320.
15. Mooij, P. (1993) The thyroid, iodine and autoimmunity. Academic Thesis, Erasmus University, Rotterdam.
16. Mooij, P., de Wit, H.J., Bloot, A.M., Wilders-Truschnig, M.M., Drexhage, H.A. (1993) Iodine deficiency induces thyroid autoimmune reactivity in Wistar rats. Endocrinology 133, 1197–1204.
17. Mooij, P., de Wit, H.J., Drexhage, H.A. (1993) An excess of dietary iodine accelerates the development of a thyroid-associated lymphoid tissue in autoimmune prone BB rats. Clin Immunol Immunopathol 69, 189–198.
18. Mooij, P., de Wit, H.J., Drexhage, H.A. (1994) A high iodine intake in Wistar rats results in the development of a thyroid-associated ectopic thymic tissue and is accompanied by a low thyroid autoimmune reactivity. Immunology 81, 309–316.
19. Mooij, P., Simons, P.J., de Haan-Meulman, M., de Wit, H.J., Drexhage, H.A. (1994) Effect of thyroid hormones and other iodinated compounds on the transition of monocytes into veiled/dendritic cells: role of GM-CSF, TNF- and IL-6. J Endocrinol 140, 503–512.
20. Peters, J.H., Gieseler, R., Thiele, B., Steinbach, F. (1996) Dendritic cells: from ontogenetic orphans to myelomonocytic descendants Immunology Today, 17, 273–278.
21. Shresta, S., Smyth, J.R. Jr., Erf, G.F. (1997) Profiles of pulp infiltrating lymphocytes at various times throughout feather regeneration in Smyth line chickens with vitiligo. Autoimmunity 25, 193–201.
22. Simons, P.J., Delemarre, F.G.A., Jeucken, P.H.M., Drexhage, H.A. (1998) Pre-autoimmune thyroid abnormalities in the biobreeding diabetes-prone (BB-DP) rat: a possible relation with the intrathyroid accumulation of dendritic cells and the initiations of the thyroid autoimmune response.
23. Sundick, R.S., Bagchi, N., Brown, T.R. (1996) The obese strain chicken as a model for human Hashimoto's thyroiditis. Exp Clin Endocrinol Diabetes 104, 4–6.
24. Todd, J.A., Farrall, M. (1996) Panning for gold: genome wide scanning for linkage in type 1 diabetes. Human Molecular Genetics 5, 1443–1448.
25. Wick, G., Brezinschek, H.P., Hala, K., Dietrich, H., Wolf, H. and Kroemer, G. (1989) The obese strain of chickens: an animal model with spontaneous autoimmune thyroiditis. Adv Immunol 47, 433–500.
26. Wilders-Truschnig, M.M., Kabel, P.J., Drexhage, H.A., Beham, A., Leb, G., Eber, O., Hebenstreit, J., Loidolt, D., Dohr, G., Lanzer, G., Krejs, G.J. (1989) Intrathyroidal dendritic cells, epitheloid cells, and giant cells in iodine deficient goiter. Am J Pathol 135, 219–225.
27. Yokochi, T., Inoue, Y., Fukada, M., Kawai, M., Yoshikawa, K., Suzuki, J., and Kato, N. (1991) Histological and functional changes in the thyroid glands of mice implanted with hybridomas secreting monoclonal autoantibody against mouse thyroglobulin. Autoimmunity 10, 125–131.

Environmental factors in healthy women at risk for autoimmune thyroid disease

W. M. Wiersinga, M. F. Prummel, T. G. A. Strieder

Dept. of Endocrinology and Metabolism, Academic Medical Center, University of Amsterdam, Amsterdam, The Netherlands.

Introduction

Autoimmune thyroid disease (AITD) is an organ-specific autoimmune disorder that runs in families and has a female preponderance. The disease is characterized by lymphocytic infiltration of the thyroid gland and by activation of the immune system as evident from activated T-lymphocytes and thyroid-specific autoantibodies in the serum. AITD manifests itself in various forms: the most prevalent are Hashimoto's disease, which frequently results in hypothyroidism, and Graves' disease, which in most cases results in hyperthyroidism. AITD is considered to be a complex, multifactorial polygenic disease.

Genes versus environment

A family history of AITD can be obtained in up to 70 % of patients with either Graves' hyperthyroidism or Hashimoto's hypothyroidism. Although Graves' disease and Hashimoto's disease run in families and both diseases may occur in the same family, the mode of inheritance is unknown and does not show a single Mendelian mode of transmission. Some reports indicate autosomal dominant inheritance of TPO antibodies in women with reduced penetrance in men (1), but not all subjects with TPO antibodies develop clinically manifest thyroid function disorders. A particular genetic background may facilitate the development of AITD, but the genes involved are largely unknown at the present time. The relevance of HLA in this respect is widely acknowledged, but the relative risk of 2 to 4 associated with possession of certain HLA haplotypes is very modest. The same holds true for the recently found association of CTLA4 polymorphism and AITD. Several international consortia have undertaken a genome-wide search using microsatellite markers to identify DNA regions conferring susceptibility to AITD. So far, a few loci have been found, some linked to Graves' disease and others to Hashimoto's disease (2, 3). No consensus exists, however, on the validity of these findings, and the results obtained await confirmation in a larger number of families. It is also still unknown whether the genetic background of Graves' disease differs substantially from that of Hashimoto's disease or whether a certain genetic make-up just confers susceptibility to AITD in general.

The quantitative contribution of the genotype to the phenotype of either Graves' hyperthyroidism or Hashimoto's hypothyroidism has been evaluated in the past. The influence of genetic factors might, however, not be as powerful as previously thought. A recent population-based study of Graves' hyperthyroidism in Danish twins reports pairwise concordance rates of 0.22 for monozygotic pairs and 0 for dizygotic pairs (4). These figures are much lower than the pairwise concordance rates of 0.76 and 0.25 for monozygotic and dizygotic twins respectively in a study from 1956 (5). Another recent population-based twin study from Denmark found no difference in the prevalence of Hashimoto's hypothyroidism between monozygotic (0.42 %) and dizygotic (0.40 %) twins; the concordance rate was 0.55 for monozygotic pairs but zero for dizygotic pairs (6).

The data do confirm that genes contribute to the development of AITD. The data indicate, however, at the same time, that the size of the genetic contribution is small (7). It follows that other – environmental – factors must play a more important role in the etiology of AITD than previously thought. Environmental insults may interact differently in different genetic backgrounds. Study of environmental factors in conjunction with genetic background might thus be most profitable.

Environmental factors

A number of environmental factors has been associated with the development of AITD, as indicated in figure 1 (8). Lasting effects of early environmental influences are clearly demonstrated in experimental animals, and have been referred to as examples of 'biological Freudianism' (9). Reduced fetal and infant growth has been identified as a determinant of several common diseases in adult life. In this respect a study of women in their 7th decade is of interest, reporting an inverse relationship between birth weight and prevalence of TgAb and TPOAb (10). The described association awaits confirmation in other studies.

The greatest known risk factor for AITD is female sex, with a 5- to 10-fold excess of disease in women. The mechanistic explanation for the link between sex and autoimmunity remains obscure. It has been proposed that cytokines are involved in the sex difference because sex steroids affect the synthesis and release of various cytokines (11). Hashimoto's disease seems not to be associated with parity, but the risk of Hashimoto's disease decreases with a later menarche and increases with a later menopause (12). The latter finding has been explained by the hyperestrogenic state

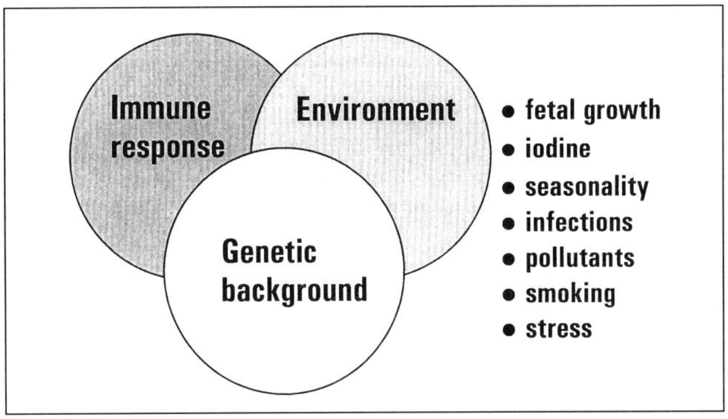

Fig. 1 Venn diagram illustrating the concept of AITD as a polygenic multifactorial disease, in which the immune response directed against thyroid antigens develops as a result of interaction between disease susceptibility and environmental factors (8).

associated with a longer reproductive span. Reproductive life events may provoke AITD, as evident from postpartum thyroiditis, which has a high incidence of 5–7 %. Permanent autoimmune hypothyroidism occurs in about one third of women who have experienced an episode of postpartum thyroiditis. It has also been reported that a fair proportion of Graves' hyperthyroidism starts in the postpartum period. In this respect, it is of interest to note that use of oral contraceptives exerts a protective effect on AITD (13).

Iodine intake is a well-known modulator of AITD. Hypothyroidism is relatively more common in iodine-deficient regions than in areas with sufficient iodine intake (14), and the overall prevalence of thyrotoxicosis is higher in iodine-deficient areas. In line with these epidemiological data are studies on the incidence of thyroid function disorders induced by iodine excess (such as generated by treatment with the antiarrhythmic drug amiodarone). Iodide-induced thyrotoxicosis is more common in iodine-deficient regions, whereas iodide-induced hypothyroidism occurs more frequently in iodide-replete areas (15,16). Fewer data are available on the consequences of incidental exposure to iodine excess (e.g. by iodine-containing X-ray contrast agents, iodine-rich foodstuffs, or kelp tablets) in subjects at risk for AITD living in iodine-sufficient areas.

Infections may trigger AITD by various mechanisms, e g. by molecular mimicry (17). A nice example is Yersinia enterocolitica, which has specific TSH binding sites. Infection with Yersinia may give rise to antibodies directed against these TSH binding sites, which are able to stimulate adenylate cyclase in human thyroid membranes by cross-reacting with the thyroidal TSH receptor. A causal relationship between Yersinia infection and Graves' disease is, however, disputed (18). It must be said that the epidemiological evidence for a relationship between infectious diseases and AITD is rather weak; the observed associations are all obtained from cross-sectional studies, and no prospective studies have been done.

Smoking is definitely an environmental factor which increases the risk for Graves' hyperthyroidism, and even more so for Graves' ophthalmopathy (19). The association has been found in numerous cross-sectional studies, but it remains incompletely understood how smoking provokes Graves' disease. An intriguing observation in a case-control study has been that smoking behavior is not related to autoimmune hypothyroidism (19).

Stressful life events have also been identified as a risk factor for Graves' hyperthyroidism (20). The evidence is derived from case-control studies in which patients with recently diagnosed Graves' hyperthyroidism were questioned on life events in the year preceding the diagnosis. Such a study design is liable to bias in view of its retrospective nature: negative life events are more likely to be remembered by patients than by healthy subjects. Another criticism of these studies has been that no correction was performed for mood disturbances (like depression) that affect memory (21). Nevertheless, the circumstantial evidence for a causal relationship between stress and Graves' disease is rather strong, as illustrated again by a rise in the incidence of Graves' hyperthyroidism in Eastern Serbia during the recent civil war (22). Studies on an association between stress and Hashimoto's hypothyroidism have not been done.

From this short review of environmental factors in AITD one may draw several conclusions. The relevance of the environment has seldom been studied in a prospective manner. The various environmental factors have been studied in isolation, i.e. no studies have been done to evaluate a possible cumulative effect of simultaneous exposure to a number of environmental insults. More is known about the environmental contribution to the development of Graves' disease than of Hashimoto's disease. The impact of environmental factors on the occurrence of AITD has never been studied in conjunction with the genetic background.

Amsterdam cohort of AITD relatives

In view of the above-mentioned comments, we embarked on a prospective study to evaluate the relative contribution of genetic and environmental factors to the development of AITD in a population at risk. Female relatives of patients with AITD are clearly at risk, and therefore we included healthy women without known thyroid disease who had two or more 1st or 2nd degree relatives with AIT (either Graves' hyperthyroidism or Hashimoto's hypothyroidism). Study subjects were recruited via our own outpatient clinics, via thyroid patient associations, and via advertisements in local newspapers. The study design is that of a prospective observational cohort study, with a follow-up of five years. The main outcome measurements are the development of either overt hypothyroidism or overt hyperthyroidism, as evident from both plasma TSH and plasma FT_4 values outside the reference range. Taking into account a number of assumptions, we calculated that a cohort of 1000 women followed for five years will generate 40 to 80 end-points (cases with overt hypo- or hyperthyroidism). The subjects are seen every year. Annual investigations include clinical examination, blood collection for measurement of thyroid hormones and thyroid antibodies, and questionnaires on iodine intake, reproductive events, infections, smoking behavior, and stressful life events.

The inception cohort consists of 1003 women. At study entrance, subclinical hypothyroidism was present in 7.6 %, overt hypothyroidism in 1.5 %, subclinical hyperthyroidism in 1.6 %, and overt hyperthyroidism in 0.3 %. TPO antibodies at a concentration greater than 100 kU/l were present in 25.9 %, TBII at a concentration greater than 12 U/l in 0.7 %. Preliminary analysis indicated a lower frequency of hyperthyroidism among subjects who had ever used oral contraceptives, and a higher frequency of hypothyroidism in subjects who had been exposed to iodine excess in the past year.

It will be fascinating to see to what extent the environment directs the clinical expression of AITD, and if the effects of environmental insults can be related to a certain genetic background.

References

1. Phillips DIW, McLachlan SM, Stephenson A, et al. Autosomal dominant transmission of autoantibodies to thyroglobulin and thyroid peroxidase. J Clin Endocrinol Metab 1990; 70: 742–746.
2. Barbesino G, Tomer Y, Concepcion E, et al. Linkage analysis of candidate genes in autoimmune thyroid disease: I. Selected immunoregulatory genes. J Clin Endocrinol Metab 1998; 83: 1580–1584.
3. Barbesino G, Tomer Y, Concepcion ES, et al. Linkage analysis of candidate genes in autoimmune thyroid disease: II. Selected gender-related genes and the X-chromosome. J Clin Endocrinol Metab 1998; 83: 3290–3295.
4. Brix TH, Christensen K, Holm NV, Harvald B, Hegedüs L. A population-based study of Graves' disease in Danish twins. Clin Endocrinol 1998; 48: 397–400.
5. Brix TH, Kyvik KO, Hegedüs L. What is the evidence of genetic factors in the etiology of Graves' disease? A brief review. Thyroid 1998; 8: 727–734.
6. Brix TH et al. Abstract. Program 72nd Annual meeting of the American Thyroid Association, Palm Beach, Florida, 1999.
7. Philippou G, McGregor AM. The aetiology of Graves' disease: what is the genetic contribution? Clin Endocrinol 1998; 48: 393–395.
8. Wiersinga WM. Environmental factors in autoimmune thyroid disease. Exp Clin Endocrinol Diab 1999; 107 (Suppl. 3): S67-S70.
9. Dubos R, Savage R, Schaedler R. Biological Freudianism. Lasting effects of early environmental influences. Pediatrics 1966; 38: 789–800.
10. Phillips DIW, Cooper C, Fall C, Prentice L, Osmond C, Barker DJP, Rees Smith B. Fetal growth and autoimmune thyroid disease. Quart J Med 1993; 86: 247–253.
11. Olsen NJ, Kovacs WJ. Gonadal steroids and immunity. Endocr Rev 1996; 17: 369–384.
12. Phillips DIW, Lazarus JH, Butland BK. The influence of pregnancy and reproductive span on the occurrence of autoimmune thyroiditis. Clin Endocrinol 1990; 32: 301–306.
13. Frank P, Ray CR. Incidence of thyroid disease associated with oral contraceptives. Brit Med J 1978; 3: 1531.
14. Laurberg P, Pedersen KM, Hreidarsson A, Sigfusson N, Iversen E, Knudsen PP. Iodine intake and the pattern of thyroid disorders: a comparative epidemiological study of thyroid abnormalities in the elderly in Iceland and in Jutland, Denmark. J Clin Endocrinol Metab 1998; 83: 765–769.

15. Martino E, Safran M, Aghini-Lombardi F, et al. Environmental iodine intake and thyroid dysfunction during chronic amiodarone therapy. Ann Int Med 1984; 101: 28–34.
16. Trip MD, Wiersinga WM, Plomp TA. Incidence, predictability, and pathogenesis of amiodarone-induced thyrotoxicosis and hypothyroidism. Am J Med 1991; 91: 507–511.
17. Tomer Y, Davies TF. Infection, thyroid disease, and autoimmunity. Endocr Rev 1993; 14: 107–120.
18. Arscott P, Rosen ED, Koenig RJ, et al. Immunoreactivity to Yersinia enterocolitica antigens in patients with autoimmune thyroid disease. J Clin Endocrinol Metab 1992; 75: 295–300.
19. Prummel MF, Wiersinga WM. Smoking and risk of Graves' disease. JAMA 1993; 269: 479–482.
20. Winsa B, Adami H-O, Bergström R, et al. Stressful life events and Graves' disease. Lancet 1991; 338: 1475–1479.
21. Harris T, Crzedo F, Brugha TS. Stressful life events and graves' disease. Brit J Psychiatry 1992; 161: 535–541.
22. Paunkovic N, Paunkovic J, Panhovic O, Paunovic Z. The significant increase in incidence of Graves' disease in Eastern Serbia during the civil war in the former Yugoslavia. Thyroid 1998; 8: 37–41.

Session III:

Environment and thyroid cancer

Chairpersons: J. Nauman, P. Langer

Prevalence and types of thyroid cancer as a function of iodine intake

U. Feldt-Rasmussen

Department of Medical Endocrinology, National University Hospital, Rigshospitalet, 2100 Copenhagen, Denmark

Abstract

Thyroid carcinomas are the most frequent endocrine malignancies. Among thyroid carcinomas the most frequent types are the differentiated forms (follicular, papillary or mixed papillary-follicular), while both anaplastic thyroid carcinoma and medullary thyroid carcinomas are rare. Animal experiments have demonstrated a clear increase in cancer incidence after prolonged iodine deficiency leading to a stimulation of the thyroid gland by e.g. thyrotropin. The overall incidence of thyroid carcinoma is not generally considered to be influenced by the iodine intake of a population. However, the distribution of the types of thyroid carcinoma does seem to be related to iodine intake, with fewer of the more aggressive follicular and anaplastic carcinomas and more papillary carcinomas in iodine rich areas. Among populations starting iodine prophylaxis, a shift with an increase in the ratio of papillary to follicular carcinoma is seen. Since a population with higher iodine intake usually has fewer benign nodules in the thyroid gland and the incidence of thyroid carcinomas is similar to an iodine deficient region, this may affect the diagnostic work-up of nodules in the thyroid gland. The present paper summarizes available data from both epidemiological studies and animal experiments.

Introduction

Thyroid carcinomas are by far the most frequent endocrine gland malignancies accounting for approximately 0.5–1.5 % of all malignancies. Thyroid carcinomas have a marked variability in aggressiveness from highly differentiated papillary carcinomas to undifferentiated anaplastic cancers occurring mainly in older people and with a very poor prognosis. Malignant tumors of the thyroid gland are of either follicular, parafollicular or stromal origin (3). The annual incidence of thyroid carcinoma is approximately 20 to 50 per million inhabitants with about 5 deaths per million inhabitants per year (10). With conventional therapy, the overall survival rate of thyroid carcinoma is high, usually exceeding 90 %, in subgroups of patients with papillary carcinomas even close to 99 %. Thyroid carcinomas may, however, relapse decades after apparently successful initial treatment, which makes life-long follow-up mandatory (10).

The overall incidence of thyroid carcinoma is generally not considered to be influenced by the iodine intake of a population, whereas the distribution of the types of thyroid carcinoma may be related to the intake of iodine. The objective of the present paper is to summarize available data on the possible relationship between iodine intake and the development of thyroid carcinoma.

Types of thyroid carcinoma

The most frequent types of thyroid carcinoma are the differentiated forms (follicular, papillary or mixed papillary-follicular), whereas other forms such as anaplastic carcinomas, lymphomas, medullary thyroid carcinomas and secondary cancers are rare. The WHO classification of malignant thyroid tumors appears in table 1.

Most malignancies of the thyroid gland are found among nodules appearing 'cold' on a thyroid scintiscan, but thyroid cancer has been described in all types of

Table 1 WHO classification of malignant thyroid tumors

- Malignant epithelial tumors
  - Follicular carcinoma
  - Papillary carcinoma
  - Mixed papillary-follicular carcinoma
  - Undifferentiated carcinoma
  - Squamous cell carcinoma
  - Medullary carcinoma (C-cells)
- Malignant non-epithelial tumors
  - Fibrosarcoma
  - Others
- Other malignant tumors
  - Sarcoma
  - Malignant lymphoma
  - Malignant hemangiothelioma
  - Malignant teratoma
- Secondary tumors
- Unclassified tumors

Table 2 Characteristics of malignant thyroid tumors

- Rapidly growing or painful thyroid nodule
- Family history of thyroid cancer
- Exposure to neck irradiation in child-hood
- Hoarseness
- Firm and/or fixed nodule
- Cervical lymphadenopathy
- Vocal cord paralysis

thyroid enlargements and the majority of 'cold' nodules are benign, leaving a great differential diagnostic problem. Clinically evident thyroid nodules and benign goiters occur frequently depending on the iodine intake in a population, with fewer nodules and goiters in iodine rich areas. Postmortem examinations and epidemiological surveys of populations with evaluation of the thyroid gland texture by ultrasound have revealed even more clinically non-detectable thyroid nodules. Most of these nodules are benign, and it is therefore a continuing challenge for the clinician to pick out the few malignant thyroid nodules.

The diagnostic work-up may be different in iodine rich compared to iodine poor regions since a single thyroid nodule has a higher a priori likelihood of malignancy in iodine sufficient areas. In general, a rapidly growing mass in the thyroid gland is likely to be malignant (table 2). However, it must be born in mind that a cyst, a hemorrhage into a cyst or adenoma, subacute thyroiditis (De Quervain), and chronic thyroiditis of the Hashimoto type may all present as rapidly growing masses and all of them may also be firm and appear fixed upon palpation. A single nodule in a male is more likely to be malignant compared to that in a female. Features strongly indicative of benign thyroid nodules include long duration without growth, multinodular or diffuse goiter, simple thyroid cyst, 'hot' nodule on thyroid scintiscan, high levels of thyroglobulin and/or thyroperoxidase, a family history of benign goiter, and a suppressed serum thyrotropin (TSH).

Experiments in iodine deficient animals

In the 1960s, experiments showed an increased development of thyroid carcinomas in various animals such as mice (13) and golden hamsters (5) fed on a low iodine diet. Iodine-deficient Fisher rats were further shown to develop chromosomal abnormalities of the thyroid cells (1). The cancers described were of both papillary (13) and follicular (5) types. In the golden hamsters, the spontaneous cancer types were both papillary and follicular, whereas the malignancies reported in the iodine-deficient animals were follicular adenocarcinomas (5). Only thyroid epithelial cells were involved. Initially, the thyroids showed hyperplasia and it was already then proposed that hyperplasia and cancer development were both due to overstimulation by TSH, which is the main growth factor for the thyroid gland, although several others exist. Some of these growth factors such as epidermal growth factor and insulin-like growth factor-I are probably required for TSH to induce its growth stimulating effect (10). The results of these early studies have later been verified in other animal experiments and a model for thyroid tumorigenesis has been proposed (4, 16).

Epidemiological studies in humans

Clinically evident thyroid nodules and benign goiters occur frequently in iodine-deficient areas. Numerous epidemiological studies and animal experiments have demonstrated a relationship between iodine intake and the occurrence of benign nodules. The search for a similar relationship between the occurrence of malignant thyroid tumors and iodine intake has, however, been subject to much controversy and conflicting results. The overall incidence of thyroid carcinoma is generally considered not to be influenced by the iodine intake in a population (10), although one study from two regions in Italy has recently demonstrated a 2-fold increase in thyroid cancer incidence in an iodine-deficient area compared to an iodine-sufficient one (2). Contrary to this, the incidence of thyroid carcinoma was also increased in two areas of high iodine intake, Iceland (15) and Hawaii (8). This was initially linked to the iodine excess but may rather be due to the basaltic volcanic nature of these islands.

Epidemiological studies have also attempted to link iodine intake with the type of thyroid cancer. In relation to the increased cancer incidence in Iceland, it was noted that papillary carcinoma was the prevailing type (15). On the other hand, radiation is also known to cause thyroid carcinoma especially of the papillary type (10). In some studies, a negative association has been found between papillary carcinoma and the presence of endemic goiter (6, 14)

More solid evidence for a change in type of thyroid carcinoma has come from the study of areas with previous iodine-deficiency before and after iodine prophylaxis. In one such study from an area in Argentina, the ratio of papillary to follicular carcinomas rose from 2.5:1 to 6.2:1 (9). Introduction of iodine prophylaxis in Switzerland increased the ratio of papillary to follicular carcinomas (11).

The importance of accurate histological typing in cancer epidemiology cannot be overemphasized, but great caution is needed in comparison of different types of thyroid tumors. The reproducibility of the WHO classification has been questioned and considerable observer variation has been reported, particularly as regards follicular and mixed papillary-follicular ones (12). Differences in the detection and inclusion of occult thyroid cancers in the studies could also play a role. Finally, it should be noted that concomitant selenium deficiency in iodine-deficient areas has not been taken into account. This will be important in future studies, since selenium deficiency in itself has recently been associated with an increased incidence of thyroid carcinoma (7).

Conclusion

Available evidence, mainly from epidemiological studies and from the introduction of iodine prophylaxis, has demonstrated a relationship between iodine intake and the types of thyroid carcinoma. On the other hand, no clear evidence exists for a relationship between the overall cancer incidence and the iodine intake. The studies are, in general, hampered by difficulty in comparing populations since many factors other than the iodine intake have to be considered, such as ethnicity, other dietary factors, the histological examination, and radiation. In future studies, selenium intake should be also taken into consideration.

References

1. Al-Saadi A. Precursor cytogenetic changes of transplantable thyroid carcinoma in iodine-deficient goiters. Cancer Research 1968; 28; 739–745.
2. Belfiore A, La Rosa GL, La Porta GA, et al. Cancer risk in patients with cold thyroid nodules: relevance of iodine intake, sex, age and multinodularity. Am J Med 1992; 93; 363–369.
3. Clark OH, Duh Q-Y. Thyroid cancer. In: The thyroid gland. Monte A. Greer, ed. Raven Press, New York 1990; 537–572.
4. Farid NR, Shi Y, Zou M. Molecular basis of thyroid cancer. Endocrine Rev 1994; 15; 202–232.
5. Fortner JG, George PA, Sternberg SS. Induced and spontaneous thyroid cancer in the Syrian (golden) hamster. Endocrinology 1960; 66; 364–376.
6. Franssila K, Saxén E, Teppo L, et al. Incidence of different morphological types of thyroid cancer in the Nordic countries. Acta Pathol Microbiol Scand Sect A 1981; 89; 49–55.
7. Glattre E, Thomassen Y, Thoresen Sϕ, et al. Prediagnostic serum selenium in a case-control study of thyroid cancer. International J of Epidemiology 1989; 18; 45–49.
8. Goodman MT, Yoshizawa CN, Kolonel LN. Descriptive epidemiology of thyroid cancer in Hawaii. Cancer 1988; 61; 1272–1281.
9. Harach HR, Escalante DA, Oñativia A, et al. Thyroid carcinoma and thyroiditis in an endemic goitre region before prophylaxis. Acta Endocrinol (Copenh) 1985; 108; 55–60.
10. Kaplan MM, ed. Thyroid carcinoma. Endocrinol and Metab Clin of North America 1990; 19; 469-766.
11. Langsteger W, Költringer P, Wolf G. The impact of geographical, clinical, dietary and radiation-induced features in epidemiology of thyroid cancer. Eur J Cancer 1993; 29A; 1547–1553.
12. Saxén E, Franssila K, Bjarnason O, et al. Observer variation in histologic classification of thyroid classification. Acta Path Microbiol Scand Sect A 1978; 86; 483–486.
13. Schaller RT, Stevenson JK. Development of carcinoma of the thyroid in iodine-deficient mice. Cancer 1966; 19; 1063–1080.
14. Williams ED. The aetiology of thyroid tumours. Clin Endocrinol Metab 1979; 8; 49–55.

15. Williams ED, Doniach I, Bjarnason O, et al. Thyroid cancer in an iodide rich area: a histopathological study. Cancer 1977; 39; 215–222.
16. Wynford-Thomas D. Molecular basis of epithelial tumorigenesis: the thyroid model. Crit Rev Oncogenesis 1993; 4; 1–23.

Thyroid cancer after exposure to ionizing irradiation: histology, staging and clinical data

Chr. Reiners, J. Biko, [1]E. P. Demidchik, [2]V. Drozd

Clinic and Policlinic for Nuclear Medicine, University of Würzburg, Germany; [1]Center for Thyroid Tumors; [2]Research and Clinical Institute of Radiation Medicine and Endocrinology, Minsk, Belarus

Abstract

Exposure of the thyroid to ionizing radiation leads to an increased cancer risk. Whereas the average excess relative risk after external exposure amounts to approximately 8 per Gy, this relative risk is lower by a factor of 2 after exposure to radioiodine. The risk is greatest in newborns and small children below the age of 5, intermediate in adolescents, and negligible in adults. Papillary thyroid cancer with a relative incidence of approximately 80 % *per se* is typical for thyroid cancer in childhood and adolescence; however, after exposure to radioiodine this relative frequency is increased close to 100 %. Bilateral involvement, multicentric growth and cancer not limited to the thyroid gland seem to be characteristic of radiation induced thyroid cancer. Approximately 1,500 cases of thyroid cancer were diagnosed between 1990 and 1998 in children below the age of 15 from Belarus, the Ukraine, and Russia after the Chernobyl accident. Histologically, 98 % of the tumors were classified as papillary thyroid cancer and tumors with stage pT1 in 26 %, pT2 in 28 %, pT3 in 1 % and pT4 in 45 %. Between 1 April 1993 and 31 March 2000, 199 children from Belarus with the most advanced stages of thyroid cancer were given 694 treatments with radioiodine in Germany. 72 % of those selected cases were staged as pT4, 97 % as pN1, and 46 % as pM1. Disseminated miliary spread was typical for lung metastases detectable in 90 of those children. Complete remissions of tumor disease were achieved in 84 % of the whole group (67 % of children with distant metastases). Fortunately, no case of progressive disease or a recurrence has been observed.

Experiences from the past

It has been known for 50 years that exposure of the thyroid to ionizing radiation in childhood produces an appreciable cancer risk (7). The thyroid gland and the bone marrow are considered the most radiosensitive cancer sites (24). Concerning thyroid cancer, many epidemiological studies in populations of children treated with external radiotherapy for benign or malignant lesions in the head and neck region have been published (14, 24, 25, 29, 30). The indications for treatment included skin hemangioma, enlarged thymus and tonsils, lymphoid hyperplasia, tuberculous adenitis, acne, and tinea capitis. A pooled analysis (24) using data from cohort studies of individuals exposed to acute external ionizing radiation before the age of 20 years found an average excess relative risk of 7.7 per Gy (95 % confidence interval (CI) 4.9–12), while the excess absolute risk was 4.4 per 10^4 person-year Gy (95 % CI 1.9–10). A linear dose-response function was found to fit the data well; the risk was about 30 % lower for fractionated doses than for unfractionated exposure. Almost no thyroid cancers prior to 5 years after irradiation have been reported; the pooled analysis suggested that the excess relative risk per Gy was greatest about 15 years after exposure, but was still elevated 40 or more years after irradiation (24).

Unlike studies concerning external irradiation, where epidemiological data on more than 50,000 exposed children and adolescents are available, only sparse data from childhood exposure to radioiodine (I-131) have been published (13, 14, 30). Cohort studies of approximately 9,000 children exposed to I-131 before the age of 20 years suggested no significant increase of thyroid cancer risk from diagnostic or therapeutic use of I-131 (13, 14). A small, but significant increase in thyroid cancer risk has been seen in children and adolescents from the Marshall Islands exposed to fallout from atomic bomb experiments, amounting to an excess relative risk of 0.3 (95 % CI 0.1–0.8). However, 80 % of this dose originated from short-lived radioiodine isotopes and external radiation rather than from I-131 (30). The situation after the atomic bomb explosions of Hiroshima and Nagasaki was similar. The data from the Japanese atomic bomb study have been used to estimate age-related excess relative risk coefficients per Gy amounting to 9.5, 3.0, 0.3 and -0.2 at ages 0–9, 10–19, 20–39 and $\geq$ 40 respectively (1).

These risk coefficients show that the risk for thyroid cancer induction by radiation from atomic bomb explosions is high in children, intermediate in adolescents and negligible in adults. Epidemiological studies of adults, showing no increased risk for thyroid cancer after external or internal irradiation, underline this hypothesis (24, 29). The publications include comprehensive studies among patients following diagnostic or therapeutic exposure to I-131 (13, 14). In general, microdosimetric considerations (2) and/or the low dose rates involved with I-131 as compared to external thyroid irradiation with kilovoltage X-rays appear to reduce the carcinogenic potency substantially (29). External irradiation seems to be 1.5–2 times more dangerous than I-131 (18). Concerning age related effects of I-131, it is important to mention that besides the higher cancer risk of children and adolescents whose thyroids are still growing, considerably higher absorbed doses for a given activity of I-131 play an important role. The doses to the thyroid (in Gy) per ingested activity of I-131 (in kBq) in a newborn and at ages 1, 5, 10, 15 and ≥ 20 amount to 9.6, 3.9, 2.2, 0.9, 0.6 and 0.4 respectively (37).

It has been claimed that malignant thyroid tumors after external irradiation typically present as papillary cancers in approximately 85 % of the exposed children and adolescents (23, 24, 30, 36). However, Samaan et al. (1987) compared two cohorts of thyroid cancer patients with and without a history of head and neck irradiation as children. They showed that the proportion of papillary cancers in those two cohorts did not differ (87 % and 84 % respectively). This indicates that papillary histology *per se* is typical of thyroid cancer in childhood and adolescence. However, Samaan's study also revealed that bilateral lobe involvement (51 %) and cancer not limited to the thyroid gland (70 %) were significantly more common in radiation induced thyroid cancer (26).

The Chernobyl accident

During the night from 25th to 26th April 1986, the most severe reactor accident in history occurred at the nuclear power plant Chernobyl 30 km south of the border between Ukraine and Belarus. The reactor core exploded and caught fire, which was not extinguished until 9 May 1986. Because of the burning graphite, enormous amounts of radioactivity were released during the first 10 days. According to recent calculations, approximately 12 x 10^{18} Bq (≅ 0.3 billion Ci) of radioactivity were released, among them 1.8 x 10^{18} Bq of I-131. The radioactivity was transported with the prevailing winds from the northern parts of the Ukraine to Belarus and the western parts of Russia, and later to Scandinavia and parts of Western Europe. Belarus was most heavily contaminated, receiving 70 % of the released activity. Extremely high contamination has been found in the regions surrounding the cities of Gomel and Brest (16).

The frequency of thyroid cancer in children from Belarus, the Ukraine and the western parts of Russia has been increasing since 1990 (5, 6, 8, 31, 32). In all, in the 3 Republics affected by radioactive fallout from the Chernobyl accident approximately 1500 cases of thyroid cancer were diagnosed between 1990 and 1998 in children below age of 15, compared with approximately 100 cases diagnosed between 1968 and 1989 (5, 6, 8, 31, 32).

The most reliable epidemiological data seem to be available from Belarus (5, 6). The relative incidence of thyroid cancer per 100.000 children below age of 15, which was 0.1–0.3 between 1986 and 1989 increased to 4.0 in 1995 (figure 1). In the re-

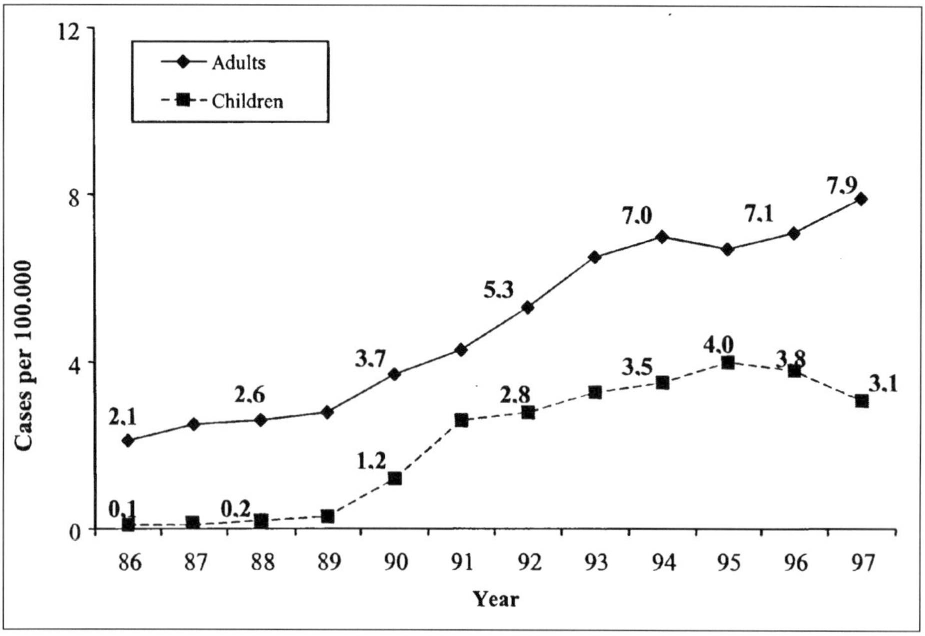

Fig. 1 Relative incidence of thyroid cancer in adults and children below the age of 15 years in Belarus between 1986 and 1997.

gion of Gomel, which was most heavily contaminated after the Chernobyl accident by radioactive fallout containing I-131 and short-lived radioisotopes of iodine, the relative incidence increased to 13.5 in 1995. Since 1996, the relative incidence of thyroid cancer in children has been decreasing (Figure 1).

Figure 1 shows that the relative incidence of thyroid cancer in adults from Belarus has also increased since 1986. However, whereas the increase in children was approximately 20-fold, comparing 1995 with the mean for 1986–1989, the increase of the relative incidence among adults between 1986 and 1997 has been only 4-fold. According to current data of the Survival Epidemiology and End Results Program (28) from the United States, the annual incidence of thyroid cancer between 1990 and 1994 was 4.9 per 100,000 inhabitants (women 6.9, men 2.8 per 100,000). Among children and adolescents below age of 20, the incidence was 0.1 per 100.000 US inhabitants. Between 1950 and 1994, the incidence of thyroid cancer in the USA increased by approximately 22% (28). This comparison shows that the incidence of thyroid cancer among children from Belarus, which was comparable to the incidence in the USA before 1990, undoubtedly increased after the Chernobyl reactor accident. By contrast, the incidence of thyroid cancer in adults from Belarus was lower by a factor of 2 in 1986 and at the end of the observation period in 1997, the incidence in Belarus was approximately 2-fold higher compared with adults from the USA. This increase in adults may also be related to the Chernobyl accident, since subjects aged

4 or older changed at exposure in 1986 would be defined as adults (older than 15 years) in 1997. On the other hand, it must be recognized that the incidence rate of 7.9 cases per 100,000 adults lies in within world wide variability of incidence rates from 0.2–8.8 for men and 0.8–18.2 for women, respectively (11).

The mean dose to the thyroid of the 500,000 children from Belarus exposed to irradiation was 0.4 Gy (25th percentile 0.08, 75 percentile 1.0 Gy) (17). After correction for the dependence of average thyroid doses on age, the radiation induced absolute thyroid risk in Gomel is about a factor of 3 higher for children up to the age of 10 years at exposure compared to older ones. Up to 10 years of age at exposure, the female: male ratio is about 1.5. After puberty, the ratio increases. Taking the data together, an excess absolute risk of 2.3 (95 % CI 1.4–3.8) per 10^4 person-year Gy for children below age of 15 can be calculated (15). This is a factor of 2 lower than the best estimate derived from the pooled study of thyroid cancer after external exposure (18). Projecting the age-adjusted average excess risk per unit thyroid dose for the period of 5–50 years following the Chernobyl accident, it has been estimated that about 15,000 cases (95 % CI 5,000–45,000) may develop (19).

574 cases of childhood thyroid cancer were detected and underwent surgery at the Center for Thyroid Tumors in Minsk between 1986 and 1997 (5, 6). 53 % of these children lived in the Gomel region. Histologically, 98 % of the tumors were classified as papillary thyroid cancer. At the time of surgical intervention in Minsk 26 % of the cases were staged as pT1 (tumors diameter < 1 cm), 28 % as pT2 (diameter 1–4 cm), 1 % as pT3 (diameter > 4 cm without invasion of surrounding tissue), and 45 % as the most advanced stage, pT4 (tumors invading soft tissue surrounding the thyroid gland). The cancer was classified histologically as multicentric in 25 % of stage pT1–2 tumors and 45 % of stage pT4 tumors. Lymph node metastases were observed at surgery in 50 % of stage pT1–3 cases and 81 % of stage pT4 patients. Distant metastases to lungs were diagnosed in Minsk immediately postoperatively in 5 % in of stages pT1–3 tumors and 24 % of stage pT4 tumors.

Treatment of thyroid cancer of children from Belarus in Germany

In April 1993, the German project "Scientists Help Chernobyl Children" was launched by the Joint Committee for Radiation Research. The project was supported by the German Minister of the Environment, Radiation Protection and Reactor Safety, as well as by the Minister of Health of Belarus. Generous funds for this project could have been raised from German Electricity Suppliers.

The project has been established in the framework of bilateral cooperation between two centers in Minsk and the University Clinics for Nuclear Medicine in Essen and later Würzburg. Surgical resection of thyroid tumors and removal of lymph nodes was performed by the surgical team of the Center for Thyroid Tumors in Minsk. Radioiodine treatment and staging with nuclear medicine procedures was the task of the Clinics for Nuclear Medicine in Essen and Würzburg respectively. Follow-up was performed in Minsk by the Center for Thyroid Tumors and the Research and Clinical Institute of Radiation Medicine and Endocrinology in Minsk.

Patients

Between 1 April 1993 and 31 March 2000, 199 children from Belarus with advanced thyroid cancer were selected for treatment in Germany (table 1).

The children traveled by plane in groups of 4 and were accompanied by a physician from Minsk. They stayed for 1 week in the Clinic and Polyclinic for Nuclear

Table 1 Children with thyroid cancer from Belarus treated with I-131 in Germany between 01.04.1993 and 31.03.2000

Patients	199 Children			
	694 Treatment courses			
Origin	85 Gomel area			
	114 Other parts of Belarus			
Gender	117 Girls			
	82 Boys			
Age	7–18 Years (11.9 ± 2.5)			
Histology	197 Papillary cancers			
	2 Follicular Cancers			
Stage	pTx – 2	pNo – 6	pMo – 107	
	pT1 – 3	pN1 – 193	pM1 – 92	
	pT2 – 47		90	Lung
	pT3 – 4		2	Bone
	pT4 – 143		1	Brain
Pretreatment	37 Radioiodine therapies in Minsk			
	5 Radioiodine therapies in Italy			
	19 Percutaneous irradiation			
	6 Chemotherapy			

Medicine of the University of Essen (after January 1 1995, in the Clinic and Polyclinic for Nuclear Medicine of the University of Würzburg). 694 courses of I-131 therapy were administered up to March 31, 2000.

43 % of the children originated from the Gomel region. The mean age of the children at the time of the reactor accident was 2.6 ± 2.2 years (78 % of the children were below age of 5). Their mean age at the time of surgery ranged from 7–18 years with a mean age of 11.9 ± 2.5 years. This corresponds to a mean latency time of approximately 9 years; the shortest time interval between exposure and surgery was 3.2 years. 59 % of the children were female, 41 % male. 99 % of the cancers were typed histologically as papillary and 1 % as follicular carcinomas.

72 % of the cases selected for treatment in Germany because of the aggressiveness of tumors were classified as stage pT4. Lymph node metastases were detected in 97 % and distant metastases in 46 %. With the exception of two cases with secondary deposits in bone, distant metastases were localized in the lungs (among those cases one child with metastases to lungs and brain). Nearly all cases with lung metastases presented as disseminated miliary spread, only 4 % of the children showed single localized nodular lesions. Only 53 % of children with lung metastases detectable by I-131 scanning showed positive thoracic radiographs; this proportion was higher (82 %) for high resolution computed tomography. 42 of the 199 children had previously received radioiodine treatment with different activities in Minsk (mainly low activities up to 1 GBq). 19 children had been irradiated percutaneously with mainly low radiation doses (up to 20 Gy). 6 children had received chemotherapy with different drugs in Minsk.

Protocol

The diagnostic protocol included ultrasonography and scintigraphy of the neck, chest radiograph, computer tests of pulmonary function, differential blood cell count, and determination of serum thyroglobulin, TSH, free T_4 and free T_3, calcium, and phosphate. In addition, X-ray computed tomography (CT), whole-body counting of incorporated radionuclides and biological dosimetry were performed in a subset of children.

For treatment, 50 MBq of I-131 per kg body weight was administered to eliminate thyroid remnants. For ablation of metastases, 100 MBq of I-131 per kg body weight was given. Simultaneously, antiemetics and emulsions for protection of gastric mucosa were given to reduce gastrointestinal side effects. 2 days after treatment, replacement therapy with levothyroxine, which had been withdrawn 4 weeks before treatment, was restarted. The mean dose was 2.5 μg of levothyroxine per kg body weight. For staging, whole body scans were performed 4 days after radioiodine administration.

Table 2 Results of radioiodine treatment in 169 children with differentiated thyroid cancer from Belarus (01.04.1993 – 31.03.2000)

N=169			Complete remission	Partial remission	No change	Progressive disease
pT1–3	N0	M0	1	–	–	–
		M1	1	1	–	–
	N1	M0	24	–	–	–
		M1	4	7	–	–
pT4	N0	M0	1	–	–	–
		M1	1	–	–	–
	N1	M0	60	–	–	–
		M1	50	19	–	–

Results of treatment

169 of 199 have received more than one course of radioiodine treatment in Germany. Results of treatment have been monitored in these cases by follow-up with I-131 scintigraphy, ultrasonography of the neck, chest radiograph, and determination of serum thyroglobulin (table 2).

142 out of 169 children (84 %) have achieved complete remission of thyroid cancer. 16 % have had partial remissions, defined as a decrease of tumor volume, serum level of tumor markers or intensity of radioiodine uptake of at least 50 %. Fortunately, progressive disease has not been observed in any patients. It is important to mention that the results given here are not the final results of treatment since, in some cases without complete remission, further courses of radioiodine are appropriate. Fortunately, only 2 children from Belarus with differentiated thyroid cancer and widespread local tumor who could not be treated with radioiodine have died because of postoperative complications.

Discussion

There is no doubt that exposure to radiation may induce thyroid cancer in children (35). According to the review of Ron et al., *"The thyroid gland in children has one of the highest risk coefficients of any organ and is the only with convincing evidence for risk at about 0.1 Gy"* (24). Linearity best describes the dose response in children exposed to radiation before age of 15. Risk decreases significantly with increasing age at exposure, with little risk apparent after age of 20. The excess relative risk seems to be higher for females that for males (24).

Latency times between radiation exposure and development of thyroid cancer range between a minimum of 3–7 years and a maximum of 40–50 years. Between 10 and 15 years, a nadir of the statistical distribution may be presumed (29). The relative incidence of thyroid cancer per 100,000 of children below the age of 15 increased in Belarus from 0.1–0.3 cases between 1986 and 1989 to 4.0 cases in 1995. This compares with approximately 0.3–0.5 cases per 100,000 of thyroid cancer among children below the age of 15, based on figures from the USA (12, 20, 28) and data from the German Cancer Registries in Hamburg and the Saarland.

Table 3 compares recent multicenter studies on childhood thyroid cancer from Italy, France and Germany (9, 21) with the statistical material available at the Center for Thyroid Tumors in Minsk, Belarus, about 574 cases of childhood cancer diagnosed after the Chernobyl accident between 1986 and 1997 (5, 6). Table 3 proves that a high proportion of papillary histology is typical for thyroid cancer in children and adolescents (26). However, among children exposed to irradiation from Belarus the percentage of papillary cancers is extremely high with 98 %, compared with children from Italy and France (82 %) and Germany (78 %). In addition, the proportions of tumors with multicentric growth (33 % versus 20 %) and pT4-stage (45 % versus 25 % and 29 % respectively) are higher among children from Belarus. Lymph node involvement is also more frequent among children from Belarus (68 %) as compared to children from Italy and France (54 %) or Germany (52 %). There is no unequivocal difference in the frequency of distant metastases (16 % versus 17 % and 25 % re-

Table 3 Thyroid cancer in children: Data from Belarus in comparison to data from Italy, France, and Germany

Study	**Belarus (6)**	**Italy and France (21)**	**Germany (9)**
Number of children	574	369	114
Mean age	9.9 years	14.6 years	13.2 years
Female : male	1.5 : 1	2,5 : 1	2,4 : 1
Papillary histology	98%	82%	78%
Multicentric growth	33%	–	20%
pT4	45%	25%	29%
pN1	68%	54%	52%
pM1	16%	17%	25%

spectively). However, the data available from Belarus may underestimate the frequency of distant metastases because routine I-131 whole body scans were performed only in a small subgroup of the patients.

To summarize, characteristics of thyroid cancer in children exposed to Chernobyl fallout seem to be papillary histology and signs of aggressive growth. However, it cannot be excluded that these differences are related to the younger age of Chernobyl children (mean 9.9 years) as compared to the mean ages of children from Italy and France (14.6 years) and Germany (13.2 years) (Table 3).

It is well known, that papillary thyroid cancers tend to spread via the lymphatic pathway to the lungs (33). Typically, this miliary type of disseminated pulmonary metastases may only be detected by whole-body scintigraphy and not by chest radiographs (27), as observed in 47 % of our children with lung metastases. 86 of the 90 children from Belarus with lungs secondary deposits treated in Germany presented with disseminated pulmonary lesions. These were ablated completely by I-131 therapy in 67 % of the children. In the remaining 33 % of patients, partial remissions were observed with decreased radioiodine uptake and a reduction in the mostly extremely elevated serum thyroglobulin levels. However, 8 of the 90 children with radioiodine uptake in lung metastases showed reductions in vital capacity, which was measured routinely during therapy. Computed tomography proved that pulmonary fibrosis had developed. Lung fibrosis is one of the possible complications of high-dose radioiodine treatment among patients with pulmonary metastases of thyroid cancer. However, 5 of the 8 cases diagnosed in our study had been treated previously with bleomycin, which is also known to induce pulmonary fibrosis. According to the literature, fibrosis may develop in up to 10 % of children with lung metastases (22).

However, in general, the prognosis of thyroid cancer among children is reported to be excellent (3, 4, 12, 20, 26, 34). Children have a better prognosis than adults. Prognosis seems to be good even where there are persistent pulmonary metastases on scintigraphy (27, 28). It is now generally accepted that treatment guidelines for children and adults should be identical (3, 4, 12, 20, 26, 34). Routine treatment should include thyroidectomy, selective removal of positive lymph nodes, and subsequent radioiodine treatment. Only for stage pT1, are total thyroidectomy and subsequent radioiodine ablation of thyroid remnants not mandatory because of the excellent prognosis of such tumors. However, it should be taken into consideration that a tumor diameter of 1 cm in a 10-year old child with a thyroid volume of approximately 10 ml is relatively larger by a factor of 2 compared with a tumor of the same size in an adult with a thyroid volume of 20 ml (10).

References

1. Akiba S, Lubin J, Ezaki E, Ron E, Ishimaru T, Asona Y, Shimizu Y, Kato H. Thyroid Cancer Incidence among Atomic Bomb Survivors in Hiroshima and Nagasaki 1958–1979. Technical Report TR 5–91, Radiation Effects Research Foundation, Hiroshima, Japan. 1991.
2. Brenner DJ. The relative effectiveness of exposure to ^{131}I at low doses. Health Physics 1999; 76:180–185.
3. Danese D, Gardini A, Farsetti A, Sciacchitano S, Andreoli M, Pontecorvi A. Thyroid carcinoma in children and adolescents. Eur J Pediatr 1997; 156:190–194.
4. Dottorini ME, Vignati A, Mazzucchelli L, Lomuscio G, Colombo L. Differentiated Thyroid Carcinoma in Children and Adolescents: A 37-Year Experience in 85 Patients. J Nucl Med 1997; 38:669–675.
5. Demidchik EP, Mrochek A, Demidchik Yu, Vorontsova T, Cherstvoy E, Kenigsberg J, Rebeko V, Sugenoya A. Thyroid Cancer Promoted by Radiation in Young People of Belarus (Clinical and Epidemiological Features). In: Radiation and Thyroid Cancer. G. Thomas, A. Karaoglou, ED Williams (Eds). World Scientific Singapore-New Jersey-London-Hong Kong 1999; 51–54.
6. Demidchik EP. Personal Communication, March 2000.
7. Duffy BJ, Fitzgerald P. Thyroid Cancer in childhood and adolescence. Report of 28 cases. J Clin Endocr Metab 1950; 10:1296–1308.
8. Epsthein OE. Personal Communication, March 2000.
9. Farahati J, Parlowsky T, Mäder U, Reiners C, Bucsky P. Differentiated thyroid cancer in children and adolescents. Langenbeck's Arch Surg 1998; 383:235–239.
10. Farahati J, Reiners C, Demidchik EP. Is the UICC/AJCC Classification of Primary Tumor in Childhood Thyroid Carcinoma Valid? J Nucl Med 1999; 40:2125.
11. Franceschi S, Boyle P, Maisonneuve P, La Vecchia C, Burt AD, Kerr DJ, MacFarlane GJ. The Epidemiology of Thyroid Carcinoma. Critical Reviews in Oncogenesis 1993; 4:25–52.
12. Gorlin JB, Sallan SE. Thyroid cancer in childhood. Endocrinol Metabol Clin North America 1990; 19:649–662.
13. Hall P, Holm LE. Late Consequences of Radioiodine for Diagnosis and Therapy in Sweden. Thyroid 1997; 7:205–208.
14. Hall P, Holm LE. Radiation-Associated Thyroid Cancer-Facts and Fiction. Acto Oncologica 1998; 37:325–330.
15. Heidenreich WF, Kenigsberg J, Jacob P, Buglova E, Goulko G, Paretzke HG, Demidchik EP, Golovneva A. Time Trends of Thyroid Cancer Incidence in Belarus after the Chernobyl Accident. Radiat Res 1999; 151:617–625.
16. International Atomic Energy Agency. One decade after Chernobyl: Summing-up the consequences of the accident. IAEA and WHO, Vienna 1996.
17. Jacob P. Thyroid cancer risk to children calculated. Nature 1998; 392:31–32.
18. Jacob P, Kenigsberg Y, Zvonova I, Goulko G, Buglova E, Heidenreich WF, Golovneva A, Bratilova AA, Drozdovitch V, Kruk J, Pochtennaja GT, Balonov M, Demidchik EP, Paretzke HG. Childhood exposure due to the Chernobyl accident and thyroid cancer risk in contaminated areas of Belarus and Russia. Brit J Cancer 1999; 80:1461–1469.
19. Jacob P, Kenigsberg Y, Goulko G, Buglova E, Gering F, Golovneva A, Kruk J, Demidchik EP. Thyroid cancer risk in Belarus after the Chernobyl accident: Comparison with external exposures. Radiat Environ Biophys 2000; 39:25–31.
20. Moir CR, Telander RL. Papillary carcinoma of the thyroid in children. Semin Pediatr Surgery 1994; 3:182–187.
21. Pacini F, Vorontsova T, Demidchik EP, Molinaro E, Agate L, Romei C, Shavrova E, Cherstvoy ED, Ivashkevitch Y, Kuchinskaya E, Schlumberger M, Ronga G, Filesi M, Pinchera A. Post-Chernobyl Thyroid Carcinoma in Belarus Children and Adolescents: Comparison with Naturally Occurring Thyroid Carcinoma in Italy and France. J Clin Endocrinol Metab 1997; 82:3563–3569.
22. Reiners C, Perret G, Sonnenschein W, John-Mikolajewski V. Radiation reactions to the lung after radioiodine therapy for thyroid cancer. In: Strahlenschutz in Forschung und Praxis, Band 36, Th. Herr-

mann, Chr. Reiners, O. Messerschmidt (Eds). Gustav Fischer Stuttgart – Jena – New York 1994; 139–146.

23. Reiners C, Biko J, Kruglova N, Demidchik EP. Therapy of thyroid carcinoma in children from Belarus after the Chernobyl accident. In: The Thyroid and Iodine. Merck European Thyroid Symposium Warsaw 1996, May 16–18. J. Nauman, D. Glinoer, LE Braverman, U Hostalek (Eds). Schattauer Stuttgart-New York 1996; 89–97.
24. Ron E, Lubin JH, Shore RE, Mabuchi K, Modan B, Pottern LM, Schneider AB, Tucker MA, Boice JD. Thyroid cancer after exposure to external radiation: A pooled analysis of seven studies. Radiat Res 1995; 141:259–277.
25. Ron E, Schneider AB. External Radiation and the Thyroid Cancer Risk in Humans. In: Radiation and Thyroid Cancer. G. Thomas, A. Karaoglou, ED Williams (Eds). World Scientific Singapore-New Jersey-London-Hong Kong 1999; 5–12.
26. Samaan NA, Schultz PN, Ordonez NG, Hickey RC, Johnston DA. A comparison of thyroid carcinoma in those who have and have not had head and neck irradiation in childhood. J Clin Endocrinol 1987; 64:219–223.
27. Samuel AM, Rajashekharrao B, Shah DH. Pulmonary Metastases in Children and Adolescents with Well-Differentiated Thyroid Cancer. J Nucl Med 1998; 39:1531–1536.
28. Surveillance, Epidemiology and End Results (SEER) Program of the USA 1973–1994, National Cancer Institute, Bethesda 1998.
29. Shore RE. Issues and epidemiological evidence regarding radiation-induced thyroid cancer. Radiation Research 1992; 131:98–111.
30. Shore RE. Human thyroid cancer induction by ionizing radiation: Summary of studies based on external irradiation and radioactive iodines. In: European Commission and the Belarus, Russian and Ukrainian Ministries on Chernobyl Affairs, Emergency Situations and Health: The Radiological Consequences of the Chernobyl Accident. A. Karaoglou, G. Desmet, GN Kelly, HG Menzel (Eds). European Commission, Brussels 1996; 669–675.
31. Tronko M, Bogdanova T, Komisarenko I, Rybakov S, Kovalenko A, Epsthein O, Oliynik V, Tereshchenko V, Likhtarev I, Kairo I, Chepurnoy M. The Post-Chernobyl Incidence of Childhood Thyroid Cancer in Ukraine. In: Radiation and Thyroid Cancer. G. Thomas, A. Karaoglou, ED Williams (Eds). World Scientific Singapore-New Jersey-London-Hong Kong 1999; 61–69.
32. Tsyb AF, Shakhtarin, Lushnikov EF, Stepanenko VF, Snykov VP, Parshkov EM, Trofimova SF. Development of Cancer and Non-Cancer Thyroid Diseases in Children and Adolescents after the Chernobyl Accident. In: Radiation and Thyroid Cancer. G. Thomas, A. Karaoglou, ED Williams (Eds). World Scientific Singapore-New Jersey-London-Hong Kong 1999; 79–87.
33. Vassilopoulou-Sellin R, Klein MJ, Smith TH, Samaan NA, Frankenthaler RA, Goepfert H, Cangir A, Haynie TP. Pulmonary metastases in children and young adults with differentiated thyroid cancer. Cancer 1993; 71; 1348–1352.
34. Vassilopoulou-Sellin R, Goepfert H, Raney B, Schultz PN. Differentiated Thyroid Cancer in Children and Adolescents: Clinical Outcome and Mortality after long-term follow-up. Head Neck 1998; 20:549–555.
35. Williams D. Editorial: Thyroid Cancer and the Chernobyl Accident. J Clin Endocrinol Metab 1996; 81:6–8.
36. Winship T, Rosvoll RV. Thyroid carcinoma in childhood: final report on a 20 year study. Clin Proc Child Hosp (Washington, DC) 1970; 26:327–349.
37. Zanzonico PB. Age-Dependent Thyroid Absorbed Doses for Radiobiologically Significant Radioisotopes of Iodine. Health Phys 2000; 78:60–67.

Oncogenes and thyroid cancer

M. Derwahl, D. Manole, B. Schildknecht

Department of Medicine, St. Willehad Hospital, Wilhelmshaven and Faculty of Medicine, Ruhr University of Bochum, Germany

Introduction

Cell proliferation is stimulated through growth factor receptors that are activated by their corresponding ligands. Activation of the receptors results in transmission of signals via a complex network of interacting pathways. Many growth factor receptors and signaling proteins are proto-oncogenes that may be converted into oncogenes by overexpression or functional or structural alterations leading to a constitutive activation of down-stream signaling and thus stimulation of excess cell proliferation (1).

Oncogenes and growth factors

Overexpression of growth factors is commonly found in various carcinomas. The underlying mechanism that causes overexpression is, however, still unknown. Most growth factors including fibroblast growth factor 1 and 2 (FGF) and vascular endothelial growth factor (VEGF) are expressed in nodular goiters, benign and malignant thyroid tumors, albeit at a higher level in neoplastic thyroid tissue (2–7). Although the pathogenetic role of these growth factors remains unclear, their angiogenic potential suggests relevance for neovascularization in the process of thyroid tumor growth.

The first link between oncogenes and growth factors was established when the amino acid sequence homology between platelet-derived growth factor (PDGF) and v-sis oncogene, a transforming protein originally detected in simian sarcoma virus (SSV), was determined (8). In thyroid cancer PDGF A and B have only been described in undifferentiated carcinoma cell lines (9). Whether they are also expressed in thyroid carcinoma samples is not known.

Oncogenes and growth factor receptors

Binding of, e.g. EGF, to its receptor leads to phosphorylation of signaling proteins by the intrinsic EGF receptor tyrosine kinase domain and in turn to an activation of dependent pathways. Overexpression of the EGF receptor has been reported in both benign and malignant thyroid tumors (12). It may occur through gene amplification, resulting in an increased number of receptors.

More than 15 years ago, a direct link between growth factor receptors and some oncogenes was detected. Analysis of the amino acid sequence of the EGF receptor revealed a close similarity with parts of the sequence deduced for the v-erb B oncogene (13). Its cellular relative c-erb B2/neu is amplified and overexpressed in different carcinomas (14). Both overexpressed normal receptors and their truncated forms may function as a constitutively "turned-on" signal for cell proliferation.

In papillary thyroid carcinomas overexpression of met, the tyrosine kinase receptor for hepatocyte growth factor (HGF) is very common (15, 16). The molecular mechanism by which the met oncogene promotes tumor growth is not fully understood. Met overexpression is often associated with rearrangement of ret and trk (15).

Ret is the membrane receptor for glial cell neurotrophic growth factor (17) and is not expressed in normal thyroid cells. The ret/PTC oncogene is generated by an interchromosomal exchange (rearrangement) that links the promotor(s) of unrelated gene(s) to the C-terminal domain of ret missing the ligand-binding and transmembrane region. The truncated ret tyrosine kinase constitutively activates the dependent growth-promoting pathways mimicking the stimulatory effect of ligand-binding. 3 major ret/PTC hybrid genes have been detected in papillary carcinomas. Ret/PTC1 is generated by a paracentric inversion of the long arm of chromosome 10 carrying the ret kinase encoding domain that is fused to the H4 gene (18). Very recently, a novel H4-Ret rearrangement form, designated Ret/PTC1L, that exhibits a lower transforming potency than Ret/PTC1 has been described (19). Ret/PTC2 is generated by a reciprocal translocation between chromosomes 10 and 17 that results in the juxtaposition of the TK domain of ret with a portion of the regulatory subunit of RI cAMP-dependent protein kinase A (20). Ret/PTC3 is also due to intrachromosomal rearrangement, and is generated by fusion with the RFG/ELEI gene (21).

A high frequency of Ret/PTC3 variants has been observed in radiation-associated papillary carcinomas, such as those appearing after the Chernobyl nuclear accident (22, 23). However, as revealed very recently, Ret/PTC oncogenes may also be operative in Hürthle cell carcinomas (24).

Other tyrosine kinase receptors may also be a target of rearrangements. TRK oncogenes are created by a rearrangement of the NTRK1 gene that encodes a receptor for nerve growth factor, linking it to different activating genes (25). TRK is activated in less than 20% of papillary carcinomas (26).

TSH and TSH receptor-dependent signaling play a major role in growth regulation of normal thyroid cells. In toxic thyroid adenomas, the dependent pathways may be constitutively, i.e. independently of ligand-binding, activated by mutations in the transmembrane or adjacent extracellular domain of the TSH receptor gene, although the mutations are not sufficient to generate these tumors (27). Because of the absence of or a very low degree of transforming potency, these mutations are very rarely found in thyroid carcinomas (28, 29).

Oncogenes and signaling pathways

Activation of tyrosine kinase receptors results in autophosphorylation of cytoplasmic tyrosine residues of the receptor and, in turn, high affinity binding of phosphorylated tyrosines to adapter molecules that initiate a chain of phosphorylation reactions. A major target of these reactions is the ras-raf-MAP (mitogen-activated protein) signaling cascade. Ras is a membrane-bound protein that belongs to the family of GTP-binding proteins (30).

All 3 ras genes (H-ras, N-ras, K-ras) are targets of point mutations in thyroid tumors. The mutations are predominantly found in follicular adenomas and carcinomas, with codon 61 of the H-ras and N-ras being preferentially affected (31). They represent early events in the pathogenesis of these tumors. Ras mutations are more frequent in iodide-deficient than in iodide-sufficient regions (32). The reason for this finding is unknown.

The central role of ras and ras-dependent signaling for the control of cellular growth is underlined by studies with FRTL-5 thyroid cells, which grow independently of TSH when transfected with mutant ras (33). However, mutant ras does not confer a transformed state on the cells, in accordance with the observation that ras mutations are already detectable in thyroid adenomas.

Besides being found in the TSH receptor gene, activating mutations have also been identified in the dependent GTP-binding protein (34). Activation of the TSH receptor results in a conformational change in the heterotrimeric G-protein complex, which consists of α-, β- and γ- subunits. The activated GTP-binding α-subunit is the target for activating mutations (Gsα mutations) that constitutively stimulate the dependent adenylate cyclase cascade, as do TSH receptor mutations. Gsα mutations are found in some toxic adenomas, and with a lower frequency in differentiated follicular carcinomas (29, 35).

Tumor suppressor genes

Each proliferating cell possesses regulatory molecular mechanisms that prevent excessive growth and thus tumor formation. Some of these mechanisms are already activated when normal cell proliferation is initiated (12). Tumor suppressor genes encode proteins that inhibit proliferation or restrict cell division (1). Whereas oncogenes act as dominant cell regulators, that is, a defect in one allele is sufficient to evoke the neoplastic phenotype, tumor suppressor genes are operative in a recessive manner.

The retinoblastoma (Rb) and p53 genes are paradigmatic of this type of gene. Both genes are involved in the regulation of cell cycle progression (36). The Rb protein controls the G1/S transition of the cell cycle. When Rb is unphosphorylated, it prevents cell cycle progression and thus entry into S phase. Phosphorylation and thus inactivation of the gene occurs at the beginning of DNA replication (37). Inactivation of Rb by allelic loss has been observed not only in retinoblastoma but also in many other carcinomas. Deletions of exon 21 of the Rb gene were found in about half of the malignant thyroid tumors examined (38, 39), with both copies of the Rb gene deleted in about one third of samples. There is, as yet, no comprehensive study of structural defects within the Rb gene in thyroid neoplasia.

p53 is a transcription factor that plays a critical role in the maintenance of genomic integrity. Exposure to agents that damage DNA enhances p53, which blocks the cell cycle at the G1 phase (40). Other functions of p53 include regulation of the mitotic spindle checkpoint (41), negative regulation of the c-fos and c-jun proto-oncogenes (42), inhibition of bcl-2 expression (see next paragraph on "Apoptosis"), and induction of several genes that encode proteins (e.g. p21) that arrest the cell cycle (43).

Inactivating point mutations of the p53 gene are frequently found in anaplastic and poorly differentiated thyroid tumors (44). In contrast to ras mutations that are found in the early stage of thyroid tumorigenesis, p53 inactivating mutations represent late events in the progression of thyroid cancer.

Genes that inhibit cyclins and their dependent kinases may also function as tumor suppressor genes. p16 specifically inhibits cyclin D1/cyclin-dependent kinase (Cdk) 4. p16 mutations have been detected in several thyroid cancer cell lines, but only rarely in cancer tissues (45). p21 is a downstream effector in p53-mediated arrest of the cell cycle (36). Almost 40 % of thyroid carcinoma samples were found to harbor p21 defects and/or p53 mutations (46).

Apoptosis

In the normal thyroid gland, cell numbers are maintained constant by a balance between proliferation and programmed cell death (apoptosis). The apoptotic process is characterized by activation of various pathways that finally lead to chromatin condensation, DNA cleavage and cytosolic shrinkage.

Since normal thyrocytes divide only 4–5 times in their lifetime, the rate of apoptosis is consequently low. However, if thyroid cells are transformed into tumor cells by mutational events, at least in the early stage of tumorigenesis, compensatory activation of apoptotic pathways is found. Experimentally, it has been shown that oncogene activation may induce apoptosis (47).

The members of the bcl-2 protein family represent important regulators of apoptosis. In thyroid adenomas and in most follicular thyroid carcinomas anti-apoptotic bcl-2 was slightly elevated, whereas expression of pro-apoptotic bax was lower in carcinomas than in adenomas (48). This may reflect a futile attempt by tumor cells to counterbalance the action of growth-promoting factors in thyroid tumorigenesis.

With the increasing dedifferentiation of thyroid carcinoma cells, there is a negative association between p53 expression and bcl-2 expression. By contrast, in normal thyroid cells, p53 down-regulates bcl-2 and induces bax expression (49).

DNA methylation

Epigenetic changes represent important molecular mechanisms that contribute to the pathogenesis of thyroid cancer. A change in the methylation pattern in promotor regions of certain genes is an important mechanism in tumorigenesis (50). DNA methylation leads to heritable inhibition of gene transcription, e.g. of tumor suppressor genes (51). In thyroid tumors, the prevalence of methylation abnormalities has been reported to be very high (52).

Adenoma-carcinoma sequence

As with all other neoplasms, thyroid tumors do not arise from a single molecular defect, but are the consequence of an array of genetic and epigenetic abnormalities (12). For both papillary and follicular thyroid carcinomas, the sequence of genetic abnormalities is not well defined. In figure 1 a model of a potential adenoma-carcinoma sequences for papillary and follicular carcinomas is depicted. The model is based on the genetic aberrations described above and chromosomal alterations including genomic instability (53), aneuploidy (54) and loss of heterozygosity (55).

Acknowledgement

This work was supported by Dr. Mildred Scheel Foundation for Cancer Research, Bonn, and Biomedic e.V., Wilhelmshaven, Germany.

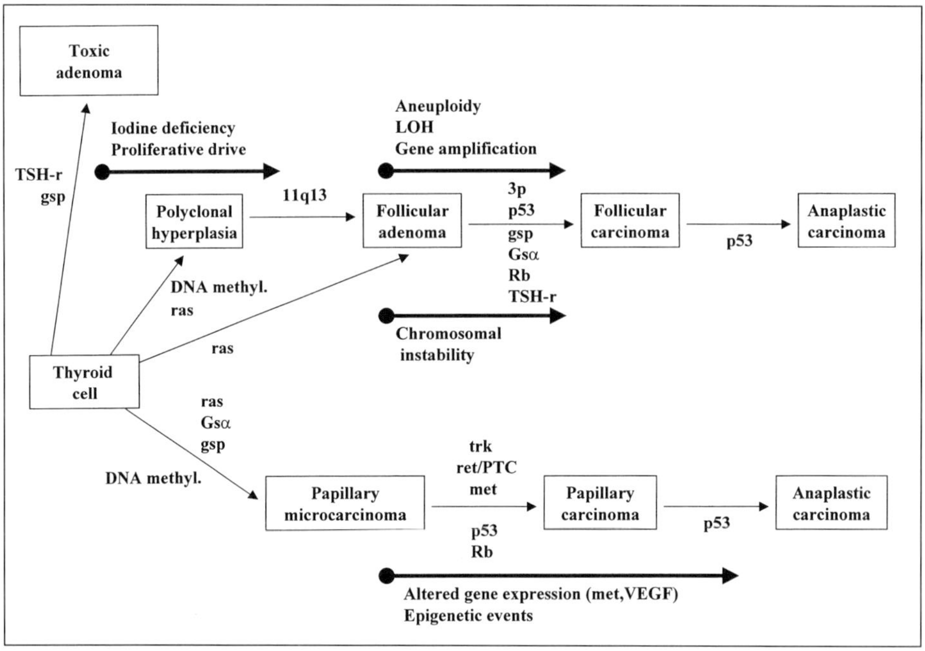

Fig. 1 Adenoma-carcinoma sequence: genetic, epigenetic and chromosomal aberrations in the pathogenesis of follicular and papillary thyroid carcinomas from the normal cell to anaplastic dedifferentiation.

References

1. Fagin JA. 1998 Molecular pathogenesis of tumors of thyroid follicular cells. In: Fagin JA, ed. Thyroid Cancer. Boston: Kluwer Academic Publishers; 59–84.
2. Shingu K, Sugenoya A, Itoh N, Kato R. 1994 Expression of basic fibroblast growth factor in thyroid disorders. World J Surg 18:500–505.
3. Eggo MC, Hopkins JM, Franklyn JA, Johnson GD, Sanders DS, Sheppard MC. 1995 Expression of fibroblast growth factors in thyroid cancer. J Clin Endocrinol Metab 80:1006–1011.
4. Viglietto G, Maglione D, Rambaldi M, et al. 1995 Upregulation of vascular endothelial growth factor (VEGF) and downregulation of placenta growth factor (PlGF) associated with malignancy in human thyroid tumors and cell lines. Oncogene 11:1569–1579.
5. Soh EY, Duh QY, Sobhi SA, et al. 1997 Vascular endothelial growth factor expression is higher in differentiated thyroid cancer than in normal or benign thyroid. J Clin Endocrinol Metab 82:3741–3747.
6. Derwahl M, Studer H. 1998 Pathogenesis and treatment of multinodular goiter. In: Fagin JA, ed. Thyroid Cancer. Boston: Kluwer Academic Publishers; 155–186.
7. Derwahl M, Broecker M, Kraiem Z. 1999 Clinical review 101: Thyrotropin may not be the dominant growth factor in benign and malignant thyroid tumors. J Clin Endocrinol Metab 84:829–834.
8. Doolittle RF, Hunkapiller MW, Hood LE, et al. 1983 Simian sarcoma virus onc gene, v-sis, is derived from the gene (or genes) encoding a platelet-derived growth factor. Science 221:275–277.
9. Broecker M, Hammer J, Derwahl M. 1998 Excessive activation of tyrosine kinases leads to inhibition of proliferation in a thyroid carcinoma cell line. Life Sci 63:2373–2386.

10. Haugen DR, Akslen LA, Varhaug JE, Lillehaug JR. 1993 Demonstration of a TGF-alpha-EGF-receptor autocrine loop and c-myc protein over-expression in papillary thyroid carcinomas. Int J Cancer 55:37–43.
11. van der Laan BF, Freeman JL, Asa SL. 1995 Expression of growth factors and growth factor receptors in normal and tumorous human thyroid tissues. Thyroid 5:67–73.
12. Studer H, Derwahl M. 1995 Mechanisms of nonneoplastic endocrine hyperplasia – a changing concept: a review focused on the thyroid gland. Endocr Rev 16:411–426.
13. Downward J, Yarden Y, Mayes E, et al. 1984 Close similarity of epidermal growth factor receptor and v-erb-B oncogene protein sequences. Nature 307:521–527.
14. Slamon DJ, Godolphin W, Jones LA, et al. 1989 Studies of the HER-2/neu proto-oncogene in human breast and ovarian cancer. Science 244:707–712.
15. Di Renzo MF, Olivero M, Ferro S, et al. 1992 Overexpression of the c-MET/HGF receptor gene in human thyroid carcinomas. Oncogene 7:2549–2553.
16. Belfiore A, Gangemi P, Costantino A, et al. 1997 Negative/low expression of the Met/hepatocyte growth factor receptor identifies papillary thyroid carcinomas with high risk of distant metastases. J Clin Endocrinol Metab 82:2322–2328.
17. Sanicola M, Hession C, Worley D, et al. 1997 Glial cell line-derived neurotrophic factor-dependent RET activation can be mediated by two different cell-surface accessory proteins. Proc Natl Acad Sci U S A 94:6238–6243.
18. Grieco M, Santoro M, Berlingieri MT, et al. 1990 PTC is a novel rearranged form of the ret proto-oncogene and is frequently detected in vivo in human thyroid papillary carcinomas. Cell 60:557–563.
19. Giannini R, Salvatore G, Monaco C, et al. 2000 Identification of a novel subtype of H4-RET rearrangement in a thyroid papillary carcinoma and lymph node metastasis [In Process Citation]. Int J Oncol 16:485–489.
20. Bongarzone I, Monzini N, Borrello MG, et al. 1993 Molecular characterization of a thyroid tumor-specific transforming sequence formed by the fusion of ret tyrosine kinase and the regulatory subunit RI alpha of cyclic AMP-dependent protein kinase A. Mol Cell Biol 13:358–366.
21. Santoro M, Dathan NA, Berlingieri MT, et al. 1994 Molecular characterization of RET/PTC3; a novel rearranged version of the RETproto-oncogene in a human thyroid papillary carcinoma. Oncogene 9:509–516.
22. Klugbauer S, Lengfelder E, Demidchik EP, Rabes HM. 1996 A new form of RET rearrangement in thyroid carcinomas of children after the Chernobyl reactor accident. Oncogene 13:1099–1102.
23. Klugbauer S, Demidchik EP, Lengfelder E, Rabes HM. 1998 Molecular analysis of new subtypes of ELE/RET rearrangements, their reciprocal transcripts and breakpoints in papillary thyroid carcinomas of children after Chernobyl. Oncogene 16:671–675.
24. Cheung CC, Ezzat S, Ramyar L, Freeman JL, Asa SL. 2000 Molecular basis off hurthle cell papillary thyroid carcinoma. J Clin Endocrinol Metab 85:878–882.
25. Greco A, Pierotti MA, Bongarzone I, Pagliardini S, Lanzi C, Della Porta G. 1992 TRK-T1 is a novel oncogene formed by the fusion of TPR and TRK genes in human papillary thyroid carcinomas. Oncogene 7:237–242.
26. Bongarzone I, Fugazzola L, Vigneri P, et al. 1996 Age-related activation of the tyrosine kinase receptor protooncogenes RET and NTRK1 in papillary thyroid carcinoma. J Clin Endocrinol Metab 81:2006–2009.
27. Derwahl M. 1996 Molecular aspects of the pathogenesis of nodular goiters, thyroid nodules and adenomas. Exp Clin Endocrinol Diabetes 104 Suppl 4:32–35.
28. Matsuo K, Friedman E, Gejman PV, Fagin JA. 1993 The thyrotropin receptor (TSH-R) is not an oncogene for thyroid tumors: structural studies of the TSH-R and the alpha-subunit of Gs in human thyroid neoplasms. J Clin Endocrinol Metab 76:1446–1451.
29. Russo D, Arturi F, Schlumberger M, et al. 1995 Activating mutations of the TSH receptor in differentiated thyroid carcinomas. Oncogene 11:1907–1911.
30. Medema RH, Bos JL. 1993 The role of p21ras in receptor tyrosine kinase signaling. Crit Rev Oncog 4:615–661.
31. Farid NR, Shi Y, Zou M. 1994 Molecular basis of thyroid cancer. Endocr Rev 15:202–232.

32. Shi YF, Zou MJ, Schmidt H, et al. 1991 High rates of ras codon 61 mutation in thyroid tumors in an iodide-deficient area. Cancer Res 51:2690–2693.
33. Fusco A, Berlingieri MT, Di Fiore PP, Portella G, Grieco M, Vecchio G. 1987 One- and two-step transformations of rat thyroid epithelial cells by retroviral oncogenes. Mol Cell Biol 7:3365–3370.
34. Lyons J, Landis CA, Harsh G, et al. 1990 Two G protein oncogenes in human endocrine tumors. Science 249:655–659.
35. Esapa C, Foster S, Johnson S, Jameson JL, Kendall-Taylor P, Harris PE. 1997 G protein and thyrotropin receptor mutations in thyroid neoplasia. J Clin Endocrinol Metab 82:493–496.
36. Doree M, Galas S. 1994 The cyclin-dependent protein kinases and the control of cell division. Faseb J 8:1114–1121.
37. Chen PL, Scully P, Shew JY, Wang JY, Lee WH. 1989 Phosphorylation of the retinoblastoma gene product is modulated during the cell cycle and cellular differentiation. Cell 58:1193–1198.
38. Zou M, Shi Y, Farid N. 1994 Frequent inactivation of the retinoblastoma gene in human thyroid carcinoma. Endocrinol J 2:193.
39. Zou M, Shi Y, Farid NR, al-Sedairy ST. 1998 Inverse association between cyclin D1 overexpression and retinoblastoma gene mutation in thyroid carcinomas. Endocrine 8:61–64.
40. Greenblatt MS, Bennett WP, Hollstein M, Harris CC. 1994 Mutations in the p53 tumor suppressor gene: clues to cancer etiology and molecular pathogenesis. Cancer Res 54:4855–4878.
41. Cross SM, Sanchez CA, Morgan CA, et al. 1995 A p53-dependent mouse spindle checkpoint. Science 267:1353–1356.
42. Levine AJ, Perry ME, Chang A, et al. 1994 The 1993 Walter Hubert Lecture: the role of the p53 tumour-suppressor gene in tumorigenesis. Br J Cancer 69:409–416.
43. el-Deiry WS, Harper JW, O'Connor PM, et al. 1994 WAF1/CIP1 is induced in p53-mediated G1 arrest and apoptosis. Cancer Res 54:1169–1174.
44. Fagin JA, Matsuo K, Karmakar A, Chen DL, Tang SH, Koeffler HP. 1993 High prevalence of mutations of the p53 gene in poorly differentiated human thyroid carcinomas. J Clin Invest 91:179–184.
45. Jones CJ, Shaw JJ, Wyllie FS, Gaillard N, Schlumberger M, Wynford-Thomas D. 1996 High frequency deletion of the tumour suppressor gene P16INK4a (MTS1) in human thyroid cancer cell lines. Mol Cell Endocrinol 116:115–119.
46. Shi Y, Zou M, Farid NR, al-Sedairy ST. 1996 Evidence of gene deletion of p21 (WAF1/CIP1), a cyclin-dependent protein kinase inhibitor, in thyroid carcinomas. Br J Cancer 74:1336–1341.
47. Bissonnette RP, Echeverri F, Mahboubi A, Green DR. 1992 Apoptotic cell death induced by c-myc is inhibited by bcl-2. Nature 359:552–554.
48. Brocker M, de Buhr I, Papageorgiou G, Schatz H, Derwahl M. 1996 Expression of apoptosis-related proteins in thyroid tumors and thyroid carcinoma cell lines. Exp Clin Endocrinol Diabetes 104 Suppl 4:20–23.
49. Branet F, Brousset P, Krajewski S, et al. 1996 Expression of the cell death-inducing gene bax in carcinomas developed from the follicular cells of the thyroid gland. J Clin Endocrinol Metab 81:2726–2730.
50. Baylin SB, Herman JG, Graff JR, Vertino PM, Issa JP. 1998 Alterations in DNA methylation: a fundamental aspect of neoplasia. Adv Cancer Res 72:141–196.
51. Herman JG, Merlo A, Mao L, et al. 1995 Inactivation of the CDKN2/p16/MTS1 gene is frequently associated with aberrant DNA methylation in all common human cancers. Cancer Res 55:4525–4530.
52. Matsuo K, Tang SH, Zeki K, Gutman RA, Fagin JA. 1993 Aberrant deoxyribonucleic acid methylation in human thyroid tumors. J Clin Endocrinol Metab 77:991–995.
53. Nikiforov YE, Nikiforova M, Fagin JA. 1998 Prevalence of minisatellite and microsatellite instability in radiation-induced post-Chernobyl pediatric thyroid carcinomas. Oncogene 17:1983–1988.
54. Joensuu H, Klemi P, Eerola E, Tuominen J. 1986 Influence of cellular DNA content on survival in differentiated thyroid cancer. Cancer 58:2462–2467.
55. Ward LS, Brenta G, Medvedovic M, Fagin JA. 1998 Studies of allelic loss in thyroid tumors reveal major differences in chromosomal instability between papillary and follicular carcinomas. J Clin Endocrinol Metab 83:525–530.

Session IV:

Environment and non-autoimmune hyperthyroidism

Chairpersons: J. Leclère, G. Gerasimov

Epidemiological evidence of iodine deficiency as risk determinant for non-autoimmune hyperthyroidism

P. Laurberg

Dept. of Endocrinology and Medicine, Aalborg Hospital, DK-9000 Aalborg, Denmark

Abstract

Iodine is an essential component of thyroid hormones, but is also a major regulator of thyroid growth and function. The most common abnormalities leading to thyroid disease are autonomous nodular growth of follicular tissue and thyroid autoimmunity. Both processes are influenced by the iodine intake level. Hence it is not surprising that the iodine intake of a population has a major effect on the epidemiology of thyroid diseases.

Epidemiological studies comparing areas with long standing low and high population iodine intake demonstrate that low iodine intake with mild to moderate iodine deficiency is associated with a high prevalence of subclinical hyperthyroidism and a high incidence of clinical hyperthyroidism in elderly subjects. This is caused by autonomous multifocal growth and function of the thyroid gland. In addition there is a high frequency of clinical goiter in elderly females. In a high iodine area, on the other hand, there is a high prevalence of subclinical hypothyroidism in the elderly and an earlier onset of autoimmune hyperthyroidism.

The population iodine intake should probably be high enough to avoid iodine deficiency related disorders, but not much higher.

Introduction

A number of mechanisms allow the normal thyroid gland to compensate for large differences in iodine intake and still deliver the optimal amount of thyroid hormone for growth and development and for maintenance of metabolism (1, 2).

The abnormal thyroid gland, on the other hand, whether affected by autoimmunity or proliferative abnormalities is less able to adapt to changes in iodine intake and thyroid hyperfunction or hypofunction may develop (3). In addition iodine intake may modulate the basic thyroid disease mechanisms involved in multifocal nodular follicular cell proliferation and thyroid autoimmunity (4, 5). Hence it is to be expected that the population iodine intake level would influence the epidemiology of thyroid disorders.

Alterations in population iodine intake and the epidemiology of hyperthyroidism

It has been demonstrated convincingly in many areas that a sudden increase in iodine intake from low to a normal or a high level is accompanied by a several- to manyfold increase in the incidence of hyperthyroidism (6, 7). The main mechanism seems to be uncontrolled thyroid hormone synthesis and release from autonomous thyroid nodules developed during the previous period of low iodine intake. Accordingly the surge of hyperthyroidism tends to diminish and gradually disappear within a number of years (7).

The mechanism behind the development of a mixture of mono- and polyclonal multifocal nodules in the thyroid gland when iodine intake is low is unclear (8). Some of the nodular alterations show an increase in activity despite suppression of serum TSH, while other areas are inactive. It is not known when in life this multifocal alteration is induced. However, once it has developed it seems to continue despite an increase in iodine intake (9, 10).

Hence recent alterations in the iodine intake level of a population may hamper the evaluation of the long-term relation between iodine intake and the epidemiology of thyroid disorders. The iodine intake has changed considerably in many countries because of iodine supplementation programs, addition of iodine to animal feeds, and the use of iodine containing chemicals in the food industry (11, 12).

Iodine intake in Iceland and Denmark

Iceland and Denmark are well suited for comparative epidemiological studies of the effect of different levels of iodine intake. In Iceland, iodine intake has been stable and high for many years, of the order of 300 μg/day (13), primarily because of a high intake of fish and the use of fish meal for domestic animal feeding. In Denmark the iodine intake has been stable and low for the lifetime of the inhabitants with mild to moderate iodine deficiency in Jutland (iodine intake 40–70 μg/day) and mild iodine deficiency in Sealand (70–110 μg/day) (14). The geographical difference is due to a difference in ground water iodine content (15). The two areas have similar levels of socioeconomic development and health care and a similar genetic background (16).

Iodine intake and the incidence of hyperthyroidism

The incidence of various types of hyperthyroidism was studied in a comparative epidemiological investigation (JUICE 1) (17). The two cohorts investigated were the entire population of Iceland (n = 229,114) and the population of a well defined area in Eastern-Jutland (n = 284,554). The population-years observed were 1,264,450. Information on new cases of hyperthyroidism was obtained by contacting all hospitals and practitioners in the areas diagnosing and treating patients with hyperthyroidism. Hyperthyroidism was significantly (1.6 times) more common in Jutland with a low iodine intake than in Iceland with a high iodine intake (Table 1). However, much larger differences are observed when evaluating the data in detail (Figure 1). Figure 1 shows the relative contribution of the four most common nosologic types of hyperthyroidism in the two areas. In Iceland, where iodine intake is high, autoimmune hyperthyroidism (Graves' disease) was absolutely dominant with few cases of solitary toxic adenoma, multinodular toxic goiter and subacute thyroiditis. In Jutland, where iodine intake is low, the most common cause of hyperthyroidism was multinodular toxic goiter. Autoimmune hyperthyroidism was less common compared to Iceland. When studying the data in detail, this difference was mainly due to a delay of 10–20 years in the onset of autoimmune hyperthyroidism in Jutland. The incidence of hyperthyroidism due to a solitary toxic adenoma or to subacute thyroiditis did not differ much between the two areas.

Age dependent incidences of hyperthyroidism are shown in Figure 2. Among young subjects, hyperthyroidism was 2–3 times more common in Iceland, primarily because of an earlier onset of autoimmune hyperthyroidism. On the other hand hy-

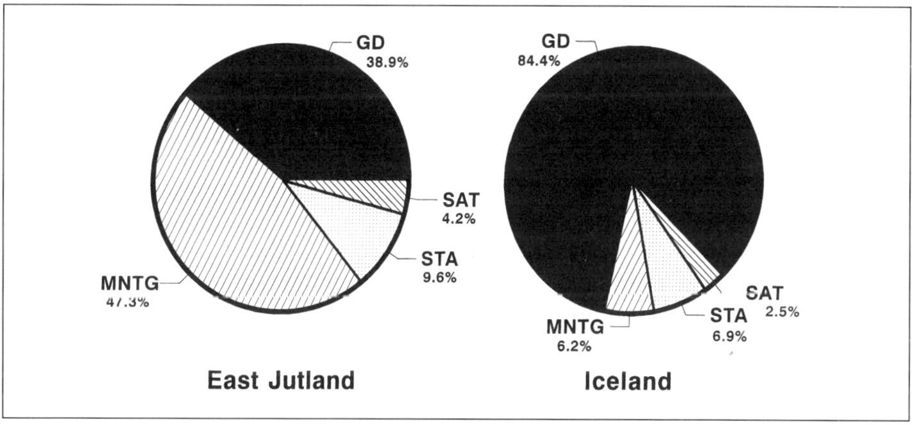

Fig. 1 The relative contribution of the four most common nosologic types of hyperthyroidism in East-Jutland with mild to moderate iodine deficiency and in Iceland with a high iodine intake. Modified from (17).

Table 1 Incidence of hyperthyroidism per 100,000 inhabitants per year.

	All types	Graves' disease	Multi-nodular goiter	Single toxic adenoma	Thyroiditis
East-Jutland	38.7	14.8	18.0	3.6	1.6
Iceland	23.6	19.7	1.5	1.6	0.6
p-value	< 0.001	< 0.05	< 0.001	< 0.05	NS

perthyroidism was much more common among elderly subjects in the low iodine intake areas, the prime cause being multinodular toxic goiter.

Iodine intake and the prevalence rate of hyper- and hypothyroidism among elderly subjects

The major difference in the incidence of hyperthyroidism in elderly subjects found in JUICE 1 led to a study comparing the prevalence rates of thyroid function abnormalities in the elderly in the two areas with high and low iodine intake (JUICE 3) (18).

Random population samples of 68 year-old subjects from Iceland and Jutland were investigated (n = 523) and thyroid function studied by measuring TSH and thy-

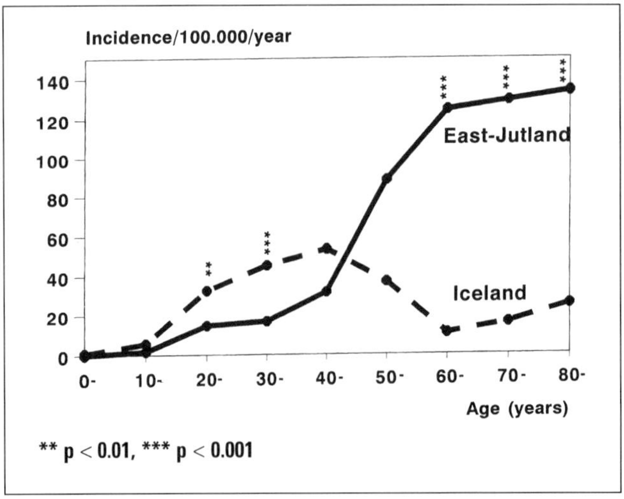

Fig. 2 Age dependent incidences of hyperthyroidism in East-Jutland (low iodine intake) and Iceland (high iodine intake). The high incidence in the young and middle aged in Iceland was mainly due to earlier onset (by 10–20 years) of autoimmune hyperthyroidism. The surge of hyperthyroidism in the elderly in East-Jutland was due to a high incidence of multinodular toxic goiter. Modified from (17).

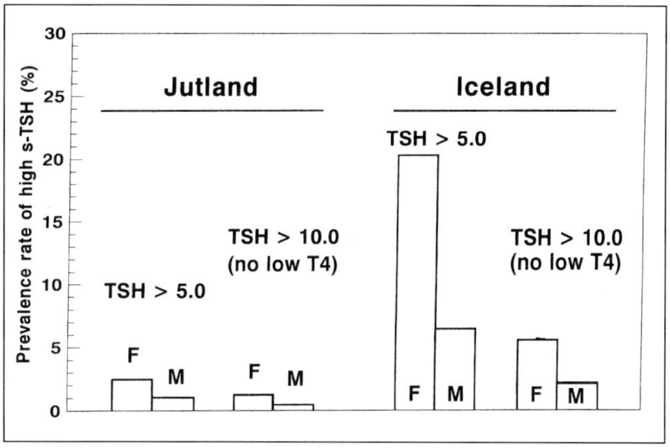

Fig. 6 Prevalence of thyroid hypofunction with elevated TSH in 68 years old subjects from East-Jutland and Iceland. High TSH was significantly more common in Iceland ($p < 0.01$). Modified from (18).

develop by two mechanisms. One is a gradual increase in size and function of the autonomous tissue over years. The other is a sudden iodine load with an increase in substrate for thyroid hormone synthesis. Accordingly hyperthyroidism is a common complication of investigations using iodine containing radio-contrast agents or of intake of iodine containing medication in low iodine intake areas (21–23). This is less common in high iodine intake areas (23).

Conclusion

The main consequences of low iodine intake with mild to moderate iodine deficiency for public health are a high prevalence of goiter and multifocal thyroid nodularity in middle aged and elderly subjects with a high incidence of multinodular toxic goiter in the elderly. On the other hand autoimmune hyperthyroidism manifest later in life, and the prevalence of impaired thyroid function is lower than in a high iodine intake area. The optimal level of iodine intake for achieving the lowest rate of thyroid abnormalities in a population remains to be defined. Iodine intake should probably be high enough to avoid iodine deficiency disorders but not much higher.

References

1. Wolff J, Chaikoff IL 1948 Plasma inorganic iodide as a homeostatic regulator of thyroid function. J Biol Chem 174:555–64.
2. Escobar Del Rey F, Mallol J, Pastor R, Morreale de Escobar G 1987 Effects of maternal iodine deficiency on thyroid hormone economy of lactating dams and pups: Maintenance of normal cerebral 3,5,3'-triiodo-L-thyronine concentrations in pups during major phases of brain development. Endocrinology 121:803–11.

3. Roti E, Vagenakis AG 1996 Effect of excess iodide: Clinical aspects. In: Braverman LE, Utiger R, eds. Werner and Ingbar's the Thyroid: A fundamental and clinical text. Philadelphia: Lippincott-Raven Publishers, p 316–27.
4. Sundick R, Bagchi N, Brown TR 1992 The role of iodine in thyroid autoimmunity: from chickens to humans: a review. Autoimmunity 13:61–8.
5. Safran M, Paul TL, Roti E, Braverman LE 1987 Environmental factors affecting autoimmune thyroid disease. Endocrinol Metab Clin North Am 16:327–42.
6. Schröder F 1989 Hyperthyreosemanifestation vor und nach alimentärer jodkomplettierung. Verlaufsuntersuchungen in Brandenburg 1983–1988. Z Gesamte Inn Med 44:229–32.
7. Connolly RJ 1973 The changing age incidence of Iodbasedow in Tasmania. Med J Aust 2:171–4.
8. Kopp P, Kimura ET, Aeschimann S, Oestreicher M, Tobler A, Fey MF, Studer H 1994 Polyclonal and monoclonal thyroid nodules coexist within human multinodular goiters. J Clin Endocrinol Metab 79:134–9.
9. Barker DJP, Philips DIW 1984 Current incidence of thyrotoxicosis and past prevalence of goiter in 12 British towns. Lancet ii:567–70.
10. Phillips DIW, Barker DJP, Rees Smith B , Didcote S, Morgan D 1985 The geographical distribution of thyrotoxicosis in England according to the presence or absence of TSH-receptor antibodies. Clin Endocrinol 23:283–287.
11. Phillips DI 1997 Iodine, milk, and the elimination of endemic goiter in Britain: the story of an accidental public health triumph. J Epidemiol Community Health 51:391–393.
12. Hollowell JG, Staehling NW, Hannon WH, Flanders DW, Gunter EW, Maberly GF, Bravermann LE, Pino S, Miller DT, Garbe PL, DeLozier DM, Jackson RJ 1998 Iodine nutrition in the United States. Trends and public health implications: Iodine excretion data from National Health and Nutrition Examination Surveys I and III (1971–1974 and 1988–1994). J Clin Endocrinol Metab 83:3401–08.
13. Sigurdsson G, Franzson L 1988 Urine excretion of iodine in an Icelandic population. Icelandic Med J 74:179–181.
14. Pedersen KM, Nøhr SB, Laurberg P 1997 Iodine intake in Denmark. Ugeskr Læger 159: 2201–06.
15. Pedersen KM, Laurberg P, Nøhr S, Jørgensen A, Andersen S 1999 Iodine in drinking water varies by more than 100-fold in Denmark. Importance for iodine content of infant formulas. Eur J Endocrinol 140:400–03.
16. Ryder LP, Andersen E, Svejgaard A 1978 An HLA map of Europe. Human Hered 28: 171–200.
17. Laurberg P, Pedersen KM, Vestergaard H, Sigurdsson G 1991 High incidence of multinodular toxic goiter in the elderly population in a low iodine intake area vs. high incidence of Graves' disease in the young in a high iodine intake area: comparative surveys of thyrotoxicosis epidemiology in East-Jutland Denmark and Iceland. J Intern Med 229:45–420.
18. Laurberg P, Pedersen KM, Hreidarsson A, Sigfusson N, Iversen E, Knudsen PR 1998 Iodine intake and the pattern of thyroid disorders: a comparative epidemiological study of thyroid abnormalities in the elderly in Iceland and in Jutland, Denmark. J Clin Endocrinol Metab 83:765–9.
19. Laurberg P, Bülow Pedersen I, Pedersen KM, Vestergaard H 1999 Low incidence rate of overt hypothyroidism compared with hyperthyroidism in an area with moderately low iodine intake. Thyroid 9:33–8.
20. Szabolcs I, Podoba J, Feldkamp J, Dohán O, Farkas I, Sajgó M, Takáts K, Góth M, Kovács L, Kressinszky K, Hnilia P, Szilágyi G 1997 Comparative screening for thyroid disorders in old age in areas of iodine deficiency, long-term iodine prophylaxis and abundant iodine intake. Clin Endocrinol 47:87–92.
21. Nolte, Muller R, Siggelkow H, Emrich D, Hufner M 1996 Prophylactic application of thyrostatic drugs during excessive iodine exposure in euthyroid patients with thyroid autonomy: a randomized study. Eur J Endocrinol 134:337–41.
22. Hintze G, Blombach O, Fink H, Burkhardt U, Kobberling J 1999 Risk of iodine-induced thyrotoxicosis after coronary angiography: an investigation in 788 unselected subjects. Eur J Endocrinol 140:264–7.
23. Martino E, Safran M, Aghini-Lombardi F, Rajatanavin R, Lenziardi M, Fay M, Pacchiarotti A, Aronin N, Macchia E, Haffajee C, et al 1984 Environmental iodine intake and thyroid dysfunction during chronic Amiodarone therapy. Ann Intern Med 110:28–34.

Molecular mechanism for induction of thyroid autonomy by iodine deficiency

C. Balázs

III. Department of Medicine, Kenézy Teaching Hospital, 4043 Debrecen, Hungary

Abstract

Thyroid autonomy is defined as the supranormal functioning of thyroid follicular cells in the absence of thyrotropin (TSH). The molecular basis for TSH- independent growth and function has been found by presenting somatic and germline activating mutations in $G_s\alpha$ and TSH-R genes. The activating mutations (constitutive mutations) may represent either activation of stimulatory factors (such as increased cAMP) in a regulation cascade or inactivation of negative factor(s) (inhibition of cAMP phosphodiesterases). It has been postulated that mutations in the TSH-R gene may account for more than 80 % of all toxic adenomas, the remaining cases being caused by $G_s\alpha$ mutations. Most mutations have been found in the third intracellular loop and the sixth transmembrane domain of the TSH-R and rarely in the other loops of transmembrane regions. The relatively large number of mutations in the TSH-R suggests that its special molecular structure might be responsible for the increased mutability rate. In general, certain mutations in the ectodomain and proximal transmembrane domain appear to be specific for germline mutations as opposed to somatic mutations. Thus, mutations at codon 183, 505, 509 and 597 are exclusive to germline mutations. However, those at codons 630 and 633 are limited to somatic mutations. On the other hand, several mutations in codons 619–633 (the mutation cluster region) represent mutational "hot-spots" for both. Furthermore, iodine may modulate ras oncogene mutations and thus play an important, but nonspecific, role in the initiation and/or maintenance of follicular adenomas. However, additional epigenetic factors are also needed. These epigenetic factors, including apoptosis (programmed cell death), are able to trigger cell suicide by a molecule called Fas found on the surface of thyrocytes. It has been observed that both TSH and iodine are able to inhibit Fas-mediated apoptosis in a dose-dependent manner. It was concluded that the molecular mechanisms of thyroid toxic autonomic nodules consist of a multistep process. The first step is high intrinsic mutability. The second step is the increased susceptibility of TSH-R or $G_s\alpha$ genes to exogenous factors involving iodine deficiency. The third step is a possible second mutational event such as activation of one of the oncogenes (e.g. ret, trk, ras) due to selection pressure of TSH-R or $G_s\alpha$ mutation and iodine-dependent apoptosis.

Introduction

Thyroid autonomy is defined as the supranormal functioning of thyroid follicular cells in the absence of thyrotropin (TSH). This disorder may appear as a single hyperfunctioning adenoma or a toxic multinodular goiter. The autonomous functional nodules develop the ability to produce more and more thyroid hormones gradually in excess leading to subclinical and finally overt hyperthyroidism. Increased secretion of thyroid hormones by the autonomous nodules leads to inhibition of TSH secretion and consequent depressed TSH serum levels result in understimulation of the non-functioning part of thyroid gland. Thyroid autonomy can manifest as monoclonal or polyclonal forms. The frequency of thyroid autonomy rises with age (13). According to the European multicenter hyperthyroidism study, Graves' hyperthyroidism peaks between the ages of 30 and 60 years, whereas the rate of hyperthyroidism due to autonomy increases after the age of 40 years (44, 29). The epidemiological studies provide clear evidence that the prevalence of thyroid autonomy is significantly higher in iodine deficient areas (1, 36). In contrast, in regions with sufficient iodine intake of the population, these thyroid diseases are relatively rare (22, 5, 30, 40). The role of iodine depletion in the pathogenesis of goiter and thyroid autonomy is rather complex (21). The classical view is that any shortage of iodine supply will decrease thyroid hormone secretion by intrathyroidal autoregulation, thereby increasing TSH long before the thyroid gland becomes significantly depleted of iodine (40). Recent molecular biological and genetic studies have provided new insights into the complex mechanism of induction of thyroid autonomy. This minireview has attempts to summarize, with no claim to comprehensiveness, some of major trends in molecular mechanism of iodine deficiency in thyroid autonomy.

Pathophysiological considerations

Thyroid follicular cells are highly differentiated, having evolved a highly efficient system for concentrating iodide for the synthesis, storage and release of thyroid hormones, under basal conditions as well as conditions of increased need. Unlike many other highly specialized cells, thyrocytes are not irreversibly terminally differentiated. When they proliferate in response to certain growth signals they may temporarily lose their ability to concentrate iodide. Surprisingly, the thyroid cell turns over, on average, no more than five or six times through adulthood (19). Due to inhomogeneity of the growth potential of thyrocytes and their variable sensitivity to stimulatory signals, a proportion of these cells may well turn over much more than five times. Cycles of cell division may be more frequent in benign or malignant tumors (50). Therefore, an appreciation of the physiological and pathophysiological factors involved in normal thyroid cell growth, signaling, and differentiation is necessary for understanding thyroid autonomy. Functional and morphologic heterogeneity of "hot" nodules has been studied by transplanting them into nude mice. "Hot" transplants had higher autonomous iodine uptake than did cold tissue in TSH suppressed hosts (39). It is well established that TSH and iodine are two opposing regulating agents. TSH exerts its action on thyrocytes via specific receptor sites restricted to the basal membranes of thyroid cells. It has become clear that the TSH-receptor (TSH-R) is a plasma membrane site able to bind G (guanine nucleotide-binding) protein for signal transduction (28). The current models of TSH-R indicate that the human TSH-R is a heptahelical glycoprotein molecule with an extremely large extracellular domain at the N-terminus, a transmembrane/intracellular region consisting of seven intramembrane helices connected by three alternating intracellular and extracellular loops, and an intracellular tail at the carboxyl terminus (56). The extracellular domain is the ligand-binding site, and its structure is highly specific for recognition and binding of TSH, distinguishing it from other G-protein-coupled receptors. The three extracellular loops are known to help the ligand to fit to the tertiary structure, while the intramembrane and intracellular domains appear to be critical for signal transduction (34). TSH has been shown to stimulate more than one signal transduction pathway via TSH-R in the regulation of both growth and differentiation (17). The binding of TSH to the TSH-R involves structural changes in the receptor, activating the G protein. This activation results in dissociation of the α_S subunit of the G protein ($G_S\alpha$), stimulating adenylate cyclase and increasing the intracellular concentration of cAMP. Furthermore, the TSH-R is able to activate the other phosphatidyl-inositol-Ca^{2+} pathway. It is generally accepted that cAMP accounts for the stimulating and mitogenic effects of TSH, mediated by the activation of cAMP-dependent kinases. It is important, however, that higher concentration of TSH and more prolonged stimulation of the cAMP cascade are necessary to induce cell proliferation than for expression of differentiated function (45).

There is accumulating evidence that iodine has complex autoregulatory functions within the thyroid gland (13). Excess iodine inhibits both the synthesis and secretion of thyroid hormones. This protective mechanism ensures that excess of the substrate does not lead to hyperthyroidism. Deficiency of iodine results in stimulation of thyrocytes by two mechanisms. It acts directly by increasing sensitivity to TSH through removal of iodine inhibition, and indirectly by an enhanced TSH level (7). Interestingly, recent data indicate that other trace elements including selenium have additional effects on iodine deficiency. Köhrle found that long-term, severe strong selenium deficiency leads to necrosis and fibrosis after large iodine loads in experimental animals (26).

Growth factors (insulin/ IGF-1), along with the TSH, are known to be involved in proliferation of thyrocytes (35). The experimental data suggest that a complex interaction between the phosphatidyl-inositol-Ca^{2+} and the adenyl-cyclase signal transduction mechanisms is important in regulation of thyroid growth by TSH and IGF-1 (13, 14). The mitogenic effect of TSH was studied in in vitro cultures and it was found that TSH stimulates, in a dose- and time-dependent manner, recruitment of noncycling G_0 cells into the cycling compartment, as well as entry into S phase and the entry of G_2 cells into mitosis. Recent data indicate that the follicular cell population of the thyroid gland has an intrinsic heterogeneity in relation to response to TSH (49). Studer at al hypothesized that a few subsets of stemlike thyrocytes possess increased growth potential compared with the majority of thyrocytes, and that this trait is stable and heritable (50). In this model, chronic TSH stimulation would select those preexisting ("stemlike") clones with the greatest proliferative potential without loss of function. Another possibility is prolonged stimulation of thyrocytes by TSH might increase the mutation rate and that the mutated cells are selected, resulting in hyperfunctioning and proliferating nodules (49). Both models predict that thyroid autonomy involves rare subsets of cells responsive to prolonged TSH stimulation, but they differ concerning the origin of follicular cell heterogeneity. These possibilities based on clinical observations and experimental data have provided a considerable impetus for molecular genetics studies to answer the question as to whether iodine deficiency may result in mutations.

Molecular genetic factors

The molecular basis for TSH- independent growth and function has been recently defined by presenting somatic and germline activating mutations in the $G_S\alpha$ and TSH-R genes (58, 46). Activating mutations (constitutive or gain mutations) may represent either activation of stimulatory factor (such as increased cAMP) in a regulation cascade or inactivation of negative factor(s) (such as inhibition of cAMP phospho-diesterases). Derwahl and co-workers defined four types of hyperfunctioning thyroid tissues: 1) toxic adenomas with activating mutations in the TSH-R or $G_S\alpha$ genes, 2) toxic adenomas without known mutations, 3) hyperplastic tissue derived from a toxic goiter resulting from a germline mutation of TSH-R, 4) nodular tissue of the same goiter (15, 27). It has been postulated that mutations in the TSH-R gene may account for more than 80 % of all toxic adenomas, the remaining cases being caused by $G_S\alpha$ mutations (55). The cause of this large excess of TSH-R mutations is not known. This suggests two possibilities: first, the constitutive activation of the adenylate-cyclase-cAMP pathway is more efficient at the receptor level than at the $G_S\alpha$ level (32, 38, 37), or secondly, the number of effective targets for activating mutations is much higher in the TSH-R (more than 20 locations) than in $G_S\alpha$ (56). Most mutations were

Table 1 Frequency of TSH receptor mutations in thyroid toxic adenomas

Authors	Positive samples	%
Paschke et al.	2/9	22
Takeshita et al.	1/38	3
Russo et al.	10/44	22
Porcellini et al.	11/40	27
Parma et al.	27/33	81
Derwahl et al.	6/20	30
Führer et al.	16/34	47

found in the third intracellular loop and the sixth transmembrane domain of the TSH-R and rarely in the other loops of transmembrane regions (16). More recently, intensive molecular biological analysis has been undertaken to determine and characterize these mutations. However, these studies resulted in conflicting data (Table 1). Porcellini and co-workers found TSH-R mutations in 7 out of 11 toxic adenomas and in 11 out of 40 cases (41, 43). Derwahl and Broeker found these mutations in only 6 out of 20 toxic adenomas, while, surprisingly, other investigators could not detect any mutations among 38 patients with toxic adenomas (14, 52). These discrepancies might be explained by methodological differences. However, the role of variations in iodine intake cannot be excluded because these observations were made in different regions. The next question was whether constitutive mutations might be detected in multinodular goiter. Holzapfel and co-workers screened six patients with toxic multinodular goiters for mutations in exons 9 and 10 of TSH-R gene and exons 7–10 of the $G_s\alpha$ gene. They found two different somatic TSH-R mutations (L632I and F631L) in one patient. In another patient, two different toxic nodules harbored the same TSH-R mutations (I630L), whereas only one TSH-R mutation (F631L) was identified in one of the two toxic nodules of a third patient. They concluded that both solitary adenomas and toxic multinodular goiters may arise from constitutively activating mutations of the TSH-R (23). Similar observations were made by Tonacchera and co-workers in 17 patients with multinodular toxic adenomas, and they transfected COS7 cells with wild type and mutated receptors as well. Most mutations were located in the sixth transmembrane segment, and all were heterozygotic and somatic. COS7 cells transfected with constructs harboring the mutant receptors (L629F, I630L, P639S) exhibited increased cAMP production compared with the wild type TSH-R. Interestingly, all mutated TSH-R constructs produced lower levels of expression at the cell surface, demonstrating that the increased cAMP production was not induced by overexpression of receptor (54). Other authors also found TSH-R mutations located on the sixth transmembrane segment and analyzed the characteristics of transfected wild type and mutant receptors (42). They found that the growth rates of thyroid cells expressing the wild type or various receptor mutants were similar in the presence of high TSH concentrations. Furthermore, they found no differences in the affinity of mutant receptors to TSH compared with wild type receptor. The relative potency of mutant receptors measured by cAMP accumulation was maintained in absence of, and in the presence of low and intermediate concentrations of TSH. They suggested that these constitutively activated receptors have a "priming" effect, which might explain why these cells proliferate more than control cells at low TSH concentrations.

Almost all studies concerning thyroid autonomy have tried to uncover integration of TSH-dependent signaling at the nuclear level and thyroid growth. The molecular mechanism whereby cAMP induces thyrocyte proliferation is unknown, but recent evidence suggests that the transcription factor cAMP response element binding protein (CREB) may serve as an important intermediate in the proliferative process. Brunetti and co-workers investigated the expression of CREB in normal thyroid and autonomous adenomas. In all tumors examined, the expression of the activated, phosphorylated form of CREB was markedly reduced compared with normal tissue. They found no correlation between CREB phosphorylation and either protein kinase A activity or protein phosphatase expression. They concluded that in human hyperfunctioning adenomas, the protein kinase C/ CREB system did not play a role in cell proliferation (9).

The relative large number of mutations in the TSH-R suggests that its special molecular structure might be responsible for the increased mutation rate. We therefore examined the TSH-R mutations database, updated January 1999 (24, 18). 15 germline mutations at 14 codons (Table 2) and 94 somatic activating mutations at 15 codons were identified in TSH-R. Two short deletions associated with constitutive activation were also recognized (Table 3). In general, activating mutations tend to be concentrated in the transmembrane helices and intervening loops. Certain mutations in the ectodomain and proximal transmembrane domain appear to be specific for germline mutations as opposed to somatic mutations. Thus, mutations at codon 183, 505, 509 and 597 are exclusive to germline mutations. However, those at codons 630 and 633 are limited to somatic mutations. On the other hand, several between codons 619 and 633 (the mutation cluster region) represent mutational "hot-spots" for both (18). It is interesting to note that two of the codons in the mutable distal transmembrane region stand out: 632 for its high frequency of C $\rightarrow$ T transition and 633 for the variety of mutations in all 3 codon positions. Furthermore, none of the TSH-R germline or somatic mutations involve CpG dinucleotides and, by implication, spontaneous deamination that might be an attribute of TSH-R codon usage. These data and observations indicate that the high frequency of mutations of TSH-R is dictated by the intrinsic characteristic of its structure.

Oncogenes such as c-ras, c-myc, c-fos and tumor suppressor genes have been detected in autonomous thyroid glands. Previously, we studied the ras protooncogene family in 25 patients with thyroid adenomas. Dietary iodine intake in Eastern Hungary is suboptimal, whereas in North America it is more than sufficient. We found that ras genes were more frequently activated in thyroid adenomas in Eastern Hun-

Table 2 TSH-receptor germline mutations (18). Ts and Tv refer to transitions and transversions respectively.

Number	Codons	Mutation	Nature
1	183	A ⟶ G	Ts
2	281	G ⟶ A	Ts
3	453	T ⟶ C	Ts
4	505	C ⟶ A	Tv
5	505	C ⟶ A	Tv
6	509	T ⟶ C	Ts
7	597	G ⟶ C	Tv
8	623	C ⟶ T	Ts
9	629	C ⟶ T	Tv
10	631	C ⟶ T	Ts
11	639	C ⟶ T	Ts
12	632	C ⟶ T	Ts
13	650	A ⟶ T	Tv
14	670	A ⟶ G	Ts
15	672	G ⟶ A	Ts

gary than in Newfoundland, and that frequency of activation was similar in the early stages (adenoma) and late stages (follicular carcinoma) of tumorigenesis. The ras oncogene mutation rate was significantly higher in the iodide-deficient area, being 85 % versus 17 % in adenomas. The most common mutation site was Ha-ras codon 61 with Gln → Arg substitution. Two ras mutations at codon 61 (Gln → Lys in N-ras and Gln → Arg in Ha-ras) were found in microfollicular adenoma specimens from Eastern Hungary. Russo and co-workers also described two cases with co-existence of TSH-R and ras mutation (47). We concluded that dietary iodine might modulate ras oncogene mutations, and that, in iodine deficient areas, ras oncogene activation might play an important, but not specific, role in the initiation and/or maintenance of follicular adenomas. However, additional factors are necessary to initiate mutations (19). Recently, Bouras and co-workers have confirmed in a large series the frequent occurrence of HA- ras codon 12 gene mutation both in adenomas and in carcinomas (6). However, there is still disagreement on this issue because other authors have failed to find an increased frequency of mutations in ras and other oncogenes, and have claimed that activating mutations are of no pathogenic relevance in driving thyroid tumorigenesis in iodine-deficient areas (4).

Table 3 TSH receptor somatic mutations (18). Ts, Tv and del refer respectively to transitions, transversions and deletions

Number	Codons	Mutation	Nature
1	281	G ⟶ T	Tv
2		G ⟶ A	Ts
3		G ⟶ C	Tv
4	453	T ⟶ C	Ts
5	486	C ⟶ G	Tv
6		A ⟶ T	Tv
7	586	T ⟶ C	Ts
8	619	A ⟶ G	Ts
9	Del 613		del
10	623	G ⟶ T	Tv
11		GC ⟶ AT	Ts
12		C ⟶ T	Ts
13	629	G ⟶ C	Tv
14		G ⟶ T	Ts
15	630	A ⟶ C	Tv
16	631	T ⟶ A	Tv
17		T ⟶ C	Ts
18		T ⟶ A	Tv
19	632	C ⟶ T	Ts
20		A ⟶ G	Ts
21	633	A ⟶ C	Tv
22		G ⟶ C	Tv
23		G ⟶ T	Tv
24		C ⟶ G	Tv
25		C ⟶ A	Tv
26	639	C ⟶ T	Ts
27	656	G ⟶ T	Tv
28	666	T ⟶ C	Ts
29	677	C ⟶ G	Ts
30	Del 658		del

An association of benign and malignant thyroid diseases with certain HLA alleles has been reported (19). While no association between HLA antigens and well differentiated thyroid cancer was reported among patients from an iodine-sufficient area (Newfoundland), HLA-DR1 was significantly more frequent among patients with thyroid adenomas from iodine-deficient Eastern Hungary (25). The explanation for these observations is not clear. To account for these variations in HLA association with thyroid adenomas in different geographic locations, it has been suggested that HLA -DR1 positive individuals are at increased risk for development of thyroid adenomas in iodine-deficient areas and this predisposition disappears in conditions of iodine sufficiency (3).

Although it is accepted that the mutations described in thyroid autonomy generally can bring about cellular hyperfunction and hyperthyroidism, it seems to be not sufficient to generate thyroid adenomas and nodules. Therefore, other epigenetic factor may contribute to thyroid cell growth and nodular genesis (11, 14).

Epigenetic factors

Epigenetic factors, alterations of gene(s) activity not involving mutations have proved to be important in the pathogenesis in the thyroid autonomy induced by iodine deficiency. Mutations of the TSH-R and $G_s\alpha$ genes support the concept that TSH-dependent cAMP synthesis is only one the important players in a complex growth regulating network and that TSH is not the dominant growth factor in benign and malignant thyroid tumors (14). Accumulating evidence concerning thyroid autonomy indicates that IGF-1-dependent and TSH-independent signaling may have important roles in the growth regulation of human thyroid gland. As mentioned above, excessive constitutive synthesis of IGF-1 by autocrine mechanisms is involved into abnormal growth of toxic adenomas (60). It appears that additional epigenetic mechanisms include increased expression of epidermal growth factor (EGF) receptors and fibroblast growth factor. Of particular relevance is that TGF-β is able to inhibit proliferation of thyrocytes and can induce resistance. This type of resistance is frequent in thyrocytes derived from nodular goiters and may contribute to autonomy (2).

Recently, apoptosis, programmed cell death, has been shown to be a physiological process for regulation of thyroid cell populations by elimination of unwanted thyrocytes (61). The total amount of thyroid tissue is maintained by a balance between proliferation and apoptosis of thyrocytes. Apoptosis involves complex processes influenced by various factors. One key to triggering this process of cell suicide is a molecule called Fas, found on the surface of many cells including thyrocytes. Feldkamp and co-workers studied the role of Fas-induced apoptosis in primary human thyrocytes in vitro. They observed a significant increase in apoptosis rates in normal

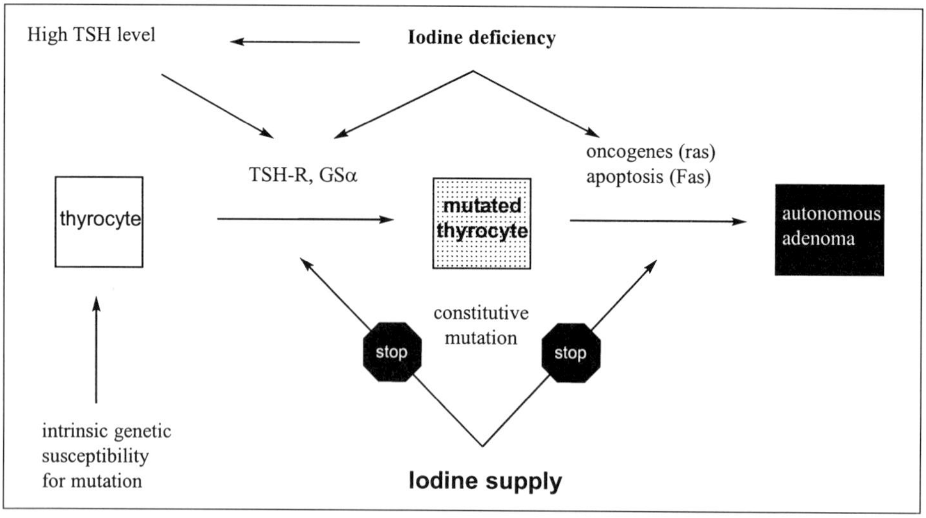

Fig. 1 The possible multistep mechanism of thyroid autonomy.

thyrocytes after incubation with anti-Fas antibody. Surprisingly, TSH was able to inhibit Fas-mediated apoptosis in a dose-dependent manner. Furthermore, low concentrations of iodine were able to inhibit apoptosis, while high concentrations of iodine increased the rate of Fas apoptosis or were cytotoxic (20, 10). Li and co-workers investigated the mechanism of apoptosis in FRTL-5 cells. FTRL-5 cells were found to undergo growth arrest in the G1 phase in the absence of TSH and TSH might thus act as a survival factor by preventing anchorage-dependent apoptosis in this in vitro system (33). Apoptosis is known to be regulated by various membrane-bound cytoplasmic proteins, including Bcl-2, BclxL and Bax (53). Recent data do not support the hypothesis that these proteins play an important role in the iodine-dependent apoptosis. Vitale and co-workers provided evidence that iodide excess induced apoptosis in an immortalized thyroid cell line (TAD-2) and primary cultures of human thyrocytes. It is important to note that this apoptosis was not influenced by inhibition of protein synthesis. In addition, inhibition of endogenous p53 activity did not affect the sensitivity of TAD-2 cells to iodide, and it was demonstrated that p53, Bcl-2, Bcl-cL and Bax protein expression did not change when these cells were treated by iodide (59).

Thyrocytes produce remarkable amounts of free oxygen radicals. Experimental data confirm that excess molecular iodide, generated by oxidation of ionic iodine by endogenous peroxidases, induces apoptosis in thyrocytes (59). This effect of reactive oxygen radicals on apoptosis might be exaggerated if the protective superoxide dismutase activity is impaired or concentrations of other potential toxic environmental elements (e.g. chromium) are increased (51, 62).

Conclusion

Finally, we conclude from the above that the pathogenesis of toxic thyroid nodules consists of a multistep process (Figure 1). The first step is high endogenous mutability, the second step is increased susceptibility of TSH-R or $G_s\alpha$ genes to exogenous factors involving iodine deficiency. The third step is a second mutational event such as activation of one of the oncogenes (e.g. ret, trk, ras) due to selection pressure of TSH-R or $G_s\alpha$ mutation and iodine-dependent apoptosis.

References

1. Aghini-Lombardi F, Antonangeli L, Martino E et al. The spectrum of thyroid disorders in an iodine-deficient community: the Pescopagano survey. J Clin Endocrinol Metab 1999; 84: 561–66.
2. Asmis LM, Kaempf J, Von Grueningen et al. Acquired and naturally occurring resistance of thyroid follicular cells to the growth inhibitory action of transforming growth factor-β1. J Endocrinol 1996; 149: 485–96.
3. Balázs Cs, Farid NR. Immunogenetics of thyroiditis and thyroid carcinoma. In: Immunogenetics of endocrine disorders. Ed. Farid NR, Alan R Liss, Inc., New York 1988:267–307.
4. Bartolone L, Vermiglio F, Finocchiraro MD, et al. Thyroid follicular oncogenesis in iodine-deficient and iodine-sufficient areas: Search for alterations of the ras, met and bFGF oncogenes and of the Rb anti-oncogene. J Endocrinol Invest 1998; 21: 680–87.
5. Bauch K. Epidemiology of functional autonomy. Exp Clin Endocrinol Diabetes 1998; 106: Suppl.4: 16–22,
6. Bouras M, Bertholon J, Detrieux-Berger N, et al. Variability of Ha-ras (codon 12) proto-oncogene mutations in diverse thyroid cancers. Eur J Endocrinol 1998; 139: 209–16.
7. Brabant G, Bergmann P, Kirsh CM et al. Early adaptation of thyrotropin and thyroglobulin secretion to experimentally decreased iodine supply in man. Metabolism 1992; 41:1093–6.
8. Brabant G, Maenhaut C, Köhrle J, et al. Human thyrotropin receptor gene: expression in thyroid tumors and correlation to markers of thyroid differentiation and dedifferentiation. Mol Cell Endocrinol 1991: 82: R7-R12.
9. Brunetti A, Chiefari Em Filetti S, Russo D. The 3'5'-cyclic adenosine monophosphate response element binding protein (CREB) is functionally reduced in human toxic adenomas. Endocrinology, 2000; 141: 722–30.
10. Chiovato L, Martino E, Tonacchera M et al. Studies on the in vitro cytotoxic effect of amiodarone. Endocrinology 1994; 134: 2277–82.
11. Chiovato L. Treatment of hyperthyroidism. In: Thyroid International, Eds. Henneman G and Krenning E. Merck, Darmstadt, 1995, 2:1–22.
12. Corvilain B, Laurent E, Lecomte M, et al. Role of the cyclic adenosine 3'5' monophosphate and the phosphatidylinositol-Ca cascades in mediating the effects of thyrotropin and iodine on hormone synthesis and secretion in human thyroid slices. J Clin Endocrinol Metab 1994; 79: 152–9.
13. Corvilain B, Sande JV, Dumont JE et al. Autonomy in endemic goitre. Thyroid 1998; 8: 107–12.
14. Derwahl M, Broecker M, Kraiem Z. Thyrotropin may not be the dominant growth factor in benign and malignant thyroid tumors. J Clin Endocrinol Metab 1999; 84: 829–34.
15. Derwahl M, Hamacker C, Russo D et al. Constitutive activation of the $G_s\alpha$ protein-adenylate cyclase pathway may not be sufficient to generate toxic adenomas. J Clin Endocrinol Metab 1996; 81:1898–1901.
16. Derwahl M. Editorial: TSH receptor and $G_s\alpha$ gene mutations in the pathogenesis of toxic adenomas. A note of caution. J Clin Endocrinol Metab 1996; 81: 2783–85.

17. Dumont JE, Lamy F, Roger P et al. Physiological and pathological regulation of thyroid cell proliferation and differentiation by thyrotropin and other factors. Physiol Rec 1992; 72: 667–97.
18. Farid NR, Kaczur V, Balázs Cs. The human thyrotropin receptor is highly mutable. Eur J Endocrinol 2000 (in press).
19. Farid NR, Shi Y, Zou M. Molecular basis of thyroid cancer. Endocr Rev 1994; 15: 202–32.
20. Feldkamp J, Pascher E, Perniok A, Scherbaum WA. Fas-mediated apoptosis is inhibited by TSH and iodine in moderate concentration in primary thyrocytes in vitro. Horm Metab Res 1999; 6: 355–58.
21. Gärtner R. Etiopathogenesis and therapy of iodine deficiency goitre. Z Arztl Fortbild (Jena) 1995; 89: 27–31
22. Hamburger JI. The autonomously functioning thyroid nodule: Goetsh's disease. Endocrine Rev 1987; 8: 439–47.
23. Holzapfel HP, Führer D, Wonerow P et al. Identification of constitutively activating somatic thyrotropin receptor mutations in a subset of toxic multinodular goiters. J Clin Endocrinol Metab 1997; 82: 4229–33.
24. Http://www.univ-leipzig-innere/TSH-R (1999)
25. Juhász F, Boros P, Balazs Cs et al. Immunogenetic and immunologic studies of differentiated thyroid cancer. Cancer 1989; 63: 1318–26.
26. Köhrle J. The trace element selenium and the thyroid gland. Biochemie 1999; 81: 527–44
27. Kopp P, van Sande J, Parma J, et al. Brief report: congenital hyperthyroidism caused by a mutation in the thyrotropin-receptor gene. N Engl J Med 1995; 332: 150–54.
28. Laugwitz KL, Allgeier A, Offermanns S, et al. The human thyrotropin receptor: a heptahelical receptor capable of stimulating members of all four G protein families. Proc Natl Acad Sci USA 1996; 93: 116–20
29. Laurberg P, Pedersen B, Pedesen I. et al. Epidemiology of thyroid dysfunction in an area with moderately low iodine intake: low incidence of hypothyroidism compared tohyperthyroidism. J Endocrinol Invest 1998; 21: 91–6.
30. Laurberg P, Pedersen KM, Hreidarsson A et al. Iodine intake and pattern of thyroid disorders: a comparative epidemiological study of thyroid abnormalities in the elderly in Iceland and in Jutland, Denmark. J Clin Endocrinol Metabolism 1998; 83: 756–69.
31. Lavard L, Sehested A, Brock Jacobsen B et al. Long-term follow-up of an infant with thyrotoxicosis due to germline mutation of the TSH receptor gene (Met453Thr). Horm Res 1999,51,43–6.
32. Ledent C, Dumont JE, Vassart G et al. Thyroid expression of an A2 adenosine receptor transgene induces thyroid hyperplasia and hyperthyroidism. EMBO J, 1992; 11: 537–42.
33. Li X, Li s, Miyagi E et al. Thyrotropin prevents apoptosis by promoting cell adhesion and cell cycle progression in FRTL-5 cells. Endocrinology 1999; 140: 5962–70.
34. Libert F, Lefort A, Gerard C et al. Cloning, sequencing and expression of the human TSH receptor: evidence for binding of autoantibodies. Biochem Biophys Res Commun 1989; 165: 1250–55.
35. Minuto F, Barreca A, delMonte P, et al. Immunoreactive insulin-like growth factors I (IGF-I) and IGF-I binding protein content in human thyroid tissue. J Clin Endocrinol Metab 1989; 68: 621–26.
36. Mostbeck A, Galva G, Bauer P et al. The incidence of hyperthyroidism in Austria from 1987 to 1995 before and after an increase in salt iodination in 1990. Eur J Nucl Med 1998; 25: 367–74.
37. Parma J, Duprez L, van Sande J et al. Diversity and prevalence of somatic mutations in the thyrotropin receptor and $G_s\alpha$ genes as a cause of toxic thyroid adenomas. J Clin Endocrinol Metab 1997; 82: 2695–2701.
38. Parma J, Duprez L, van Sande J et al. Somatic mutations in the thyrotropin receptor gene cause hyperfunctioning thyroid adenomas. Nature 1993; 365: 649–51.
39. Peter HJ, Gerber H, Studer H et al. Pathogenesis of heterogeneity in multinodular goiter. A study on growth and function of thyroid tissue transplanted onto nude mice. J Clin Invest 1985; 76: 1992–2002.
40. Pinchera A, Rago T, Vitti P. Physiopathology of iodine deficiency. Ann 1st Super Sanita 1998; 34: 301–5.
41. Porcellini A, Cuillo I, Laviola L et al. Novel mutations of thyrotropin receptor gene in thyroid hyperfunctioning adenomas. J Clin Endocrinol Metab 1994; 79: 657–661.
42. Porcellini A, Ruggiano G, Pannain S, et al. Mutations of thyrotropin receptor isolated from thyroid

autonomous functioning adenomas confer TSH-independent growth to thyroid cells. Oncoges. 1997; 15: 781–89.
43. Porcellini A, Tassi V, Cuillo I et al. Study of the prevalence of TSH receptor mutations in a large series of consecutive hyperfunctioning thyroid adenomas. Thyroid 1995, (Suppl) S8.
44. Reinwein D, Benker G, König MP et al. Hyperthyroidism in Europe. Clinical and laboratory data of a prospective multicentric survey. J Endocrinol Invest 1986; 9: 1–36.
45. Roger P, Taton M, Van Sande J et al. Mitogenetic effects of thyrotropin and adenosine 3',5'-monophosphate in differentiated normal human thyroid cells in vitro. J Clin Endocrinol Metab 1988; 66 :1158–65.
46. Russo d, Arturi F, Chiefari E et al. Thyrotropin receptor: a role for thyroid tumourgenesis? Forum Trends in Experimental and Clinical Medicine 1999; 9: 166–75.
47. Russo D, Arturi, Chiefari E et al. Activating mutations of the TSH receptor on differentiated thyroid carcinomas. Oncogene 1995; 11: 1907–11.
48. Shi Y, Zou M, Schmidt H, et al. High rates of ras codon 61 mutation in thyroid tumors in an iodide-deficient area. Cancer Res 1991; 51: 2690–93.
49. Studer H, Derwahl M. Mechanism of nonneoplastic endocrine hyperplasia – a changing concept: a review focused on thyroid gland. Endocrine Rev 1995; 15: 411–26.
50. Studer H, Peter HJ, Gerber H. Natural heterogeneity of thyroid cells: the basis for understanding thyroid function and nodular goiter growth. Endocr Rec 1989; 10: 125–35.
51. Sugawara M, Kita T, Lee ED et al. Deficiency of superoxide dismutase in endemic goiter tissue. J Clin Endocrinol Metab 1988; 67: 1156–61.
52. Takeshita A, Nagayama Y, Yokoyama N et al. Rarity of oncogenic mutations in the thyrotropin receptor of autonomously functioning thyroid nodules in Japan. J Clin Endocrinol Metab 1995; 80: 2607–11.
53. Taylor ST, Hickman JA, Dive C. Epigenetic determinants of resistance to etoposide regulation of Bcl-XL and Bax by tumor microenvironmental factors. J Natl Cancer Inst 2000; 92: 18–23.
54. Tonacchera M, Chiovato L , Pinchera A, et al. Hyperfunctioning thyroid nodules in toxic multinodular goiter share activating thyrotropin receptor mutations with solitary toxic adenoma. J Clin Endocrinol Metab 1998; 83: 492–98.
55. Van Sande J, Parma J, Tonacchera M et al. Genetic basis of endocrine disease and germline mutations of the TSH receptor gene in thyroid diseases. J Clin Endocrinol Metab 1995; 80: 2577–85.
56. Vassart G, Dumont JE. The thyrotropin receptor and regulation of thyrocyte function and growth. Endocr Rev 1992; 13: 596–611.
57. Vassart G, Parma J, Van Sande et al. The thyrotropin receptor and the regulation of thyrocyte function and growth: update. Endocrin Rev 1994; 3: 77–80.
58. Vassart G. New pathophysiological mechanism of hyperthyroidism. Horm Res 1997; 48 (Suppl4): 47–50
59. Vitale M, DiMatola T, D'Ascoli F et al. Iodide excess induces apoptosis in thyroid cells through an p53-independent mechanism involving oxidative stress. Endocrinology 2000; 141: 598–605.
60. Williams DW, Williams ED, Wynford-Thomas D. Evidence for autocrine production of IgF-1 in human thyroid adenomas. Mol Cell Endocrinol 1989; 61: 139–43.
61. Williams N. Thyroid disease: A case of cell suicide? Science 1997; 275: 926–27.
62. Ye J, Wang S, Leonard SS et al. Role of reactive oxygen species and p53 in chromium(VI) induced apoptosis. J Biol Chem 1999; 274: 34974–80.

Iodine excess and hyperthyroidism

E. Roti

Istituto di Endocrinologia, Università di Milano, Scuola di Specializzazione in Endocrinologia, Università di Parma, Via Gramsci 14, 43100 Parma, Italy

Introduction

Iodine is an essential requirement for thyroid hormone synthesis and in the adult the recommended daily iodine intake is 150 μg. In the United States, the median urinary iodine excretion is 14.5 μg/dL. Approximately 5.3 % of the population has urinary iodine (UI) > 50 μg/dL and 1.3 % UI > 100 μg/dL (1). The thyroid gland has intrinsic regulatory mechanisms that maintain normal thyroid function even in the presence of iodine excess. When large amounts of iodine are given to subjects with normal thyroid function, a transient decrease in the synthesis of the thyroid hormones occurs for approximately 48 h. This acute inhibitory effect of iodine on thyroid hormone synthesis is termed the acute Wolff-Chaikoff effect and is due to increased intrathyroidal iodine concentrations. The escape from or adaptation to the acute Wolff-Chaikoff effect is a decrease in the thyroid iodide trap, thereby decreasing the intrathyroidal iodide concentrations (2) due to a decrement of Na+/I symporter (NIS) mRNA and protein expression (3). Excess iodine ingestion (up to 150 mg/day) also decreases the release of thyroxine (T_4) and triiodothyronine (T_3) from the thyroid resulting in small decreases in serum T_4 and T_3 concentrations with compensatory increases in basal and TRH stimulated TSH concentrations, all values remaining well within the normal range (4–9). These iodine-treated subjects remained euthyroid although they ingested the excess iodide and serum thyroid hormone and TSH values returned to basal levels when the iodide was discontinued. These subtle changes in thyroid function were accompanied by increased thyroid volume assessed by echography (8, 9) and a decrease in thyroid blood flow determined by color Doppler flow imaging (10). The smallest quantity of iodine exceeding that consumed with the diet in the United States that does not affect thyroid function is 500 μg/day (11). The administration of 1 mg iodine per week for 6 weeks followed by the administration of 2 mg iodine weekly for another 6 weeks did not affect thyroid function (12). Other studies have suggested that the administration of 500 μg iodine daily induced a small but significant increment of basal and TRH stimulated serum TSH concentrations (13, 14). Ingestion of 1500 μg iodine per day for 15 days by euthyroid subjects invariably resulted in a significant decrease in serum free T_4 (FT_4) concentrations and FT_4 Index with a significant compensatory rise in basal and TRH stimulated serum TSH concentrations (11, 13, 14). Pharmacological quantities of iodine are almost always due to the administration of inorganic and organic compounds.

Sources of excess iodine

Various drugs and food preservatives contain a large quantity of iodide that is either absorbed directly or released after metabolism of the drug. Many vitamin preparations are supplemented with about 150 μg iodine, a quantity that is considered the physiologic daily requirement. Iodophors contain large quantities of iodine and are used as udder antiseptics in the dairy industry, resulting in contamination of the milk with iodine. Iodine is also concentrated by the mammary gland and secreted into the milk and, therefore, may influence thyroid function in the newborn, fed cow's milk. Many iodine-rich products, such as kelp, are available in natural food stores. In some areas of Japan, bread is made exclusively from seaweed, exposing the population to large quantities of iodine.

Iodides are present in high concentration in various proprietary and prescribed expectorants, including iodinated glycerol, Organidin, although iodine has been removed from the latter medication in the United States. Another potential source of excess iodine is the use of contrast media in radiological studies. Preparations used for computed tomography, arteriography, or pyelography are cleared from the plasma relatively quickly, but the iodine released during these procedures affects thyroid function. However, a dye commonly used for arteriography, meglumine ioxaglate (Hexabrix), did not affect serum T_4, T_3, or free T_4 index up to 56 days after catheterization although serum TSH was not measured (15). Occasionally, drinking water may be also a source of excess iodine intake such as in some Chinese counties where the drinking water had an iodine concentration of 300–462 μg/l causing urinary iodine excretion as high as 900 μg/l in the population residing in those areas (16, 17). A partial list of medications and other preparations containing large quantities of iodine is given in Table 1.

Iodide-induced hyperthyroidism

Iodide-induced hyperthyroidism is not a single etiologic entity. Since the initial description by Coindet in 1821 (18) and the subsequent definition by Breuer and Kocher in 1904, iodine-induced hyperthyroidism has been reported among patients with a variety of underlying thyroid diseases. As shown in Table 2 iodide-induced hyperthyroidism may occur in patients with iodine deficiency goiter, in euthyroid Graves' disease patients after antithyroid drug therapy, in patients with multinodular

Table 1 Commonly used iodine-containing drugs

Drugs	Iodine content
Oral or local	
Amiodarone	75 mg/tab
Benziodarone*	49 mg/l00-mg tab
Calcium iodide (e.g., Calcidrine Syrup)	26 mg/ml
Diiodohydroxyquin (e.g., Yodoxin)	134 mg/tab
Echothiophate iodide ophthalmic solution (e.g., Phospholine)	5–41 μg/drop
Hydriodic acid syrup	13–15 mg/ml
Iodochlorhydroxyquin (e.g., Entero-Vioform)	104 mg/tab
Iodine-containing vitamins	0.15 mg/tab
Iodinated glycerol (e.g., Organidin,** Iophen)	15 mg/tab, 25 mg/ml
Idoxuridine ophthalmic solution (e.g., Herplex)	18 μg/drop
Isopropamide iodide (e.g., Darbid.Combid)	1.8 mg/tab
Kelp	0.15 mg/tab
KI (e.g., Quadrinal)	145 mg/tab, 24 mg/ml
Lugol's Solution	6.3 mg/drop
Niacinamide hydroiodide + KI (e.g., Iodo-Niacin)	115 mg/tab
Ponaris nasal emollient	5 mg/0.8 ml
SSKI	38 mg/drop
Parenteral preparations	
Sodium iodide, 10% solution	85 mg/ml
Topical antiseptics	
Diiodohydroxyquin cream (e.g., Vytone)	6 mg/g
Iodine tincture	40 mg/ml
Iodochlorhydroxyquin cream (e.g., Vioform)	12 mg/g
Iodoform gauze (e.g., NuGauze)	4.8 mg/100 mg gauze
Povidone iodine (e.g., Betadine)	10 mg/ml
Radiology contrast agents	
Diatrizoate meglumine sodium (e.g., Renografin-76)	370 mg/ml
Iodized oil	380 mg/ml
Iopanoic acid (e.g., Telepaque)	333 mg/tab

Table 1 (continued)

Drugs	Iodine content
Ipodate (e.g., Oragrafin)	308 mg/cap
Iothalamate (e.g., Angio-Conray)	480 mg/m
Metrizamide (e.g., Amipaque)	483 mg/ml (before dilution)

*Not FDA approved.
**Iodine was removed from Organidin and Tuss Organidin in 1995
(Adapted from Braverman LE. Iodide-induced thyroid disease. In: Ingbar SH, Braverman LE. Eds. Werner's The Thyroid. 5th ed. Philadelphia: JB Lippincott. 1986:734)

goiters who reside in areas of iodine repletion or deficiency, and in people with no evidence of underlying thyroid disease (19–22). Recently the pathogenesis and the epidemiology of iodide-induced hyperthyroidism have been thoroughly reviewed (19, 23).

Iodide-induced hyperthyroidism in endemic iodine-deficient areas

Iodine prophylaxis has almost eliminated endemic goiter in many countries. The incidence of iodide-induced hyperthyroidism in areas previously considered iodine deficient varied from zero in Austria to 7% in Sweden after iodination programs. The incidence of iodine-induced hyperthyroidism in an endemic goiter area has been estimated to be up to 1.7% (24). The natural course of the disease was mild, and it resolved spontaneously.

Most patients who develop hyperthyroidism suffer from multinodular thyroid disease. Most are euthyroid before iodine administration, but they may have non-sup-

Table 2 Iodine-induced hyperthyroidism (Adapted from Braverman LE. Iodide-induced thyroid disease. In: Ingbar SH, Braverman LE, eds. Werner's The Thyroid, 5th ed. Philadelphia JB Lippincott. 1986:734)

- Iodine supplementation for endemic iodine-deficiency goiter
- Iodine administration to patients with euthyroid Graves' disease, especially those in remission after antithyroid drug therapy
- Nontoxic nodular goiter
- Autonomous nodule
- Nontoxic diffuse goiter
- Iodine administration to patients with no recognized underlying thyroid disease, especially in area of mild to moderate iodine deficiency

pressible radioactive iodine uptakes, low or undetectable serum TSH values and the serum TSH may fail to respond to TRH. Single oral doses of 200, 400, and 800 mg iodine administered to adult goitrous subjects residing in the Sudan induced four cases of hyperthyroidism. However, in the three groups of subjects, serum TSH concentrations below 0.1 mU/l were present in 5.9 % to 16.7 % of the cases 12 months after iodine administration (25). Similar data have been reported 2 years after iodized salt distribution in Zaire. Among 190 adult subjects with nodular goiter, 14 subjects (7.4 %) developed severe thyrotoxicosis (26). Thyroid stimulating antibodies were absent in all. Surprisingly these alterations lasted for more than 1 year (27). In Zimbabwe, following the iodination of salt at a level of 30 to 90 ppm, a threefold increase of iodide-induced hyperthyroidism was observed (28). Furthermore, in that population, fatal outcomes occurred mainly from cardiac complications. Delange et al (29) have suggested that iodine-induced hyperthyroidism occurs only when iodine deficient populations are exposed to a recent, <2 years, excessive increment of alimentary iodine intake.

It appears, therefore, that masked thyroid autonomy becomes evident when iodine repletion permits the autonomous tissue to synthesize and release excessive quantities of thyroid hormone. The importance of thyroid autonomy for the development of iodide-induced hyperthyroidism is strengthened by a report of iodide-induced hyperthyroidism in a woman with multinodular goiter treated with suppressive doses of T_4 and simultaneously exposed to high quantities of iodide (30). Attempts have been made to link these events with thyroid autoimmunity, but the results are conflicting. Long-acting thyroid stimulator (LATS) or LATS protector was found in some patients but not in others (24). In another study, no change in the incidence of thyroid autoantibodies was found after oral iodized oil administration (31).

These observations suggest that the increased incidence of hyperthyroidism in endemic areas after iodide exposure is due to an increased supply of iodine to patients with underlying macro- or micronodular disease with autonomous thyroid nodules or underlying latent Graves' disease. This is consonant with studies from Belgium and Greece (32, 33), in which the administration of small quantities of iodide (0.5 mg/d) to patients with autonomous nodules induced frank hyperthyroidism. In Austria salt iodination was doubled in 1990 to 20 mg KI per kg salt. Before that time, UI excretion ranged from 42 to 72 μg I/g creatinine (34). This change was accompanied by an increase in the incidence of overt Plummer's disease from 30.5 to 41.7 cases per 100,000 in 1992 and a more marked increment of overt Graves' disease from 10.4 to 20.9 cases per 100,000 in 1993.

Iodine-induced hyperthyroidism in iodine-sufficient areas

In regions with nonendemic euthyroid goiter, the incidence of iodine-induced hyperthyroidism is low. The prevalence of goiter in the United States is about 3.1 %. It is surprising that only a few cases have been reported since the initial report from Boston (35), where four of eight patients with goiter developed severe iodine-induced hyperthyroidism after administration of 180 mg iodide daily for several weeks. Iodine-induced hyperthyroidism has also been reported in other patients residing in the United States (21, 36). It is likely that the susceptible patients had non-suppressible thyroids.

Iodine-induced hyperthyroidism was identified in 13 of 60 hospitalized thyrotoxic elderly subjects in Australia (37, 38) and in Germany (39), after non-ionic contrast radiography. These subjects did not have positive TPO Ab and a thyroid scan revealed the presence of a multinodular goiter. In a prospective study conducted in elderly subjects, it was observed that frank hyperthyroidism was uncommon following the administration of nonionic agents, whereas subclinical hyperthyroidism was observed (40). It has been suggested that, to reduce the incidence of iodide-induced hyperthyroidism, patients with thyroid autonomy should be given prophylactic methimazole or perchlorate, starting the day before and continuing for 2 weeks after radiological contrast medium administration (41). Other authors have reported that in euthyroid, not at risk, subjects iodine-induced hyperthyroidism after coronary angiography was rare and therefore prophylactic therapy was not recommended (42). Iodide-induced thyrotoxicosis has also been described in three travelers (traveler's thyrotoxicosis) following the ingestion of iodinated preparations for water purification (43, 44). In all three cases TPO Ab were present at the time of the diagnosis of thyrotoxicosis. The large difference in the rate of occurrence of iodide-induced hyperthyroidism between iodine-deficient and iodine-replete areas is difficult to explain.

It is possible that people with increased iodine intake are "resistant" to iodine-induced hyperthyroidism because the sensitivity of the autoregulatory mechanism has changed, rendering the thyroid better able to handle the excessive quantities of iodide. In populations residing in regions of endemic goiter and exposed to excess iodide for long periods, iodide-induced hyperthyroidism is rare.

Latent Graves' disease

Antithyroid drug therapy for Graves' disease reduces thyroidal iodine content. Overt hyperthyroidism can develop only if sufficient iodine is available. It has been reported that a small increase in dietary iodine or other iodide ingestion increases the frequency of recurrence of hyperthyroidism after antithyroid drug therapy. The difference in Graves' remission rates between the United States and Europe is attributed, at least in part, to the higher iodine intake in the United States (45). Furthermore, the response to thionamide drugs is more rapid in Graves' disease patients who reside in iodine-deficient areas and the dose required to control the disease is smaller (46). It is evident, therefore, that large quantities of iodide administered to patients with latent Graves' disease may result in frank hyperthyroidism.

Consonant with this view are the observations in Graves' disease patients treated with antithyroid drugs. In one study (47), simultaneous administration of methimazole and ipodate reduced the effectiveness of the antithyroid drug. In another study, iodide administration to patients rendered euthyroid after antithyroid drug therapy was accompanied by frank hyperthyroidism in some and an absent TSH response to TRH in others (48). Excess iodide administered to hyperthyroid patients with Graves' disease significantly increased thyrotropin receptor antibody levels, suggesting that this phenomenon was responsible for iodine-induced thyroid dysfunction in predisposed subjects (49).

Unusual episodes of iodine-induced hyperthyroidism have been observed in a few patients suffering from severe burns treated with povidone iodine (50) and in a patient who had metastatic thyroid carcinoma (51).

Amiodarone-induced thyroid disease

Amiodarone, a benzofuranic derivative containing 75 mg iodine per 200-mg tablet, is widely used for the long-term treatment of cardiac arrhythmia. About 9 mg iodine is released daily during the metabolism of the drug (300-mg dose), which has a prolonged half-life of at least 100 days. Amiodarone-induced hyperthyroidism occurs in about 10% of patients residing in iodine-deficient areas (52, 53). In the United States, amiodarone-induced hyperthyroidism is far less common. These differences are attributed to increased ambient iodine intake in the United States preceding the administration of the drug (52, 54).

Amiodarone-induced thyrotoxicosis results from two different mechanisms. The iodine released during the metabolism of the drug is responsible for the thyrotoxicosis in most cases. Predisposing factors included micro- and macronodular goiter, which are common in the older patients who most often require amiodarone. Thyroid autoimmunity has also been incriminated as a predisposing factor and antithyroid antibodies have been found in some patients (55) but not in others (56). In an interesting study, the prevalence of serum thyroid-stimulating antibodies and TSH-binding inhibiting antibodies was similar to that seen in patients with spontaneous hyperthyroidism (56). Amiodarone may also induce destructive thyroiditis resulting in thyrotoxicosis as suggested by clinical, histologic, and in vitro studies (56–58). The ultra-

Table 3 Features of Amiodarone-Induced Thyrotoxicosis. Modified from Bartalena L et al. (62)

	Iodine-induced thyrotoxicosis (type I)	**Destructive thyrotoxicosis (type II)**
Underlying thyroid abnormality	Yes	No
Thyroidal RAIU	Low, normal or elevated	Low
Serum IL-6 concentrations	Slightly elevated	Markedly elevated
Cytologic findings	?	Abundant colloid, hystiocytes, vacuolated cells
Pathogenic mechanism	Excessive thyroid hormone synthesis	Excessive thyroid hormone release (destructive thyroiditis)
Response to thionamides	Poor	No
Response to perchlorate	Yes	No
Response to glucocorticoids	?	Yes
Subsequent hypothyroidism	Unlikely	Possible
Effect of excess iodine administration following the thyrotoxic phase	Likely iodine-reinduced hyperthyroidism	Possible iodine-induced hypothyroidism

structural changes of rat thyroid gland induced by amiodarone are different from those induced by excess iodine and are mediated by disruption of subcellular organelle function with marked dilation of the endoplasmic reticulum (60). The clinical and laboratory characteristics of amiodarone-induced thyrotoxicosis are presented in Table 3.

Evaluation of thyroid function is difficult in patients receiving amiodarone therapy. Serum T_4 may be elevated and serum T_3 decreased because of the blocking effect of the drug on type 5'-deiodinase, and TSH normal or slightly elevated in euthyroid subjects receiving the drug. Hyperthyroidism is best confirmed by suppressed serum TSH and elevated serum T_3 and free T_3 concentrations as well as by an increase in sex hormone-binding globulin (61). The distinction between iodine-induced hyperthyroidism (type I) and destructive thyrotoxicosis (type II) may be achieved by measurement of serum interleukin-6, which is invariably elevated in the destructive form (62) and by fine-needle biopsy, which shows cytological findings consistent with thyroiditis (58). The thyroid radioiodine uptake is always low in the destructive form and is often low in iodine-induced thyrotoxicosis but may be normal or rarely elevated. In the latter, ^{131}I therapy is a therapeutic option.

Distinction between the two forms is important for determining the most efficacious form of therapy. Amiodarone should usually be discontinued. Large doses of antithyroid drugs are recommended for iodine-induced hyperthyroidism. If this treatment fails, potassium perchlorate (250 mg three times daily) should be added (63, 64). This drug blocks the thyroid iodide trap, thereby decreasing the intrathyroidal iodide content.

In patients with destructive thyrotoxicosis, administration of large doses of corticosteroids is rapidly effective (58, 65). Normal serum T_3 concentrations were achieved after an average of eight days. Relapses are frequent as the prednisone dose is tapered (66). Surgery has been successfully used for the treatment of amiodarone-induced thyrotoxicosis (67).

After recovering from amiodarone-induced destructive thyrotoxicosis, patients may develop permanent hypothyroidism (58, 68) as a result of fibrosis of the gland (69). The iodine-perchlorate discharge test was positive in 60 % of euthyroid patients who had recovered from amiodarone-induced destructive thyrotoxicosis (70). Chronic administration of 300 mg iodide daily to these patients induced a marked increase in basal and TRH-stimulated serum TSH concentrations, which returned to normal after iodide withdrawal.

Adult patients with beta-thalassemia have also been shown to be particularly prone to develop both hyper- and hypothyroidism during amiodarone therapy for heart failure or cardiac arrhythmias (71). In view of the high incidence of thyroid dysfunction, amiodarone should be administered with caution to patients with pre-existing goiter or a history of thyroid disease. Before starting amiodarone treatment, a careful examination is required; TSH and TPO Ab values are mandatory. During amiodarone treatment, measurement of serum TSH concentrations is required approximately every six months in order to detect the development of mild thyroid disorders.

Acknowledgement

This work was supported in part by Grants 93.00405.CT04, 94.02481, CT04, 9500940, CTO4 from Consiglio Nazionale delle Ricerche (Rome, Italy) Grant "Patologia della Tiroide: Indagine dei Fattori Etiopatogenetici" of Ministero Pubblica Istruzione 40 % (Rome, Italy).

Portions of this Chapter are identical to recent works by the Roti E and Braverman LE titled "Iodine Deficiency and Thyroid Function" in the Thyroid and Iodine, Eds. Nauman J, Glinoer D, Braverman L.E. and Hostalek, U. Proceedings of the Merck European Thyroid Symposium, Warsaw, Poland pp 0.7–18 1996; Braverman L.E., Roti E. 1996 Effects of Iodine on Thyroid Function. Acta Med. Austriaca 23: 4–9; Roti E, Vagenakis AG, Effects of excess iodide: Clinical aspects in the Thyroid 7th Ed., Eds. Braverman LE, Utiger RD, Lippincott Raven, Philadelphia pp0.316–327, 1996; Roti E, Braverman LE, in Disease of the Thyroid Ed. Braverman LE, Human Press, Totowa pp. 369–387, 1997.

References

1. Hollowell JG, Staehling NW, Hannon WH, Flanders DW, Gunter EW, Maberly GF, Braverman LE, Pino S, Miller DT, Garbe PL, DeLozier DM, Jackson RJ. Iodine Nutrition in the United States. Trends and Public Health Implications: Iodine excretion data from National Health and Nutrition Examination Surveys I and III (1971–1974 and 1988–1994). J Clin Endocrinol Metab 1998; 83; 3401–3408.
2. Wolff J, Chaikoff IL, Goldberg, Meier J.R. The temporary nature of the inhibitory action of execess iodide on organic iodine synthesis in the normal thyroid. Endocrinology 1949; 45; 504–513.
3. Eng PHK, Cardona GR, Fang SL, Previti M, Sharon A, Carrasco N, Chin WW, Braverman LE. Escape from the acute Wolff-Chaikoff effect is associated with a decrease in thyroid sodium/iodide symporter messenger ribonucleic acid and protein. Endocrinology 1999; 140; 3404–3410.
4. Vagenakis AG, Downs P, Braverman LE, Burger A, Ingbar SH. Control of thryroid hormone secretion in normal subjects receiving excess iodides. J Clin Invest 1973; 52; 528–532.
5. Safran M, Braverman LE. Effect of chronic douching with polyvinylpyrrolidone iodine on iodine absorption and thyroid function. Obstet Gynecol 1982; 60; 35–40.
6. Ader AW, Paul TL, Reinhardt W, Safran M, Pino S, Mc Arthur W, Braverman LE. Effect of mouth rinsing with polyvinylpyrrolidone-iodine mixtures on iodine absorption and thyroid function. J Clin Endocrinol Metab 1988; 66; 632–635.
7. Philippou G, Koutras DA, Piperingos G, Souvatzoglou A, Moulopoulos SD. The effect of iodide on serum thyroid hormone levels in normal persons, hyperthyroid patients, and in hypothyroid patients on thyroxine replacement. Clin Endocrinol (Oxf) 1992; 36; 573–578.
8. Le Mar HJ, Georgitis WJ, Mc Dermott MT. Thyroid adaptation to chronic tetraglycine hydroperiodide water purification tablet use. J Clin Endocrinol Metab 1995; 80; 220–223.
9. Namba H, Yamashita S, Kimura H, Yokoyama N, Otsuru A, Izumi M, Nagataki S. Evidence of thyroid volume increase in normal subjects receiving excess iodide. J Clin Endocrinol Metab. 1993; 76; 605- 608.
10. Arntzenius AB, Smit LJ, Schipper J, van der Heide D, Meinders AE. Inverse relation between iodine intake and thyroid blood flow: color Doppler flow imaging in euthyroid humans. J Clin Endocrinol Metab 1991; 73; 1051–1055.
11. Paul T, Meyers B, Witorsch RJ, Pino S, Chipkin S, Ingbar SH, Braverman LE. The effect of small increases in dietary iodine on thyroid function in euthyroid subjects. Metabolism 1988; 37; 121–124.
12. Jonckheer MH, Michotte Y, Van Steirteghem AC, Deconinck F. The adaptation of the human thyroid gland to a physiological regimen of iodide intake: evidence for a transitory inhibition of thyroid hormone secretion modulated by the intrathyroidal iodine stores. J Endocrinol Invest 1983; 6; 267–272.
13. Gardner DF, Centor RM, Utiger RD. Effects of low dose oral iodide supplementation on thyroid function in normal men. Clin Endocrinol (Oxf) 1988; 28; 283–288.
14. Chow CC, Phillips DIW, Lazarus JH, Parkes AB. Effect of low dose iodide supplementation on thyroid function on potentially susceptible subjects: are iodide levels in Britain acceptable? Clin Endocrinol (Oxf) 1991; 34; 413–416.
15. Grainger RG, Pennington GW. A study of the effect of sodium/meglumine ioxaglate (Hexabrix) on thyroid function. Br J Radiol 1981; 54; 768–772.
16. Li M, Liu DR, Qu CY, Zhang PY, Qian QD, ZhangCD, Jia QZ, Wang MX, Eastman CJ, Boyages SC, Collins JK, Jupp JJ, Maberly GF. Endemic goitre in Central China caused by excessive iodine intake. Lancet 1987; 2; 257–259.
17. Zhao J, Chen Z, Maberly G. Iodine-rich drinking water of natural origin in China. Lancet 1998; 352; 202.
18. Coindet JF. Nouvelles recherches sur les effects de l'iode, et sur les precautions a suivre dans le traitement de goitre par le nouveau remede. Bibl Univ Sci Belles Lettres Arts 1821; 16; 140–152.
19. Braverman LE. Iodine and the thyroid: 33 years of study. Thyroid 1994; 4; 351–356.
20. Vagenakis AG, Braverman LE. Adverse effects of iodides on thyroid function. Med Clin North Am 1975; 59; 1075–1088.
21. Fradkin JE, Wolff J. Iodide-induced thyrotoxicosis. Medicine 1983; 62; 1–20.

22. McGregor AM, Weetman AP, Ratanachaiyavong S, Owen GM, Ibbertson IK, Hall R. In: Hall R, Kobberling J, ed. Thyroid disorders associated with iodine deficiency and excess. Serono Symposia Series. New York: Raven Press, 1985: 209–216.
23. Stanbury JB, Ermans AE, Bourdoux P, Todd C, Oken E, Tonglet R, Vidor G, Braverman LE, Medeiros-Neto G. Iodine-induced hyperthyroidism: occurrence and epidemiology. Thyroid 1998; 8; 83–100.
24. Martin MC, Lima N, Knobel M, Medeiros-Neto G. Natural course of iodine-induced thyrotoxicosis (Jod-Basedow) in endemic goiter area: a 5 year follow up. J Endocrinol Invest 1989; 12; 239–244.
25. Elnagar B, Eltom L, Karlsson FA, Ermans AM, Gebre-Medhin M, Bourdoux PP. The effects of different doses of oral iodized oil on goiter size, urinary iodine, and thyroid related hormones. J Clin Endocrinol Metab 1995; 80; 891–897.
26. Ermans AM, Gullo D, Mugisho SG, Shibangu MT, Tonglet R, Iurato P, Mukalay MW, Mahangaiko E, Bourdoux P. Iodine supplementation must be monitored at the population level in iodine deficient areas (abstract) Thyroid 1995; 5 (suppl 1): S:137.
27. Bourdoux P, Ermans AM, Mukalay WA, Filetti S, Vigneri R. Iodine induced thyrotoxicosis in Kiwu Zaire. Lancet 1996; 347; 552–553.
28. Todd CH, Allain T, Gomo ZAR, Hasier JA, Ndiweni M, Oken E. Increase in thyrotoxicosis associated with iodine supplements in Zimbabwe. Lancet 1995; 346; 1563–1564.
29. Delange F, de Benoist B, Alnwick D. Risks of iodine-induced hyperthyroidism after correction of iodine deficiency by iodized salt. Thyroid 1999, 9; 545–556.
30. Reith PE, Granner DK. Iodine-induced thyrotoxicosis in a woman with a multinodular goiter taking levothyroxine. Arch Intern Med 1985; 145; 355–357.
31. Lazarus JH, Parkes AB, John R, N'Diaye M, G Prysor-Jones S. Endemic goitre in Senegal – thyroid function etiological factors and treatment with oral iodized oil. Acta Endocrinol (Copenh) 1992; 126; 149–154.
32. Ermans AM, Camus M. Modifications of thyroid function induced by chronic administration of iodide in the presence of "autonomous" thyroid tissue. Acta Endocrinol (Copenh) 1972; 70; 463–475.
33. Livadas DP, Koutras PA, Souvatzoglou A, Beckers C. The toxic effects of small iodine supplements in patients with autonomous thyroid nodules. Clin Endocrinol (Oxf) 1977; 7; 121–127.
34. Mostbeck A, Galvan G, Bauer P, Eber O, Atefie K, Dam K, Feichtinger H, Fritzsche H, Haydl H, Köhn H, König B, Koriska K, Kroiss A, Lind P, Markt B, Maschek W, Pesl H, Ramschak-Schwarzer S, Riccabona G, Stockhammer M, Zechmann W . The incidence of hyperthyroidism in Austria from 1987 to 1995 before and after an increase in salt iodization in 1990. Eur J Nucl Med 1998; 25; 367–374.
35. Vagenakis AG, Wang CA, Burger A, Maloof F, Braverman LE, Ingbar SH. Iodide induced thyrotoxicosis in Boston. N Engl J Med 1972; 287; 523–527.
36. Rajatanavin R, Safran M, Stoller W, Mordes JP, Braverman LE. Five patients with iodine-induced hyperthyroidism. Am J Med 1984; 77; 378–384.
37. Martin FIR, Brian WT, Colman PG, Deam DR. Iodine-induced hyperthyroidism due to nonionic contrast radiography in the elderly. Am J Med 1993; 95; 78–82.
38. Martin FI, Deam DR. Hyperthyroidism in elderly hospitalized patients. Clinical features and outcome. Med J Aust 1996; 164; 200–203.
39. Steidle B. Iodine-induced hyperthyroidism after contrast media. Animal experimental and clinical studies. In: Taenzer V, Wend S (eds). Recent developments in non-ionic contrast media. New York: Thieme 1989:6
40. Conn JJ, Sebastian MJ, Deam D, Tam M, Martin FIR. A prospective study of the effect of ionic media on thyroid function. Thyroid 1996, 6; 107–110.
41. Nolte W, Müller R, Siggelkow H, Emrich D, Hübner M. Prophylactic application of thyrostatic drugs during excessive iodine exposure in euthyroid patients with thyroid autonomy: a randomized study. Eur J Endocrinol 1996; 134; 337–341.
42. Hintze G, Blombach O, Fink H, Burkhardt U, Kobberling J. Risk of iodine induced thyrotoxicosis after coronary angiography: an investigation in 788 unselected subjects. Eur J Endocrinol 1999, 140; 264–267.
43. Liel Y, Alkan M. Transitory thyrotoxicosis induced by iodinated preparations for water purifications. Arch Intern Med 1996; 156; 807–810.

44. Mueller B, Diem P, Bürgi U. "Travelers' Thyrotoxicosis" revisited. Arch Intern Med 1998; 158; 1723.
45. Solomon BL, Evanl JE, Burman KD, Wartofskly L. Remission rates with antithyroid drug therapy: continuing influence of iodine uptake? Ann Intern Med 1987; 107; 510–512.
46. Azizi F. Environmental iodine intake affects the response to methimazole in patients with diffuse toxic goiter. J Clin Endocrinol Metab 1985; 61; 374–377.
47. Roti E, Gardini E, Minelli R, Bianconi L, Braverman LE. Sodium ipodate and methimazole in the long-term treatment of hyperthyroid Graves' disease. Metabolism 1993; 42; 403–408.
48. Roti E, Gardini E, Minelli R, Bianconi L, Salvi M, Gavaruzzi G, Braverman LE.. Effects of chronic iodine administration on thyroid status in euthyroid subjects previously treated with antithyroid drugs for Graves' hyperthyroidism. J Clin Endocrinol Metab 1993; 76; 928–932.
49. Wilson R, McKillop JH, Thomson JA. The effect of preoperative potassium iodide therapy on antibody production. Acta Endocrinol (Copenh) 1990; 123; 531–534.
50. Rath TH, Meissl G, Weissel M. Induction of hyperthyroidism in burn patients treated topically with povidone-iodine. Burns 1988; 14; 320–322.
51. Yoshinari M, Tokuyama T, Okamura K, Sato K, Kusuda K, Fujishima M. Iodide-induced thyrotoxicosis in a thyroidectomized patient with metastatic thyroid carcinoma. Cancer 1988; 61; 1674–1678.
52. Lombardi A, Martino E, Braverman LE. Amiodarone and the thyroid. Thyroid Today 1990; 23; 1–7.
53. Harjai KJ, Licata AA. Effects of amiodarone on thyroid function. Ann Intern Med 1997; 126; 63–73.
54. Martino E, Aghini-Lombardi F, Mariotti S, Bartalena L, Lenziardi M, Ceccarelli C, Bambini G, Safran M, Braverman LE, Pinchera A. Amiodarone iodine-induced hypothyroidism risk factors and follow up in 28 cases. Clin Endocrinol (Oxf) 1987; 26; 227–237.
55. Monteiro E, Galvao-Teles A, Santos ML, Mourao L, Correira MJ, Tuna JL, Ribeiro C. Antithyroidal antibodies as an early marker for thyroid disease induced by amiodarone. Br Med J 1986; 292; 227–228.
56. Safran M, Martino E, Aghini-Lombardi F, Bartalena L, Balzano S, Pinchera A, Braverman LE. Effect of amiodarone on circulating antithyroid antibodies. Br Med J 1988; 297; 456–457.
57. Chiovato L, Martino E, Tonacchera M, Santini F, Lapi P, Mammoli C, Braverman LE, Pinchera A. Studies on the in vitro cytotoxic effect of amiodarone. Endocrinology 1994; 134; 2277–2282.
58. Roti E, Minelli R, Gardini E, Bianconi L, Braverman LE. Thyrotoxicosis followed by hypothyroidism in patients treated with amiodarone. Arch Intern Med 1993; 153; 886–892.
59. Smyrk TC, Goellner JR, Brennan MD, Carnej JA. Pathology of the thyroid in amiodarone-associated thyrotoxicosis. Am J Surg Pathol 1987; 11; 197–204.
60. Pitsiavas V, Smerdely P, Li M, Boyages SC. Amiodarone induces a different pattern of ultrastructural change in the thyroid to iodine excess alone in both the BB/W rat and the Wistar rat. Eur J Endocrinol 1997; 137; 89–98.
61. Bambini G, Aghini-Lombardi F, Rosner W, Saeed Khan M, Martino E, Pinchera A, Braverman LE, Safran M. Sex hormone-binding globulin in amiodarone-treated patients: a marker for tissue thyrotoxicosis. Arch Intern Med 1987; 147; 1781–1785.
62. Bartalena L, Grasso L, Brogioni S, Aghini-Lombardi F, Braverman LE, Martino E. Serum interleukin-6 in amiodarone-induced thyrotoxicosis. J Clin Endocrinol Metab 1994; 78; 423–427.
63. Martino E, Aghini-Lombardi F, Mariotti S, Lenziardi M, Baschieri L, Braverman LE, Pinchera A. Treatment of amiodarone associated hyperthyroidism by simultaneous administration of potassium perchlorate and methimazole. J Endocrinol Invest 1986; 9; 201–207.
64. Reichert LJ, Derooy HA. Treatment of amiodarone induced hyperthyroidism with potassium perchlorate and methimazole during amiodarone treatment. Br Med J 1989; 298; 1547–1548.
65. Brousolle C, Ducotett X, Martin C, Barbier Y, Bornet H, Noel G, Orgiazzi J. Rapid effectiveness of prednisone and thionamides combined therapy in severe amiodarone iodine-induced thyrotoxicosis: comparison of two groups of patients with apparently normal thyroid glands. J Endocrinol Invest 1989; 12; 37–42.
66. Bartalena L, Brogioni S, Grasso L, Bogazzi F, Burelli A, Martino E. Treatment of amiodarone-induced thyrotoxicosis, a difficult challenge: Results of a prospective study. J Clin Endocrinol Metab 1996; 81; 2930–2933.
67. Farwell AP, Abend SL, Huang SK, Patwardhan N, Braverman LE. Thyroidectomy for amiodarone-induced thyrotoxicosis. JAMA 1990; 263; 1526–1528.
68. Minelli R, Gardini E, Bianconi L, Salvi M, Roti E. Subclinical hypothyroidism, overt thyrotoxicosis

and subclinical hypothyroidism: the subsequent phases of thyroid function in a patient chronically treated with amiodarone. J Endocrinol Invest 1992; 15; 853–855.
69. Roti E, Bianconi L, De Chiara F, Minelli R, Tosi C, Gardini E, Salvi M, Braverman LE. Thyroid ultrasonography in patients with a previous episode of amiodarone induced thyrotoxicosis. J Endocrinol Invest 1994; 17; 259–262.
70. Roti E, Minelli R, Gardini E, Bianconi L, Gavaruzzi G, UgolottiG, Neri TM, Braverman LE. Iodine-induced subclinical hypothyroidism in euthyroid subjects with a previous episode of amiodarone-induced thyrotoxicosis. J Clin Endocrinol Metab 1992; 75; 1273–1277.
71. Mariotti S, Loviselli A, Murenu S, Sau F, Valentino L, Mandas A, Vacquer S, Martino E, Balestrieri A, Lai ME. High prevalence of thyroid dysfunction in adult patients with beta-thalassemia major submitted to amiodarone treatment. J Endocrinol Invest 1999; 22; 55–63.

From genotype to phenotype in non-autoimmune hyperthyroidism

P. Rodien

Médecine C, Centre Hospitalier Universitaire d'Angers, 4 rue Larrey, 49033 Angers Cédex 01, France

Abstract

It is thought that the mechanism of activation of G-protein coupled receptor by the agonist relies on release from structural constraints, allowing the "relaxed" receptor to activate the G-protein. By analogy with experimental work on the a1b adrenergic receptor, showing that mutations may result in constitutive activation of the receptor, it was hypothesized that similar but spontaneous somatic mutations of the thyrotropin receptor might be the cause of thyroid toxic adenomas. This hypothesis has been confirmed. Furthermore, cases of familial non-autoimmune hyperthyroidism and non-autoimmune neonatal hyperthyroidism have been shown to be caused by germline mutations of the thyrotropin receptor. Besides constitutive activation of the thyrotropin receptor, a case of sensitization of the thyrotropin receptor to hCG by a mutation in the extracellular domain has been identified as the cause of familial gestational hyperthyroidism. All these phenotype-to-genotype studies have been helpful in understanding the mechanisms of activation of glycoprotein hormones. A model has been proposed using data obtained from these mutations. In this model, the extracellular domain of the receptor exerts an inhibitory action on the transmembrane domain, and this interaction must be disrupted to allow activation of the receptor. However, this model has not been demonstrated yet, and we still have to move from genotype to phenotype, that is from structure to function.

Background

The TSH receptor (TSH-R) is a member of the large, and still enlarging, family of G-protein coupled receptor (1). Based on bacteriorhodopsin three-dimensional structure, and later on rhodopsin, these receptors are thought to be organized in seven transmembrane domains, linked by three extracellular loops, and three intracellular loops. The TSH-R with the other glycoprotein hormone receptors, LH/CG and FSH receptors, define a subfamily of G-protein coupled receptors, based on the existence of a very large extracellular domain (1). This extracellular domain is known as the ligand binding domain (1, 2). The intracellular loops of the receptor are the structural basis for coupling to trimeric G-protein, and subsequently to the production of second messenger.

In human thyroid cells, the TSH-R is coupled to Gsα and Gq proteins, and thus to the cAMP and inositol phosphates pathways (3, 4). Activation of the cAMP pathway is responsible for proliferation of the thyrocytes, as well as for differentiation, i.e. expression of thyroperoxidase, thyroglobulin, and sodium-iodide symporter. Abnormally sustained high cAMP production can be obtained by stimulation of the TSH-R by stimulating antibodies in Graves' disease, and can be observed spontaneously in autonomous thyroid toxic adenomas.

Demonstration of this putative pathogenic mechanism was achieved by production of transgenic mice. By targeting the adenosine A2 receptor in the thyroid gland, under the control of the thyroglobulin promoter, Ledent et al (5) were able to trigger continuous production of cAMP in thyrocytes. The observed phenotype was a large goiter associated with hyperthyroidism and compromising the survival of the animal in the absence of treatment.

The putative mechanism of some diseases associated with hyperthyroidism, as deduced from in vitro experiments, could thus be demonstrated in vivo. However, if hyperproduction of cAMP could be reasonably regarded as responsible for hyperthyroidism, the initial causative anomaly leading to this hyperproduction remained unknown.

The hypothesis: from constitutive adrenergic receptors to constitutive thyrotropin receptor

The experimental work of the group of Lefkowitz on the adrenergic receptor can be regarded as pioneering our understanding of the physiology of G-protein coupled receptors.

By producing artificial mutations of the third intracellular loop of the α1b adrenergic receptor, this group produced a constitutively activated receptor, producing inositol triphosphate, its second messenger, in the absence of the natural ligand (6). The receptor had become autonomous and independent. The second, but major, result of those experiments, was the unexpected finding that mutation of a particular residue in this third intracellular loop, alanine 293, in to each of the possible amino acids, always induced an activated state of the mutated receptor. From these experiments, a new model for activation of G-protein coupled receptors was deduced (7). In this model, receptors are thought to exist spontaneously in at least two different conditions, the unactivated or silent state, with maximal structural constraints, and the activated, relaxed state, with minimal structural constraints. The receptor spontaneously oscillates between the two extreme states. In the absence of the ligand, the majority of receptor molecules are maintained in the constrained conformation (inactive receptor), whereas ligand binding to the receptor favors displacement of the equilibrium toward the relaxed conformation (activated receptor).

Mutation of the adrenergic receptor is thought to activate the receptor by relieving the structural constraints, and alanine 293 appears as the keystone, a lock, maintaining these structural constraints.

Since all G-protein coupled receptors are thought to have the same spatial organization, and to share the same mechanisms of activation, it was predicted that the same kind of mutation in the TSH-R could also lead to a constitutively activated TSH-R.

Somatic activating mutations in thyroid toxic adenomas

The initial verification of the hypothesis came from the study of toxic autonomous thyroid adenoma (8). The autonomy of the tumor, demonstrated by increased uptake and organification of radioactive iodide on scintiscan, contrasting with suppression of the rest of the thyroid gland, and associated with a suppressed TSH, is characteristic of the condition. It shows that hyperactivity of the nodule is an intrinsic feature of the tumor rather than being caused by any extra tumoral stimulus (TSH, TSH-R antibodies).

Genomic DNA was extracted from the tumor and used as a template for amplification of part of the coding sequence of the TSH-R gene. This amplified DNA was then sequenced and mutations were found in the third intracellular loop, as expected, in particular, a mutation of the residue corresponding to alanine 293, alanine 623 (7, 8). The heterozygote mutations present in the tumor were absent from peripheral blood and from normal thyroid tissue surrounding the adenoma.

Further studies rapidly revealed that no limited hot spot could be delineated, since many mutations were described, scattered throughout the whole transmembrane domain (9–13).

By introducing the mutations into an expression vector encoding the wild-type TSH-R sequence, the gain of function of the mutated receptor was demonstrated by transient transfection experiments in COS 7 cells. Although the mutant usually shows lower expression at the cell surface, cAMP accumulation in absence of TSH is higher than that observed with the wild-type receptor. The mutant is said to be constitutively active.

In contrast to the constantly higher cAMP production (by definition) the diacylglycerol-inositol phosphate pathway is rarely constitutively activated. The response to bovine TSH, in terms of cAMP Production was usually conserved, and apparent affinity for bovine TSH, was usually enhanced.

The frequency of activating mutations of TSH-R as a cause of toxic adenomas has been a matter of controversy. Some groups have reported mutations in only a few cases, whereas frequencies as high as 50–82 % were reported by others (9–14). It appears, that these mutations are the major cause of toxic adenomas in European countries, where borderline to moderate iodine deficiency is common. Interestingly, in a few cases, different somatic mutations were found in different independent toxic nodules in the same multinodular goiter (15).

Germline activating mutations in familial non-autoimmune hyperthyroidism

Since somatic mutations activating the receptor may lead to focal autonomous growth and hyperfunction, it was postulated that the same kind of mutation present in each of the thyrocytes would lead to diffuse hyperfunctioning goiter. This would occur with a germline mutation and would lead to inherited disease. In the early 1980s, Thomas et al. (16) reported the case of a family, in which hyperthyroidism, which was sometimes recurrent, was observed in three generations. This hyperthyroidism was associated with diffuse goiter, in the absence of Graves' ophthalmopathy. Blood tests failed to detect any kind of thyroid antibodies, especially TSH-R antibodies. Thyroid tissue from patients undergoing thyroidectomy showed no sign of an autoimmune process on histology.

The same germline mutation of the TSH-R receptor was found in all affected members of this family, as well as another mutation was found in another unrelated family (17). Increased constitutive activity of the mutated TSH-R compared with the wild-type receptor was also demonstrated. Several additional pedigrees have been reported since this first publication, and in all cases hyperthyroidism is transmitted as an autosomal dominant trait (reviewed in 13).

The description and identification of these first cases of germline TSH-R activating mutations, besides elucidating of a puzzling condition, have some important consequences. Diagnosis of this hereditary disease is important, because one of its characteristics is frequent relapse of goiter and hyperthyroidism in the absence of aggressive ablative therapy. Secondly, identification of such cases allows presymptomatic diagnosis and thus early treatment, provided a careful follow-up is established.

A related disease: neomutations of the TSH-R

Some cases of neonatal hyperthyroidism have been reported in which no evidence of autoimmune thyroid disease could be demonstrated in either the neonate or the mother. In these cases, hyperthyroidism is usually severe and requires intensive and immediate antithyroid therapy. Goiter is usually present. Exophthalmos was reported in one case (18), without any clear explanation. In these cases, germline activating mutations of TSH-R have been demonstrated also (19, 20). However, the mutation was not found in the parents.

Non-autonomous, but hyperactive TSH-R: familial gestational hyperthyroidism due to hypersensitivity to hCG

Normal early pregnancy is marked by a decrease of plasma TSH around 10–12 weeks of gestation, in response to a moderate increase in free T_4 (21). This increase in thyroid hormones is due to the thyrotropic activity of hCG, because of structural homology between hCG and TSH, similar to homology between hCG and other glycoprotein hormones. These hormones are composed of a heterodimer, in which a common a subunit is associated with different b subunits responsible for the specificity of the hormone. Although different, the b subunits have some homology also, giving rise to some cross-stimulation of the three different receptors for glycoprotein hormones, namely the TSH-R, LH/CG-R, and FSH-R (22). However cross-stimulation is not usually observed at physiological concentrations of the hormones, except in the case of pregnancy where hCG reaches concentrations high enough to cause modest stimulation of the TSH-R. The resulting moderate hyperthyroxinemia, occurring at the same time as the peak of hCG secretion, is of short duration, and does not require any treatment since clinical signs are usually absent, and, when present, rapidly regress once the hCG concentration drops. In some cases, however, true hyperthyroidism is observed, sometimes requiring transient antithyroid drug treatment. These cases are usually observed when hCG secretion is abnormally high or sustained, and hyperthyroidism is associated with, or may present as, hyperemesis gravidarum (23).

We had the opportunity to study an atypical case of gestational hyperthyroidism, not caused by autoimmune disease or a toxic adenoma. The unusual features in this case were represented by

- Recurrence of hyperthyroidism and hyperemesis gravidarum in each pregnancy,
- Normal hCG level,
- Requirement for antithyroid drug treatment throughout pregnancy,
- A similar clinical history in the mother of the patient.

A heterozygous mutation of the TSH-R was found in the patient and her mother, with exchange of lysine 183 in the extracellular domain to arginine.

Hypersensitivity of the mutant TSH-R to hCG was demonstrated *in vitro*. Interestingly, the gain of sensitivity was modest, but sufficient to allow for cross-stimulation, taking into consideration the plasma concentration of hCG even during a normal pregnancy (24).

From genotype to phenotype?

A recurrent theme when dealing with pathogenic mutation in human disease is to try to correlate genotype and phenotype, in the hope of providing a genetic prognosis following the genetic diagnosis.

When trying to sort the activating mutations of the TSH-R according to their potency, it appeared initially that there was a separation between the somatic mutations observed in toxic adenomas and germline mutations observed in familial toxic thyroid hyperplasia. An interesting observation was the apparently higher constitutive activity of most somatic mutations compared with germline hereditary mutations. In fact, it is known that an autonomous adenoma must reach a critical size before it causes to hyperthyroidism. This leads naturally to the hypothesis that potent somatic mutations lead to a more severe phenotype, as represented by stronger stimulation of proliferation. These mutations, if transmitted as germline mutations, would lead to severe in utero and neonatal hyperthyroidism, and would then be lethal in the absence of modern neonatal intensive care. In agreement with this hypothesis, germline neomutations of the "adenoma type" resulting in congenital hyperthyroidism are always extremely severe and require immediate therapy.

However, there is at least one exception to this "rule". In one family affected by hereditary non-autoimmune hyperthyroidism, a mutation already encountered in toxic adenomas was observed. The phenotype was not especially severe, since hyperthyroidism was diagnosed in children after several years of life (25). On the other hand, a correlation between genotype and phenotype is suggested by this observation, since, in this family, mitral valve prolapse cosegregated with the mutation and hyperthyroidism. However, the relationship between the two features is far from clear, and a specific consequence of this mutation is unlikely.

As previously mentioned, finding of a germline activating mutation of TSH-R is of value in familial non-autoimmune hyperthyroidism, since this allows for presymptomatic diagnosis and makes careful follow-up mandatory. However, if this genetic diagnosis can accurately identify "at risk" members of the family, it certainly does not predict who will develop the condition, when, and how severe the hyperthyroidism will be. In fact in some families, several asymptomatic subjects were identified has having the mutation, and the age of onset of hyperthyroidism was not uniform (16, 17).

Nevertheless, what can be predicted from the genetic diagnosis is that, when present, hyperthyroidism will tend to relapse following conservative treatment.

From phenotype to genotype? (Why natural mutagenesis teaches us more than directed artificial mutagenesis)

In structural studies, directed mutagenesis is a potent tool, allowing identification of functional domains, as well as different regions of a molecule interacting together.

However, in the case of TSH-R an intriguing observation has been the diversity and the spatial dispersion of activating mutations. Based on previous results obtained in other G-protein coupled receptor, directed mutagenesis looking for domains important in TSH-R activation would certainly have targeted the third intracellular loop, because of the existence of activating mutations in this region. However, it can be concluded from the results that the third intracellular loop is *the* key region of the TSH-R. By contrast, by looking for spontaneous mutations selected in vivo by the phenotype they induce, the TSH-R appears to be an easily activated receptor and locking domains or activation domains appear much more difficult to delineate.

Furthermore, some specific activating mutations have forced us to imagine a novel model of activation-silencing of the glycoprotein hormone receptor. Deletion of part of the receptor would not be expected to activate the receptor; however, this mechanism has proven to be possible with deletions of extra as well as intracellular loops found in toxic adenomas (9, 26).

The deletion along with the point mutation found in extracellular loops suggested that one of the structural constraint to relieve to activate the TSH-R may rely on structures located on the extracellular side of the receptor rather than on the intracellular side alone, i.e. the third intracellular loop. Based on experimental data from the effects of tryptic cleavage of part of the extracellular domain (26), it appears that disruption of interactions between the extracellular domain and the extracellular loops may be a mechanism of activation of TSH-R (27). Further evidence came from spontaneous mutagenesis, with the finding in toxic adenomas of different activating mutations of one residue of the extracellular domain, serine 281 (28). Some of these mutations were so mild, that it is unlikely that any experimenter would have designed them.

Similarly, exchanging a lysine to arginine would not be expected to lead to a dramatic phenotype, such as that observed in familial gestational hyperthyroidism. Furthermore, since lysine 183 is conserved in the human LH-R, as well as surrounding residues, it is improbable that targeted mutagenesis designed to identify residues important for ligand specificity would have involved this region of the extracellular domain.

Perspectives and conclusions

The search for activating mutations of the TSH-R has been triggered by studies on other G-protein coupled receptors, and can thus be regarded as a walk *from genotype to phenotype* (What phenotype would that kind of mutation of the TSH-R give?). Nevertheless, the search for mechanisms leading to cAMP overproduction in the thyrocyte, and the consequent hyperthyroidism, can rather be regarded as a walk *from phenotype to genotype* (What is the cause of this phenotype?).

It seems quite clear now that no direct and clear correlation between the genotype and the observed phenotype can be found. However, identification of germline activating or sensitizing mutations is of clinical value, especially for therapeutic management and identifying the risk of relapse of the disease.

In contrast, diagnosis of somatic activating mutations in toxic adenomas is of no help to the clinician. However, description of such a large panel of activating mutations, scattered throughout the whole receptor, has been of great benefit to the researcher. A proposed model for activation of TSH-R by disruption of putative inhibitory interactions between the extracellular domain and the extracellular loops has some basis in these natural mutations. The model, however, has not been unambiguously demonstrated yet.

References

1. Parmentier M, Libert F, Maenhaut C, Lefort A, Gerard C, Perret J, Van Sande J, Dumont JE, Vassart G. Molecular cloning of the thyrotropin receptor. Science 1989; 246: 1620–1622.
2. Nagayama Y, Wadsworth HL, Chazenbalk GD, Russo D, Seto P, Rapoport B. Thyrotropin-luteinizing hormone/chorionic gonadotropin receptor extracellular domain chimeras as probes for TSH receptor function. Proc Natl Acad Sci USA 1991; 88: 902–905.
3. Vassart G, Dumont JE. The thyrotropin receptor and the regulation of thyrocyte function and growth. Endocrinol Rev 1992; 13: 596–611.
4. Dumont JE, Lamy F, Roger P, Maenhaut C Physiological and pathological regulation of thyroid cell proliferation and differentiation by thyrotropin and other factors. Physiol Rev 1992; 72: 667–97.
5. Ledent C, Dumont JE, Vassart G, Parmentier M. Thyroid expression of an A2 adenosine receptor transgene induces thyroid hyperplasia and hyperthyroidism. EMBO J, 1992; 11: 537–542.
6. Kjelsberg MA, Cotecchia S, Ostrowski J, Caron MG, Lefkowitz RJ. Constitutive activation of the a1B-adrenergic receptor by all amino acid substitutions at a single site. J Biol Chem 1992; 267: 1430–1433.
7. Samama P, Cotechia S, Costa T, Lefkowitz RJ. A mutation-induced activated state of the beta 2-adrenergic receptor. Extending the ternary complex model. J Biol Chem 1993; 268: 4625–4636.
8. Parma J, Duprez L, Van Sande J, Cochaux P, Gervy C, Mockel J, Dumont JE, Vassart G. Somatic mu-

tations in the thyrotropin receptor gene cause hyperfunctioning thyroid adenomas. Nature 1993; 365: 649–651.

9. Parma J, Duprez L, Van Sande, Hermans J, Rocmans P, Van Vliet G, Costagliola S, Rodien P, Dumont JE, Vassart G. Diversity and prevalence of somatic mutations in the thyrotropin receptor and Gs alpha genes as a cause of toxic thyroid adenomas. J Clin Endocrinol Metab 1997; 82: 2695–2701.
10. Führer D, Holzapfel HP, Wonerow P, Scherbaum WA, Paschke R. Somatic mutations in the thyrotropin receptor gene and not in the Gsa protein gene in 31 toxic thyroid nodules. J Clin Endocrinol Metab 1997; 82: 3885–3891.
11. Porcellini A, Ciullo I, Laviola L, Amabile G, Fenzi G, Avvedimento VE. Novel mutations of thyrotropin receptor gene in thyroid hyperfunctioning adenomas. Rapid identification by fine needle aspiration biopsy. J Clin Endocrinol Metab. 1994; 79: 657–661.
12. Parma J, Van Sande J, Swillens S, Tonacchera M, Dumont J, Vassart G. Somatic mutations causing constitutive activity of the thyrotropin receptor are the major cause of hyperfunctioning thyroid adenomas: identification of additional mutations activating both the cyclic adenosine 3',5'-monophosphate and inositol phosphate-Ca2+ cascades. Mol Endocrinol 1995; 9: 725–733.
13. Duprez L, Parma J, Van Sande J, Rodien P, Dumont JE, Vassart G, Abramowicz M. TSH receptor mutations and thyroid disease. TEM 1998; 9: 133–140.
14. Tonacchera M, Cetani F, Van Sande J, Vassart G, Dumont J. Oncogenic mutations in thyroid adenoma: methodological criteria. Eur J Endocrinol 1996; 135: 444–446.
15. Duprez L, Hermans, J, Van Sande J, Dumont E, Vassart G, Parma J. Two autonomous nodules of a patient with multinodular goiter harbor different activating mutations of the thyrotropin receptor gene. J Clin Endocrinol Metab. 1997; 82: 306–308
16. Thomas JL, Leclere J, Hartemann P, Duheille J, Orgiazzi J, Petersen M, Janot C, Guedenet JC. Familial hyperthyroidism without evidence of autoimmunity. Acta Endocrinol (Copenh) 1982 100: 512–518.
17. Duprez L, Parma J, Van Sande J, Allgeier A, Leclere J, Schwartz C, Delisle MJ, Decoulx M, Orgiazzi J, Dumont JE, Vassart G. Germline mutations in the thyrotropin receptor gene cause non-autoimmune autosomal dominant hyperthyroidism. Nature Genet 1994; 7: 396–401.
18. De Roux, Polak M, Couet J, Leger J, Czernichow P, Milgrom E, Mishrahi M. Neomutation of the thyroid-stimulating hormone receptor in a severe neonatal hyperthyroidism. J Clin Endocrinol Metab 1996, 81: 2023–2026.
19. Kopp P, Van Sande J, Parma J, Duprez L, Gerber H, Joss E, Jameson JL, Dumont JE, Vassart G. Brief report: congenital hyperthyroidism caused by a mutation in the thyrotropin receptor gene. N Engl J Med 1995; 332, 150–154.
20. Holzapfel HP, Wonerow P, Von Petrykowski W, Henschen M, Scherbaum WA, Paschke R. Sporadic congenital hyperthyroidism due to a spontaneous germline mutation in the thyrotropin receptor gene. J Clin Endocrinol Metab 1997; 82: 3879–3884.
21. Glinoer D. The regulation of thyroid function in pregnancy: pathways of endocrine adaptation from physiology to pathology. Endocr Rev 1997; 18: 404–433.
22. Grossmann M, Weintraub BD, Szkudlinski MW. Novel insights into the molecular mechanisms of human thyrotropin action: structural, physiological, and therapeutic implications for the glycoprotein hormone family. Endocr Rev 1997; 18:476–501.
23. Goodwin TM, Montoro M, Mestman JH, Pekary AE, Hershman JM. The role of chorionic gonadotropin in transient hyperthyroidism of hyperemesis gravidarum. J Clin Endocrinol Metab 1992; 75: 1333–1337.
24. Rodien P, Brémont C, Raffin-Sanson ML, Parma J, Van Sande J, Costagliola S, Luton JP, Vassart G, Duprez L. Familial gestational hyperthyroidism caused by a mutant thyrotropin receptor hypersensitive to human chorionic gonadotropin. N Engl J Med 1998; 339: 1823–1826.
25. Khoo DHC, Parma J, Rajasoorya C, HO SC, Vassart G. A germline mutation of the thyrotropin receptor gene associated with thyrotoxicosis and mitral valve prolapse in a Chinese family. J Clin Endocrinol Metab 1999; 84: 1459–1462.
26. Wonerow P, Schöneberg T, Schultz G, Gudermann T, Paschke R. Deletions in the third intracellular loop of the thyrotropin receptor. A new mechanism for constitutive activation. J Biol Chem 1998; 273: 7900–7905.

27. Van Sande J, Massart C, Costagliola S, Allgeier A, Cetani F, Vassart G, Dumont JE. Specific activation of the thyrotropin receptor by trypsin. Mol cell Endocrinol 1996; 119: 161–168.
28. Duprez L, Parma J, Costagliola S, Hermans, Van Sande J, Dumont E, Vassart G. Constitutive activation of the TSH receptor by spontaneous mutations affecting the N-terminal extracellular domain. FEBS Lett 1997; 409: 469–474.

Session V:

Environment and non-autoimmune thyroiditis

Chairpersons: F. Péter, A. Lewinski

Subacute thyroiditis

I. Szabolcs

Division of Endocrinology, Department of Medicine and Geriatrics, Faculty of Health Sciences, Semmelweis University, POB 112, 1389 Budapest, Hungary

Introduction

First described by *de Quervain* (1904) (19) and even earlier by *Mygind* (1895) (68), subacute thyroiditis (SAT) is a self-limiting disorder of the thyroid gland characterized by a sudden onset of neck pain and tenderness, malaise and variable changes in thyroid function tests, usually lasting several weeks to several months. In most cases the diagnosis is obvious if the patient has the typical picture of the disease when first seen. Treatment with steroids will usually effectively ameliorate symptoms.

Perhaps because of the simplicity of diagnosis and treatment, or the low prevalence of the disease, or the impression that nothing had been left to research in this field, scientific interest in subacute thyroiditis is rather low. Over the last two decades no more than 20–30 papers have been yearly published on this topic. At the same time, many aspects of SAT remain unclear, as listed in Table 1.

Epidemiology

Some data are summarized in Table 2. The incidence of the disease in the community is unknown. In earlier papers, subacute thyroiditis was reported not to be a rare cause of hyperthyroidism. However, it is more probable that only 1–2 % of patients seen in a thyroid outpatient clinic will have SAT. It is not known if the incidence depends on the iodine intake. In children, SAT is a rarity (28). The female-male ratio 3–10:1. Some authors have reported that SAT occurs more often during the summer, others do not (Table 2).

Etiology

The history of SAT following upper respiratory tract infections strongly suggests a connection with viral infection. An epidemic of thyrotoxicosis due to atypical subacute thyroiditis in Holland affecting 23 individuals (18) and the report of 11 patients

Table 1 Unclear aspects of SAT

- there are no exact data on the prevalence of the disease and of its possible dependence on iodine supply
- the viral etiology suggested by older literature is challenged by recent data
- even accepting the etiological role of viral infection, the precipitating factors and the mechanism of onset remain unclear
- there are no clear data on the natural course of the disease
- there are only few data on the role of adhesion molecules, cytokines and growth factors in SAT so that no complex pathogenetic scheme of the events leading to formation and resolution of the granulomatous disease as well as to the repair of the thyroid follicles could have been worked out up to now
- randomized studies are lacking concerning the effectiveness of steroid versus nonsteroidal anti-inflammatory drug treatment and the necessary duration of administration
- the recurrence of the disease is still not predictable in individual patients.

with SAT diagnosed during a mumps epidemic and anti-mumps antibodies but no clinical evidence of mumps (21) support this view. However, mumps virus was cultured from the thyroid tissue of only two patients. *Volpé et al.* (1967) (101) found some circulating viral antibody in 58 out of 71 patients with SAT and a "significant" (at least 4-fold) change of the titer in 32. The methods were complement fixation or neutralization tests. Viral antibodies included those against influenza, Coxsackie, adenovirus, ECHO and mumps viruses. Coxsackie virus antibodies have most commonly correlated with the course of the illness. However, these results have been challenged by recent data: *Luotola et al.* (1998) (59) could find no association of SAT with Coxsackie virus infection by antibody determination, virus isolation, RT-PCR or antigen detection. *Mori et al.* (1998) (67) measured serum virus-specific antibodies to measles, rubella, mumps, type 1 herpes, chicken pox, human parvovirus B 19 and cytomegalovirus (CMV) in 10 patients with SAT. Despite more than 70 % of patients having IgG to each virus in more, no significant changes in the IgG titers were observed except those to measles, rubella, chicken pox or CMV in only 10 % of patients, respectively. They also failed to detect Epstein-Barr virus and cytomegalovirus DNA in thyroid aspirates. Thus, no single agent seems to be causative in the syndrome of SAT. Except for single cases of mumps, invasion of the thyroid by viruses is not proven. Further studies are clearly required to establish the definitive role of viral infection in the pathogenesis of SAT.

Genetics

There has been a strong association between HLA-Bw35 and subacute thyroiditis in all ethnic group tested (Caucasians, Chinese and Japanese) (1, 7, 29, 49, 71, 87, 90,

Table 2 Epidemiological studies on SAT

Author, year	Number of cases	Gender ratio F:M	Incidence compared to	Preponderance of cases	Prevalent months of onset
Woolner et al. 1957 (107)	162		1:8 to Graves' disease	3–5 decades	
Reviewed by Greene 1971 (30)	12		0.01 % of all hospital admissions		
Kitaoka et al. 1985 (47)	1127	10.6:1		40 year of age	July
Martino et al. 1987 (63)	80	3.2:1		Mean: 44 years	66 % Jun-Sep; 46 % Jul-Aug
Oksa et al. 1989 (74)					no seasonal distribution
Kitchener and Chapman 1989 (48)	105		9.9 % of subjects scanned for hyperthyroidism		
Iitaka et al. 1998 (40)	1697		1.89 % of patients with thyroid disorders in hospital		
Cap et al. 1999 (14)	32		1.52 % of FNA performed in 2100 patients		

113). HLA-Bw 35 was positive in 33 out of 39 German patients with SAT (84.6 %) (7). In a study of Japanese patients, the frequency of HLA-Bw35 was 67.4 % (versus 14.1 % in the controls, $p<0.001$). Associations with other class I (Cw1 and Cw3) and class II (DRw8) HLA antigens were also found but they were much weaker: Cw1 in SAT 14.6 % and 32.1 % in the control ($p<0.01$), Cw3 in SAT 65.2 % and 46.5 % in the control ($p<0.01$), DRw8 in SAT 38.2 % and 21.9 % in the control ($p<0.05$) (49). The relative risk of the disease in the carriers of HLA-Bw35 is high, ranging from 8–56.6. It is presumed that the HLA-Bw35 augments the immune response in SAT, thus permitting expression of the disease. However, HLA-Bw35 is probably only a precipitating factor in SAT, since according to *Smallridge et al.* (1986) (87) and *Peretianu et al.* (1990) (77), the presence or absence of HLA-Bw35 did had no influence on the clinical features or outcome of the disease.

Pathology

The gland may be subtle or markedly enlarged. Usually the enlargement appears asymmetrical or focal by palpation, but sometimes the whole gland is involved. Histologically, the changes are patchy and depend on the stage of the disease. Early in the active inflammatory stage, the follicles may be entirely disrupted and replaced by neutrophils forming microabscesses. Later the more characteristic granulomatous foci appear (Figure 1) in the form of aggregations of cells around damaged follicles admixed with multinucleate giant cells enclosing naked pools or fragments of colloid. Electron microsopy and immunocytochemical studies suggest that the giant cells are of either histiocytic or follicular cell origin (65, 80, 81). In the later stages of the disease, a chronic inflammatory infiltrate and fibrosis may replace the foci. A certain degree of fibrosis appears to be characteristic of de Quervain's thyroiditis (82). Different histological stages may be found in the same gland, suggesting waves of destruction over a period of time. In a recent study (50) apoptotic nuclei were found in granulomas, especially in macrophages/histiocytes and lymphocytes, and in regenerating follicular cells. The death antagonist protein Bcl-2 and the death agonist pro-

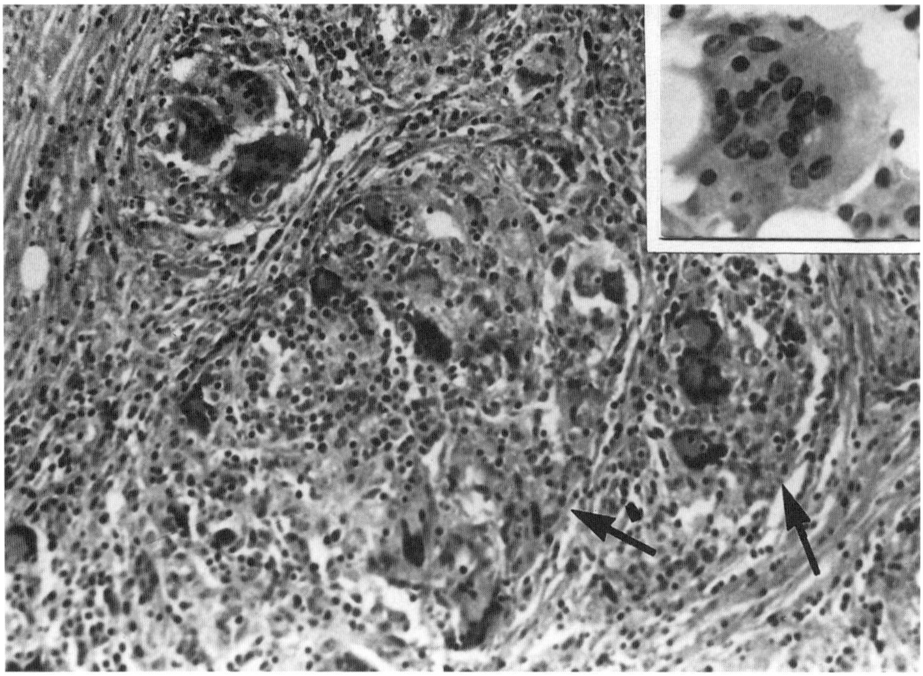

Fig. 1 Histology of subacute thyroiditis, HE, 120x magnification. Arrows indicate granulomas. Inset: multinucleated giant cell, HE, 350x magnification (courtesy of I. Lellei, Dep. of Pathology, Faculty of Health Sciences, Semmelweis University, Budapest).

teins Bak and Bax were strongly expressed in the granulomas and regenerating follicular cells suggesting that apoptosis may be involved both in the development of and recovery from SAT. The mechanism of inflammation is poorly understood. Interleukin-6 (IL-6) produced by macrophages and monocytes is the main mediator of the acute phase response. Its substantial increase in SAT seems to be related to the inflammatory disorder and not to thyrotoxicosis (4, 108). Elevation of the acute phase protein CRP may be IL-6 mediated. Increased granulocyte colony-stimulating factor (G-CSF) is one of the mediators increasing the number of neutrophils in SAT (79). An elevated circulating soluble intracellular adhesion molecule/1 concentration found in SAT may also reflect the degree of inflammatory activity in the thyroid gland (76). By contrast, IL-12, a mediator of Th1-type immune response was not elevated in SAT (34).

Interleukin-2 + tumor necrosis factor alpha + alpha interferon-treatment caused painless but antibody negative thyroiditis in 6 patients (99). *Amenomori et al.* (1998) (2) observed destructive thyroiditis in about 10 % of patients with chronic hepatitis C treated with interferon. Individual case reports also support their data (22, 51, 92). These observations indirectly indicate the importance of cytokines in the pathogenesis of SAT.

Toda et al. (1999) (94) investigated the immunohistochemical expression of growth factors in SAT. Their data suggest:

- First, that at the granulomatous stage of subacute thyroiditis, growth factor-rich monocytes/macrophages infiltrating into follicle lumina trigger the granulomatous reaction, and that the reaction is mediated by vascular endothelial cell growth factor (VEGF), basic fibroblast growth factor (bFGF), platelet-derived growth factor-BB (PDGF), and transforming growth factor-β1 (TGF-β1) produced by stroma cell types;
- Secondly, that at the regenerative stage, epidermal growth factor (EGF) serves follicle regeneration through its mitogenic effect on thyrocytes, although some cofactors with EGF are involved in folliculogenesis. The decreased expression of TGF-β1, a fibrogenic factor, contributes to thyroid tissue repair;
- And thirdly, that VEGF and bFGF are more responsible for angiogenesis at both stages than other factors.

Also, the serum VEGF level was higher among patients with untreated SAT than among those with Graves' disease or Hashimoto's thyroiditis (41).

Autoimmunity may play a role in SAT. The tissue damage leads to expression of thyroid antibodies and these may in turn influence the clinical status of the disease. Cytotoxic T cells are important in thyroid destruction. However, the autoimmune events are probably not primary but represent nonspecific response to the inflammatory process and are transient (15, 26, 44, 45, 73, 98).

Volpé et al. (1967) (101) detected antibodies against thyroglobulin (Tg) or the microsomal component in the acute stage of SAT among 25.3 % of their patients, and in 42.8 % over a period of three to four months, but in 21 of these 30 patients the antibodies subsequently disappeared. *Bliddal et al.* (1985) (11) investigated 10 patients with SAT: Tg antibodies were present in four, while microsomal antibodies were negative. TPO-Ab have not previously been studied systematically in SAT: these antibodies are probably transient, and they disappear after several months (55). In our practice, we do not determine thyroid antibodies in the acute stage of SAT but only six months later in order to identify possible misdiagnosed cases of subacute autoimmune thyroiditis. Subacute thyroiditis may trigger autoreactive B cells to produce TSH receptor antibodies, as occurred in 38 out of 1697 patients with SAT (40). In most of these cases the TSH receptor antibodies did not influence thyroid status, but *Tamai et al.* (1991) (91) found a higher proportion of antibody positivity among SAT patients who developed hypothyroidism requiring thyroxine therapy for 1.2–3.5 yr.

Graves' disease after SAT is extremely rare. In some of the reported cases (5, 8, 25, 32, 103, 106) HLA typing indicated that the patient had a genetic predisposition to Graves' disease as well as to SAT.

Diagnosis and differentiation of SAT

Diagnostic features of subacute thyroiditis are listened in Table 3. The clinical manifestations of SAT vary from the typical presentation with subacute onset, painful tender goiter and fever to cases with painless goiter (6–10 %) (38, 48) or with localized SAT presenting as cold nodules suggestive of thyroid cancer (6, 10, 33, 53, 64). Several case reports indicate that atypical SAT should be considered in cases of FUO (fever of unknown origin) (3, 24, 37, 56, 62, 59), and radiogallium scintigraphy appears to be very useful in detecting these cases (17, 58, 66, 83).

With typical presentation, the diagnosis is not difficult. In an extensive study by *Iitaka et al.* 1998 (40) (1697 patients with SAT) seven diagnostic criteria were used:

1. painful tender goiter
2. elevated erythrocyte sedimentation rate (ESR)
3. depressed radioiodine uptake
4. transient hyperthyroidism
5. ultrasonographic findings compatible with SAT
6. pathological findings by fine needle aspiration cytology (FNA) compatible with SAT
7. absent or low titers of thyroid autoantibodies

All patients met the first two criteria and at least 2 other criteria.

The features of atypical versus typical SAT are summarized in Table 4, based on data of *Yamashita et al.* (1993) (112). SAT should be differentiated from a variant of

Table 3 Diagnostic features of subacute thyroiditis and approximate frequency of their manifestation (modified from Lazarus 1996 (54))

	Characteristics	**Frequency**
History and physical examination	preceding upper respiratory infection	1/3
	fever	most
	sore throat	1/3
	painful thyroid swelling	most
	symptoms of thyrotoxicosis	1/2
	migrating thyroid tenderness	1/2
Laboratory	high erythrocyte sedimentation rate	most
	leukocytosis	1/2
	FT4 or FT3 elevated	2/3
	TSH suppressed	most
	elevated Tg	most
	thyroid antibody +	1/5, transitory
	HLA-Bw35 +	2/3
Radiological	US: generalized or multiple or single	
	hypoechogenicity	most
	low isotope uptake	most
	67-Gallium scan positive	most
Clinical course and outcome	transient hypothyroidism (second phase of the disease)	half
	recurrence	1/3
	definitive hypothyroidism	< 1/10

"most" means about 90 % of the cases

autoimmune lymphocytic thyroiditis called silent (painless) thyroiditis (reviewed by Lazarus 1996). The most helpful distinguishing features are absence of pain, normal erythrocyte sedimentation rate, and fine needle aspiration cytology (FNA). The course of the disease is very similar to SAT and proceeds from a thyrotoxic phase through a hypothyroid phase to spontaneous remission with euthyroidism. Localized SAT may be difficult to differentiate from thyroid cancer (72, 112). Pain and tenderness, fever, high erythrocyte sedimentation rate and leukocytosis, the tendency to spread to the contralateral lobe, and prompt remission on corticosteroid treatment help to make in differentiation, as does fine needle aspiration cytology (FNA).

Typically, the natural course of subacute thyroiditis has three phases. Following

Table 4 Characteristics and clinical course of atypical SAT (summarized data of Yamashita et al. 1993 (112)

	Atypical SAT (N=11)	Typical SAT (N=94)
Neck pain as initial symptom	18%	69%
Elevated thyroid hormone levels	42%	76%
Suppressed TSH	46%	85%
Misdiagnosed as having papillary thyroid cancer	9/11	
Clinically	9/11	
By US	4/11	
Admitted to hospital because of suspected cancer	8/11	
Surgery performed	4/11	

initial thyrotoxicosis (2–11 week), about half of the cases develop mild hypothyroidism (2–3 months). In the majority of cases, this is followed by a third phase with recovery to euthyroidism (30, 52)

Biochemical measurements

In the early stage of SAT elevated T_4 (FT_4) or T_3 was found in 46–100 % of the patients (7, 43, 93, 104) but mean free hormone levels were lower than in Graves' disease (85, 114). *Madeddu et al.* (1982) (60) reported, that 6/9 patient with unilobular or nodular SAT had normal free hormone levels, whereas all three patients with diffuse enlargement of the thyroid had elevated hormone levels.

With rare exceptions, TSH is suppressed in SAT patients indicating hyperthyroidism. However, using third generation TSH assay with higher analytical sensitivity *Ito et al.* (1997) (43) found that only 22 % of SAT patients (versus 86 % in Graves' disease) had TSH values below the detection limit. *Kasagi et al.* (1999) (46) have reported very similar data (undetectable TSH in SAT: 12.5 %, in Graves' disease: 82 %). The data suggest that duration of thyrotoxicosis in SAT is too short to cause complete suppression of TSH, and thus the conclusion that third-generation TSH assays may be useful for differentiation between SAT and Graves' disease.

Similarly, sex hormone binding globulin (SHBG) was elevated in only 1 out of 12 patients with SAT (versus 57 out of 82 patients with Graves' disease) (100). Red blood cell zinc concentration was depressed in only one out of ten patient with SAT (versus all ten patients with Graves' disease) (115). These parameters also indicate the shorter duration of hyperthyroidism in SAT but are rarely used in the differential diagnosis.

Serum Thyroglobulin (Tg) was elevated in 92 % of patients with SAT in the early stage. In some patients, serum Tg decreased after corticosteroid treatment, but in others levels peaked about 2 months after disease onset (61). *Smallridge et al.* (1986) (87) also observed the highest Tg concentrations 1–3 months after onset of symptoms, and in some cases elevated Tg levels persisted over 2 or more years. Thus, Tg measurements seem not to be useful in follow up of patients with SAT or for predicting disease recurrence. Interestingly, *Druetta et al.* (1999) (20) found T_4 and T_3 residues on circulating Tg to be a common feature of SAT, and speculate that, in some patients with SAT, extrathyroidal production of T_4 from serum Tg may contribute to transient thyrotoxicosis.

(For autoimmune parameters see above)

Ultrasonography

Ultrasonography (US) is useful in the diagnosis of SAT. At first presentation, practically all patients have abnormalities (generalized hypodensity, single or multiple hypodense areas). Using color flow Doppler sonography, patients with SAT have normal thyroid vascularity (absent or minimal intraparenchymal spots) and normal intraparenchymal peak systolic velocity (12) (see Figures 2a and 2b). In the recovery stage of SAT, vascularization became slightly increased and normalized after follow-up for 1 year (36). In one preliminary study, which requires confirmation, lymphadenopathy seemed to be a specific US index of SAT (88). US is also useful in the follow up of SAT (9, 95). In the series of *Bennedbaek and Hegedüs* (1997) (9), the initial median thyroid volume was 40 ml (range 20–289) and fell to 13 ml (range 9–40 ml) after a median follow-up period of 18 months. Nevertheless, 60 % of the patients had persistent morphological abnormalities. Thyroid function was not related to US changes. Recurrence (in 35 % of the patients) was related to the further extension of hypoechoic areas and an increase in thyroid volume. Thus, US seems to be of some value in the prediction of recurrence. In other studies with longer follow up, the rate of persistence of US abnormalities was less frequent: 39 % after a mean follow up of 46.5 months (7) and 11.8 % after a mean follow up of 23 months (13). However, these were earlier studies and detection of small intrathyroidal foci depends significantly on the quality of the transducer used.

Isotope scanning

In 1949 *Werner, Quimby and Schmidt* (105) described the characteristic low 131-I uptake of subacute thyroiditis and this has been recognized as one of the most dependable findings in the acute stage of the disease ascribed mainly to inflammatory follicular cell damage (reviewed by Greene 1971 (30)). Technetium-99m pertechnea 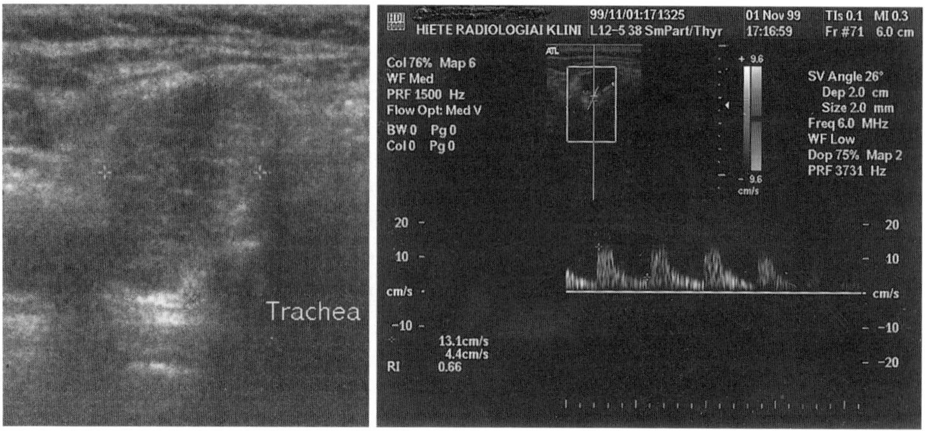 b

Fig. 2a: Ultrasonography of subacute thyroiditis: hypoechogenicity of the right lobe. **b:** Normal vascularity and normal intraparenchymal peak systolic velocity in subacute thyroiditis (courtesy of A. Szabó, Dep. of Radiology, Faculty of Health Sciences, Semmelweis University, Budapest).

tate has now almost entirely replaced radioiodine scanning. With rare exceptions (86), uptake is suppressed in the acute stage of SAT and returns to normal or becomes slightly elevated in the recovery stage, similar to the radioiodine uptake. Several other scanning agents, however, show prolonged retention in the acute stage of SAT, and they may directly reflect inflammatory changes in the thyroid associated with SAT. These agents are:

- Technetium-99m-tetrafosmin (35)
- 201-Thallium-chloride (96)
- 67-Gallium-citrate (17, 58, 66, 83)

In clinical practice, however, there is rarely a need to use these special scanning agents to make a diagnosis of SAT. In fact, in our practice, if we see a patient with painful tender goiter, fever, high erythrocyte sedimentation rate, hyperthyroid laboratory status and with ultrasonographic and FNA findings characteristic of SAT, we do not perform thyroid scanning at all.

Evaluation of the thyroid iodine content by X-ray fluorescence technique utilizing a 241-Americium source in 17 patients with SAT showed that thyroid iodine content decreased from 9.8 to a nadir of 3.8 mg and this persisted for 2 years or more (87). *Fragu et al.* (1982) (23) obtained similar results: in six out of 13 patients with SAT, iodine content was still below normal values 12 months after clinical remission. These data suggest that the course of subacute thyroiditis might be longer than would appear from the clinical data, the hormonal assays, or the radioactive uptake data.

Magnetic resonance imaging was used in three patients with SAT: On T1-weighted images, regions of abnormality with irregular margins and slightly high intensity were demonstrated. On T2-weighted images markedly increased intensity was shown in the same sites (75).

Fine needle aspiration cytology

Fine needle aspiration cytology (FNA) is less important for diagnosing SAT than for ruling out other thyroid conditions if the clinical presentation is not typical. Thus, FNA is not performed in all cases. The findings for reaching a confident cytological diagnosis are simultaneous presence in the same aspirate of the following cells:

1. follicular cells with intravacuolar granules and/or plump transformed follicular cells
2. epitheloid granulomas
3. multinucleated giant cells (see Figure 3)
4. acute and chronic inflammatory dirty background
5. the absence of following cells: fire-flare cells, hypertrophic cells, oncocytic cells, and transformed lymphocytes.

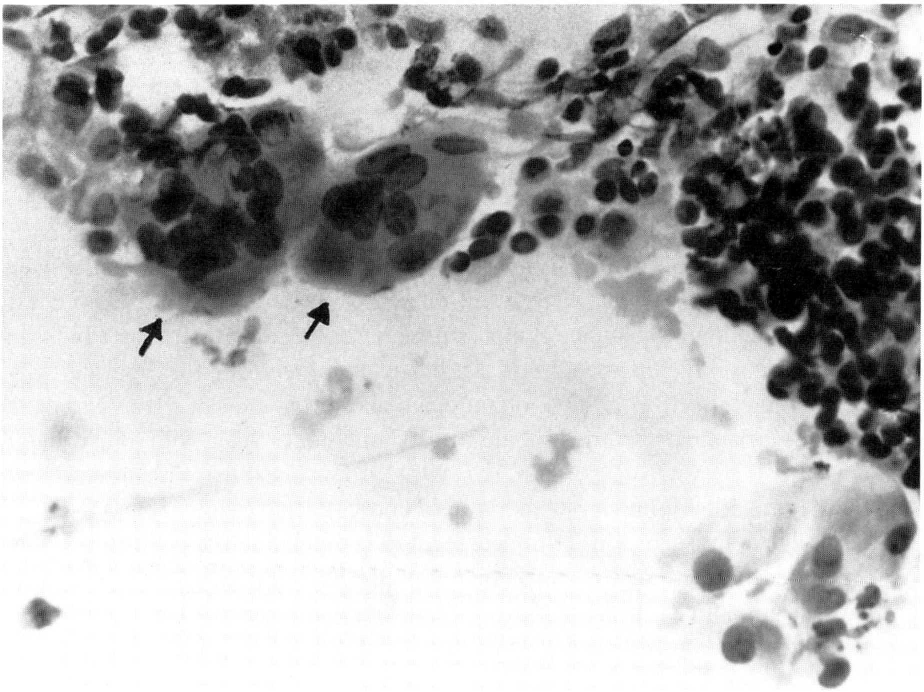

Fig. 3 Fine needle aspiration cytology: multinucleated giant cells, indicated by arrows (courtesy of Zs. Bánrévi, Dep. of Pathology, Faculty of Health Sciences, Semmelweis University, Budapest).

The absence of one or more of these requirements does not exclude SAT but does increase the number of thyroid conditions in the differential diagnosis (27).

Cytology is usually performed on initial presentation of the patient and is not necessary afterwards. Thus, serial FNA, as done by *Lu et al.* (1997) (57) is not recommended but interesting: the initial cytological findings showed chiefly enlarged, degenerate follicular cells with prominent nucleoli, lymphocytes, colloid substance, giant cells and neutrophils. In parallel with regression of sonographic hypoechogenicity, acute inflammatory cells and enlarged, degenerative follicular cells disappeared and cohesive follicles appeared. Multinucleate giant cells are typical of SAT but may also be found in papillary carcinoma, other granulomatous thyroid diseases, and benign nodular goiter, so that the accompanying cell population makes the cytological diagnosis (84). FNA is not always diagnostic. Over a period of 12 years, *Ofner et al.* (1994) (72) performed 252 FNAs among patients with clinical suspicion of SAT, but they also had 31 cases with preoperative FNA who were diagnosed histologically as SAT. Absence of typical cytological features and the appearance of atypical thyroid follicular cells, led to a suspicion of malignancy in 13 out of these 31 patients on FNA. It was concluded that the cytopathologist requires accurate clinical information relating to the possibility of SAT to avoid unnecessary surgery.

Treatment and outcome

Subacute thyroiditis is supposedly a self-limiting inflammatory process and indeed, in some patients with the mild form of the disease no medication is required. According to the older literature (reviewed by Greene 1971) (30), treatment with corticosteroids or salicylates and other nonsteroidal anti-inflammatory drugs effectively ameliorates symptoms of the disease but does not alter the basic disease process. There are no randomized studies comparing the effectiveness of corticosteroids and nonsteroidal anti-inflammatory drugs. Most authors agree (30, 102) that corticosteroids are more effective for ameliorating pain and fever, and salicylates and nonsteroidal anti-inflammatory drugs should be used only for patients with mild or moderate disease. However, *Topuzovic et al.* (1997) (97) reported that they observed recurrences more often following withdrawal of corticosteroid treatment and therefore the mean time before achieving complete restitution of the thyroid was longer among patients on corticosteroids (6.4 ± 2.7 months) than among patients receiving nonsteroidal anti-inflammatory drugs (3.6 ± 1.0 months). *Yamamoto et al.* (1979) (109) reported, that duration of thyroid swelling was shorter among patients treated with prednisolone than among those receiving aspirin, but the high ESR, thyroid tenderness and fever subsided over similar periods. Serum T_4 and T_3 and thyroglobulin declined more rapidly after prednisolone (109, 110).

The recommended initial steroid dose is 40–60 mg prednisolone (or equivalent dose of another corticosteroid) with a gradual reduction in dosage thereafter, but the optimal duration of the treatment in unknown: the recommendations range from several weeks to 3 months and over (52, 54, 70, 97, 102). If the period of corticosteroid administration is too short, there is a higher risk of recurrence during reduction of the steroid dose or just after withdrawal.

The reported recurrence rates range between 11 and 47% (30, 31, 70, 89, 102). Recurrence is an indication for more prolonged corticosteroid treatment but the doses required to control the symptoms are usually much lower than in the initial phase of the disease.

There are no practical recommendations concerning how long nonsteroidal anti-inflammatory drugs should be given in SAT. Schemes of combined treatment are also lacking. A single report describes effective of the hyperthyroidism in SAT rather than the SAT itself by sodium iodopate (16). In the very rare cases of repeated relapses despite appropriate treatment, thyroidectomy should be considered (102).

There is a tendency for laboratory parameters to normalize under corticosteroid or nonsteroidal anti-inflammatory treatment but not in all cases. C-reactive protein (CRP) returned to normal in the majority of patients after just one week of steroid therapy, but thyroglobulin and ESR had normalized in only half the cases by the time of cessation of therapy (89). Serum sialic acid levels were found by these authors to be a good marker of restitution and recurrence in SAT.

Most patients recover completely after SAT and in the older literature (reviewed by Greene 1971) (30), permanent hypothyroidism was reported to be extremely rare as outcome of SAT. More recently, *Ishizuki et al.* (1992) (42) have reported 4 cases of hypothyroidism out of 26 patient investigated 5–30 years after SAT. However, these Japanese patients as well as the control subjects without SAT in their history, had a high (over 40%) prevalence of thyroid antibody positivity. Thus, they might have had an autoimmune predisposition to develop hypothyroidism either.

Late recurrences after SAT are extremely rare: *Iitaka et al.* 1996 (39) found 48 out of 3344 patients with SAT who had a second episode of the disease after 14.5 ± 4.5 years and 5 patients who had a third episode after 7.6 ± 2.4 years. Recurrence is still not predictable in the individual patient (30, 77, 87, 111).

References

1. Aiginger P, Weissel M, Fritzsche H, Kroiss A, Hoffer R, Mayr WR. HLA antigens and de Quervain's thyroiditis. Tissue Antigens 1978;11: 59–60.
2. Amenomori M, Mori T, Fukuda Y, Sugawa H, Nishida N, Furukawa M, Kita R, Sando T, Komeda T, Nakao K. Incidence and characteristics of thyroid dysfunction following interferon therapy in patients with chronic hepatitis C. Intern Med 1998;37:246–252.
3. Bajo Bajo A, Santoz Perez ME, Ramos Delgado E. Subacute thyroiditis: a possible cause of prolonged fever syndrome in primary care. Aten Primaria (Spain) 1994;14:694–696.
4. Bartalena L, Brogioni S, Grasso L, Martino E. Increased serum interleukin-6 concentration in pa-

tients with subacute thyroiditis: relationship with concomitant changes in serum T_4-binding globulin concentration. J Endocr Invest 1993;16:213–218.
5. Bartalena L, Bogazzi F, Pecori F, Martino E. Graves' disease occurring after subacute thyroiditis: report of a case and review of the literature. Thyroid 1996;6:345–348.
6. Bartels PC, Boer RO. Subacute thyroiditis (de Quervain) presenting as a painless "cold" nodule. J Nucl Med 1987;28:1488–1490.
7. Benker G, Olbricht T, Windek R, Wagner R, Albers H, Lederbogen S, Hoff HG, Reinwein D. The sonographical and functional sequelae of de Quervain's subacute thyroiditis. Acta Endocrinol (Cobenh) 1988;117:435–441.
8. Bennedbaek FN, Gram J, Hegedus L. The transition of subacute thyroiditis to Graves' disease as evidenced by diagnostic imaging. Thyroid 1996;6:457–459.
9. Bennedbaek FN, Hegedus L. The value of ultrasonography in the diagnosis and follow-up of subacute thyroiditis. Thyroid 1997;7:45–50.
10. Bianda T, Schmid C. De Quervain's subacute thyroiditis presenting as a painless solitary thyroid nodule. Postgrad Med J 1998;74:602–603.
11. Bliddal H, Bech K, Feldt-Rasmussen U, Hoier-Madsen M, Thomsen B, Nielsen H. Humoral autoimmune manifestation in subacute thyroiditis. Allergy 1985;40:599–604.
12. Bogazzi F, Bartalena L, Brogioni S, Burelli A, Manetti L, Tanda ML, Gasperi M, Martino E. Thyroid vascularity and blood flow are not dependent on serum thyroid hormone levels: studies in vivo by color flow Doppler sonography. Eur J Endocrinol 1999;140:452–456.
13. Brander A. Ultrasound appearances in de Quervain's subacute thyroiditis with long-term follow up. J Intern Med 1992;232:321–325.
14. Cap J, Ryska A, Rehorkova P, Hovorkova E, Kerekes Z, Pohnetalova D. Sensitivity and specificity of the fine needle aspiration biopsy of the thyroid: clinical point of view. Clin Endocrinol 1999;51:509–515.
15. Chartier B, Bandy P, Wall JR. Fc receptor-bearing blood mononuclear cells in thyroid disorders: increased levels in patients with subacute thyroiditis. J Clin Endocrinol Metab 1980;51:1014.
16. Chopra IJ, van Herle AJ, Korenman SG, Viosca S, Younai S. Use of sodium iopodate in management of hyperthyroidism in subacute thyroiditis. J Clin Endocrinol Metab 1995;80:2178–2180.
17. Coolens JL, Sprengers D, Van Parys G, De Roo M. Subacute thyroiditis detected by 67 gallium-citrate scintigraphy. Acta Clin Belg 1986;41:328–332.
18. de Bruin TW, Rieckhoff FP, de Boer JJ. An outbreak of thyrotoxicosis due to atypical subacute thyroiditis. J Clin Endocrinol Metab 1990;70:396–402.
19. de Quervain F. Die akute nich eitrige Thyreoiditis und die Beteiligung der Schilddrüse an akuten Intoxikationen und Infektionen überhaupt. Mitteilungen aus den Grenzgebieten der Medizin und Chirurgie 1904; Supplement 2, Bd 1–165.
20. Druetta L, Bornet H, Sassolas G, Rousset B. Identification of thyroid hormone residues on serum thyroglobulin: a clue to the source of circulating thyroglobulin in thyroid diseases. Eur J Endocrinol 1999;140:457–467.
21. Elyan E, Zmucky R, Sheba C. Mumps virus and subacute thyroiditis. Evidence of a causal association. Lancet 1957;1:1062–1063.
22. Falashi P, Martocchia A, D'Urso R, Proietti A. Subacute thyroiditis during interferon-alpha therapy for chronic hepatitis C. J Endocrine Invest 1997;20:24–28.
23. Fragu P, Rougier P, Schlumberger M, Tubiana M. Evolution of thyroid 127I stores measured by X-ray fluorescence in subacute thyroiditis. J Clin Endocrinol Metab 1982;54:162–166.
24. Friedman ND, Spelman DW. Subacute thyroiditis presenting as pyrexia of unknown origin in a patient with human immunodeficiency virus infection. Clin Infect Dis 1999;29:1352–1353.
25. Fukata S, Matsuzuka F, Kobayashi A, Hirai K, Kuma K, Sugawara M. Development of Graves' disease after subacute thyroiditis: two unusual cases. Acta Endorinol (Copenh) 1992;126:495–496.
26. Galluzzo A, Giordano C, Andronico F, Filardo C, Andronico G, Bompiani G. Leucocyte migration test in subacute thyroiditis: hypothetical role of cell mediated immunity. J Clin Endocrinol Metab 1980;50:1038–1041.
27. Garcia Solano J, Gimenez Bascunana A, Sola Perez J, Campos Fernandez J, Marinez Parra D, Sanchez Sanchez C, Montalban Romero S, Perez-Guillermo M. Fine-needle aspiration of subacute

granulomatous thyroiditis (De Quervain's thyroiditis): a clinico-cytologic review of 36 cases. Diagn Cytopathol 1997;16:214–220.
28. Geva T, Theodor R. Atypical presentation of subacute thyroiditis. Arch Dis Child 1988;63:845–846.
29. Goto H, Uno H, Tamai H, Kuma J, Hayashi Y, Matsubayashi S, Sasazuki T. Genetic analysis of subacute (de Quervain's) thyroiditis. Tissue Antigens 1985;26:110–113.
30. Greene JN. Subacute thyroiditis. Am J Med 1971;51:97–108.
31. Grozariu L, Stroe M, Vladutiu T, Yepez-Escobar NG, Simionescu L, Szantay I, Dimitru E, Florescu O. Late hypothyroidism following subacute thyroiditis. Exp Clin Endokrinol 1986;87:48–52.
32. Grunenberger F, Chenard MP, Weber JC, Jaeck D, Schlienger JL. Relapse of Graves' disease after subacute thyroiditis. Thyroid 1998;8:683–685.
33. Hardoff R, Luboshitzky R. Transient cold nodule of the thyroid due to localized subacute thyroiditis. Clin Nucl Med 1989;12:919–920.
34. Hidaka Y, Okumura M, Fukata S, Shimaoka Y, Takeoka K, Tada H, Kuma K, Amino N. Increased serum concentration of interleukin-l2 in patients with silent thyroiditis and Graves' disease. Thyroid 1999;9:149–153.
35. Hiromatsu Y, Ishibashi M, Miyake I, Nonaka K. Technetium-99m tetrafosmin imaging in patients with subacute thyroiditis. Eur J Nucl Med 1998;25:1448–1452.
36. Hiromatsu Y, Ishibashi M, Miyake I, Soyejima E, Yamashita K, Koike N, Nonaka K. Color Doppler ultrasonography in patients with subacute thyroiditis. Thyroid 1999;9:1189–1193.
37. Hoffman HS. Subacute thyroiditis as fever of unknown origin. Conn Med 1996;60:438–439.
38. Hwang CS, Jap TS, Ho LT, Ching KN. Subacute thyroiditis – 61 cases review. Chuang Hua I Hsueh Tsa Chih (Taipei) 1989;43:113118.
39. Iitaka M, Momotani N, Ishii J, Ito K. Incidence of subacute thyroiditis recurrence after a prolonged latency: 24-year survey. J Clin Endocrinol Metab 1996;81:466–469.
40. Iitaka, M, Momotani N, Hisaoka T, Yoshimura Noh J, Ishikawa N, Ishii J, Katayama S, Ito K. TSH receptor antibody-associated thyroid dysfunction following subacute thyroiditis. Clin Endocrinol 1998;48:445–453.
41. Iitaka M, Miura S, Yamanaka K, Kawasaki S, Kitahama S, Kawakami Y, Kakinuma S, Oosuga I, Wada S, Katayama S. Increased serum vascular endothelial growth factor levels and intrathyroidal vascular area in patients with Graves' disease and Hashimoto thyroiditis. J Clin Endocrinol Metab 1998;83:3908–3912.
42. Ishizuki Y, Hirooka Y, Murata Y, Togashi K. The functional outcome of patients with subacute thyroiditis. Nippon Naibunpi Gakkai Zasshi 1992;68:154–165.
43. Ito M, Takamatsu J, Yoshida S, Murakami Y, Sakane S, Kuma K, Ohsawa N. Incomplete thyrotroph suppression determined by third generation thyrotropin assay in subacute thyroiditis compared to silent thyroiditis or hyperthyroid Graves' disease. J Clin Endocrinol Metab 1997;82616–619.
44. Iwatani Y, Amino N, Hidaka Y, Kaneda T, Ichihara K, Tamaki H, Matsuzuka F, Fukata S, Kuma K, Miyai K. Decreases in alpha beta T cell receptor negative T cells and CD8 cells, and an increase in CD4+ CD8+ cells in active Hashimoto's disease and subacute thyroiditis. Clin Exp Immunol 1992;87:444–449.
45. Karlsson FA, Totterman TH, Jansson R. Subacute thyroiditis. activated HLA-DR and interferon-gamma expressing T cytotoxic/suppressor cells in thyroid tissue and peripheral blood. Clin Endocrinol 1986;25:487–493.
46. Kasagi K, Kousaka T, Misaki T, Iwata M, Alam MS, Konishi J. Comparison of serum thyrotropin concentration determined by a third generation assay in patients with various types of overt and subclinical thyrotoxicosis. Clin Endocrinol 1999;50:185–189.
47. Kitaoka H, Sakurada T, Fukazawa H, Suzuki M, Kaise N, Kaise K. et al. An epidemiological study of subacute thyroiditis in northern Japan. Nippon Niabunpi Gakkai Zasshi 1985;61:554–570.
48. Kitchener MI, Chapman IM. Subacute thyroiditis: a review of 105 cases. Clin Nucl Med 1989;14:439–442,
49. Kobayashi N, Tamai H, Nagai K, Matsubayashi S, Matsuzuka F, Kuma K, Goto H, Uno K, Sasazuki T, Nagataki S. Studies on the pathogenesis of subacute thyroiditis. Nippon Naibunpi Gakkai Zasshi 1985;61:737–743.
50. Koga M, Hiromatsu Y, Jimi A, Toda S, Koike N, Nonaka K. Immunohistochemical analysis of Bcl-

2 Bax, and Bak expression in thyroid glands from patients with subacute thyroiditis. J Clin Endocrinol Metab 1999;84:2221–2225.
51. Kreiss Y, Cohen O, Pras E, Achiron A. Subacute thyroiditis in a patient with MS treated with interferon beta-1a. Neurology 1999;53:1606.
52. Kujat C, Dyck R, Brederhoff J, Pfannenstiel P. Diagnoostik und Therapie der subakuten Thyreooiditis. Dtsch Med Wschr 1991;116:1439–1443.
53. Lachaume E, Lecomte P, Chadenas D, Baulieu JL, Ozoux JP, Beutter P. Pseudotumoral form of subacute nodular thyroiditis. Presse Med 1991;20:2107.
54. Lazarus JH. Silent thyroiditis and subacute thyroiditis. In: Werner and Ingbar's The Thyroid. Eds: Braverman LE and Utiger RD. Seventh Edition. Lippincott-Raven, Philadelphia-New York, 1996, pp0.577–591.
55. Lio S, Pontecorvi A, Caruso M, Monaco F, D'Armiento M. Transitory subclinical and permanent hypothyroidism in the course of subacute thyroiditis (de Quervain). Acta Endocrinol (Copenh) 1984;106:67–70.
56. Loscertales P, Cabeza F, Boldova JI. Subacute thyroiditis: an entity to be considered in the context of fever of unknown origin. Rec Clin Esp 1991;189:301.
57. Lu CP, Chang TC, Wang CY, Hsiao YL. Serial changes in ultrasound-guided fine needle aspiration cytology in subacute thyroiditis. Acta Cytol 1997;41:238–243.
58. Lucero Ocana MJ, Moya Mir MS, Lopez Jimenez LE, Gonzalez Quintela A, Roman Garcia J. Subacute thyroiditis as a cause of prolonged fever diagnosed by gallium scan. Rev Clin Esp 1987;181:57–58.
59. Luotola K, Hyoty H, Salmi J, Miettinen A, Helin H, Pasternack A.Evaluation of infectious etiology in subacute thyroiditis – lack of association with Coxsackie virus infection. APMIS 1998;106:500–504.
60. Madeddu G, Langer M, Costanza C, Casu AR, Arras ML, Campus S. Alteration of thyroid function in the early stage of subacute thyroiditis. Acta Endocrinol (Cobenh) 1980;4:479–484.
61. Madeddu G, Casu AR, Costanza C, Marras G, Arras ML, Marrosu A, Langer M. Serum thyroglobulin levels in the diagnosis and follow-up of subacute ‚painful' thyroiditis. A sequential study. Arch Intern Med 1985;145:243–247.
62. Martinez Ortiz JJ. De Quervain's subacute granulomatous thyroiditis: cause of fever of unknown origin. An Med Interna (Spain) 1992;9:309–310.
63. Martino E, Buratti L, Bartlena L, Mariotti S, Cupini C, Aghini-Lombardi F, Pinchera A. High prevalence of subacute thyroiditis during summer season in Italy. J Endocrinol Invest 1987;10:321–323.
64. Meier DA. Transient cold nodule of the thyroid due to localized subacute thyroiditis. Clin Nucl Med 1991;16:139.
65. Mizukami Y, Michigishi T, Kawato M, Matsubara F. Immunohistochemical and ultrastructural study of subacute thyroiditis, with special reference to multinucleated giant cells. Hum Pathol 1987;18:929–935.
66. Miyake H, Tanaka R, Takeoka H, Kiyosue H, Wakisaga M, Ueno S, Mori H. Unsuspected painless thyroiditis detected by radiogallium scintigraphy. Kaku Igatu (Japan) 1992;29:1475–1478.
67. Mori K, Yoshida K, Funato T, Ishii T, Nomura T, Fukuzawa H, Sayama N, Hori H, Ito S, Sasaki T. Failure in detection of Epstein-Barr virus and cytomegalovirus in specimen obtained by fine needle aspiration biopsy of thyroid in patients with subacute thyroiditis. Tohoku J Exp Med 1998;186:13–17
68. Mygind H. Thyroiditis acuta simplex J Laryng 1895;8:181.
69. Nair S, Joshi VR. Acute thyroiditis – an important cause of F.U.O. J Assoc Physicians India. 1992;40:351.
70. Niklaus-Muller E, Mullhaupt B, Perschak H. Steroidtherapie und BSR Verlauf bei Thyreoiditis de Quervain. Schweiz Rundsch Med Prax 1994;83:95–100.
71. Nyulassy S, Hnilica P, Buc M. et al. Subacute (de Quervain's) thyroiditis: association with HLA-Bw35 antigen and abnormalities of the complement system, immunoglobulins and other serum proteins. J Clin Endocrinol Metab 1977;45:270–274.
72. Ofner C, Hittmair A, Kroll I, Bangerl I, Zechamnn W, Totsch M, Ladurner D, Bocker W, Schmid KW. Fine needle aspiration cytodiagnosis of subacute (de Quervain's) thyroiditis in an endemic goitre area. Cytopathology 1994;5:33–40.

73. Ohashi H, Okugawa T, Itoh M. Circulating activated T cell subsets in autoimmune thyroid diseases: differences between untreated and treated patients. Acta Endocrinol 1991;125:502–509.
74. Oksa J, Jarvenpaa P, Metsahonkala L, Pasternack A, Leinikki P. No seasonal distribution in subacute de Quervain's thyroiditis in Finland. J Endocrinol Invest 1989;12:495.
75. Otsuka N, Nagai K, Morita K, Fukunaga M, Okazaki S, Onishi M, Nanba K, Sato M, Taketa K. Magnetic resonance imaging of subacute thyroiditis. Radiat Med (Japan) 1994;12:273–276.
76. Ozata M, Bolu E, Sengul A, Altinsoy HI, Turan M, Corakci A, Hacibektasoglu A, Gundogan MA. Soluble intercellular adhesion molecule-1 concentrations in patients with subacute thyroiditis and in patients with Graves' disease with or without ophthalmopathy. Endocr J 1996;43:517–525.
77. Peretianu D, Balmes E, Gudovan E, Ursu HI, Oprescu S, Ilinca D. The diagnostic and prognostic value of HLA B 35 antigen in viral subacute thyroiditis. Endokrinologie 1990;28:63–66.
78. Roti E, Minelli R, Gardini E, Bianconi L, Braverman LE. Iodine-induced hypothyroidism in euthyroid subjects with previous episode of subacute thyroiditis. J Clin Endocrinol Metab 1990;70:1581–1585.
79. Sakane S, Murakami Y, Sasaki M, Yamano Y, Takamatsu J, Kuma K, Ohsawa N. Serum concentration of granulocyte colony-stimulating factor (G-CSF) by a highly-sensitive chemiluminescent immunoassay during the clinical course of subacute thyroiditis. Endocr J (Japan) 1995;42:391–396.
80. Satoh M. Ultrastructure of the giant cell in de Quervain's subacute thyroiditis. Acta Pathol Jpn 1976;:26:133–137.
81. Schmid KW, Ofner C, Ramsauer T, Hittmair A, Totsch M, Ladurner D, Bocker W. Ca 19–9 expression in subacute (de Quervain's) thyroiditis: an immunohistochemical study. Mod Pathol 1992;5:268–272.
82. Schnyder B, Hedinger C. Occurrence of fibrosis in subacute de Quervain thyroiditis. Schweiz Med Wochenschr 1986;116:1093–1097.
83. Seder J, Shimshak R, Williams R. Reversible 67Ga-citrate uptake in the thyroid with subacute thyroiditis. Clin Nucl Med 1979;4:158–160.
84. Shabb NS, Tawil A, Gergeos F, Saleh M, Azar S. Multinucleated giant cells in fine-needle aspiration of thyroid nodules: their diagnostic significance. Diagn Cytopathol 1999;21:307–312.
85. Shigemasa C, Abe K, Taniguchi S, Mitani Y, Ueta Y, Urabe K, Adachi T, Tanaka T, Yoshida A, Mashiba H. Serum free thyroxine and thyroxine-binding globulin concentrations in early phase of subacute thyroiditis. Endocinol Jpn 1987;34:821–829.
86. Shigemasa C, Teshima S, Taniguchi S, Ueta Y, Mitani Y, Yoshida A. Pertechnetate thyroid uptake is not always suppressed in patients with subacute thyroiditis. Clin Nucl Med 1997;22:109–114.
87. Smallridge RC, De Keyser FM, Van Herle AJ, Butkus NE, Wartofsky L. Thyroid iodine content and serum thyroglobulin: cues to the natural history of destruction-induced thyroiditis. J Clin Endocrinol Metab 1986;62:1213–1219.
88. Solivetti FM, Nasrollah N, Paganelli C, De Majo A. Lymphoadenopathy as specific ultrasonography index of subacute thyroiditis. Preliminary data. Radiol Med (Torino) 1998;96:596–598.
89. Tajiri J, NoguchiS, Morita M, Tamaru M, Murakami T, Murakami N. Serum sialic acid levels in the diagnosis and follow-up of subacute granulomatous thyroiditis. Endocr J (Japan) 1993;40:83–87.
90. Tamai H, Goto H, Uno H, Sasayuki T, Kuma K, Hazashi Z, Matsubazashi S. HLA in Japanese patients with subacute (de Quervain's) thyroiditis. Tissue Antigens 1984;24:58–59.
91. Tamai H, Nozaki T, Mukuta T, Morita T, Matsubayashi S, Kuma K, Kumagai LF, Nagataki S. The incidence of thyroid stimulating blocking antibodies during the hypothyroid phase in patients with subacute thyroiditis. J Clin Endocrinol Metab 1991;73:245–250.
92. Tanabashi S, Kawasc Y, Ukita M, Shiroko T, Kametani M, Kimuda H. A case of chronic hepatitis complicated by subacute thyroiditis during beta-interferon treatment. Nippon Shokakibyo Gakkai Zasshi 1996;93:496–500.
93. Teixeira VL, Romaldini JH, Rodrigues HF, Tanaka LM, Farah CS. Thyroid function during the spontaneous course of subacute thyroiditis. J Nucl Med 1985;5:457–460.
94. Toda S, Nishimura T, Yamada S, Koike N, Yonemitsu N, Watanabe K, Matsumura S, Gärtner R, Sugihara H. Immunohistochemical expression of growth factors in subacute thyroiditis and their effects on thyroid folliculogenesis and angiogenesis in collagen gel matrix culture. J Pathol 1999;188:415–422.
95. Tokuda Y, Kasagi K, Iida Y, Yamamoto K, Hatuba H, Hidaka A, Konishi J, Ishii Y. Sonography of

subacute thyroiditis: changes in the findings during the course of the disease. J Clin Ultrasound 1990;18:21–26.
96. Tonami N, Bunko H, Kuwajima A, Hisada K. Increased localization of 201 Tl-chlorid in subacute thyroiditis. Clin Nucl Med 1979;4:3–5.
97. Topuzovic N, Smoje J, Karner I. The therapeutical approach in subacute (de Quervain's) thyroiditis. J Nucl Med 1997;38:1665.
98. Tottenman TH, Gordin A, Hayry P, Anderson LC, Makinen T. Accumulation of thyroid antigen-reactive T lymphocytes in the gland of patients with subacute thyroiditis. Clin Exp Immunol 1978;32:153–158.
99. Vassilopoulou-Sellin R, Sella A, Dexeus FH, Theriault RL, Pololoff DA. Acute thyroid dysfunction (Thyroiditis) after therapy with interleukin-2. Horm Met Res 1992;24:434–438.
100. Vierhapper H. Bieglmayer C, Nowotny P, Waldhäusl W. Normal serum concentration of sex hormone binding-globulin in patients with hyperthyroidism due to subacute thyroiditis. Thyroid 1998;8:1107–1111.
101. Volpé R, Row VV, Ezrin C. Circulating viral and thyroid antibodies in subacute thyroiditis. J Clin Endocrinol 1967;27:1275–1284.
102. Volpe R. The management of subacute (de Quervain's) thyroiditis. Thyroid 1993;3:253–255.
103. Wartofsky L, Schaaf M. Graves' disease with thyrotoxicosis following subacute thyroiditis. Am J Med 1987;83:761–764.
104. Weihl AC, Daniels GH, Ridgway EC, Maloof F. Thyroid function tests during the early phase of subacute thyroiditis. J Clin Endocrinol Metab 1977;6:1107–1114.
105. Werner SC, Quimby EH, Schmidt C. The use of tracer doses of radioactive iodine, ^{131}I, in the study of normal and disordered thyroid function in man. J Clin Endocr 1949;9:342.
106. Werner SC. Graves' disease following acute (subacute) thyroiditis. Arch Intern Med 1979;139:1313–1315.
107. Woolner LB, McConahey WM, Beahrs OH. Granulomatous thyroiditis (de Quervain's thyroiditis) J Clin Endocr 1957;17:1202.
108. Yamada T, Sato A, Aizawa T. Dissociation between serum interleukin-6 rise and other parameters of disease activity in subacute thyroiditis during treatment with corticosteroids. J Clin Endocrinol Metab 1996;81:577–579.
109. Yamamoto M, Saito S, Kaise K, Kaise N, Yoshida K, Yoshinaga K. Changes in thyroid hormones by treatment with aspirin and prednisolone in subacute thyroiditis with hyperthyroidism. Tohoku J Exp Med 1979;127:85–95.
110. Yamamoto M, Saito S, Sakurada T, Fukazawa H, Yoshida K, Kaise K, Kaise N, Nomura T, Itagaki Y,Yonemitsu K. et al. Effect of prednisolone and salicylate on serum thyroglobulin level in patients with subacute thyroiditis. Clin Endocrinol 1987;27:339–344.
111. Yamamoto M, Saito S, Sakurada T, Tamura M, Kudo Y, Yoshida K, Kaise K, Kaise N, Fukazawa H, Itagaki Y, Yoshinaga K. Recurrence of subacute thyroiditis over ten years after the first attack in three cases. Endocr Jap 1988;35:833–839.
112. Yamashita T, Okamoto T, Kawada J, Iihara M, Tanaka R, Kanaji Y, Obara T. Characteristics and clinical course of patients with subacute thyroiditis without typical signs and symptoms. Nippon Naibunpi Gakkai Zasshi 1993;69:1057–1061.
113. Yeo PP, Chan SH, Aw TC, Lui KF, Rauff A, Mathew T, Chanh CG, Doraisingham S, Lim P, Cheah JS. HLA and Chinese patients with subacute (de Quervain's) thyroiditis. Tissue Antigens 1981;2:249–250.
114. Yoshida K, Sakurada T, Kaise N, Kaise K, Kitaoka H, Fukazawa H, Yamamoto M, Saito S, Yoshinaga K. Serum free thyroxine and triiodothyronine concentrations in subacute thyroiditis. J Clin Endocrinol Metab 1982;55:185–188.
115. Yoshida K, Kiso Y, Watanabe T. Kaise K, Kaise N, Fukazawa H, Yamamoto M, Sakurada T, Yoshinaga K. Erythrocyte zinc concentration in patients with subacute thyroiditis. J Clin Endocrinol Metab 1990;70:788–791.

Irradiation and non-autoimmune thyroiditis

F. Pacini

Department of Endocrinology and Metabolism, Section of Endocrinology, University of Pisa, Pisa, Italy

Introduction

Radiation is a mitogen that may cause damage to the cell DNA. When sufficiently severe, the damage may result in cell death. When the damage is less severe, the consequences on the cell depend upon which gene and cell system is affected.

The thyroid gland is particularly sensitive to the effect of radiation and the evidence that external radiation may damage the thyroid gland is overwhelming. External thyroid radiation, whether delivered for treatment of benign non-thyroidaldiseases or for the treatment of solid and hematological malignancies, carries an increased risk of developing hypothyroidism (in the presence or absence of associated thyroid autoimmunity) and thyroid carcinomas.

Internal radiation (131-iodine) has also been associated with thyroid disease in cases of accidental contamination, as in the case of the Chernobyl nuclear reactor accident (15). When radioactive isotopes of iodine are given for therapeutic purposes, such as for Graves' disease or toxic nodular goiter, the radiation dose is deliberately high with the intent of killing thyroid cells. Indeed, the risk of hypothyroidism at 2 years increases linearly with thyroid dose for radioactive concentrations ranging from 0.9 to 8.3 MBq/g. Thus, the subsequent hypothyroidism cannot be regarded as an unwanted secondary thyroid disease, but rather as the aim of the therapy. No convincing evidence of subsequent thyroid disorders has been provided following administration of 131-iodine for diagnostic use.

This paper will review the current understanding of non-autoimmune hypothyroidism developing after exposure of the thyroid gland to external or internal radiation. One aspect that should be taken into account when studying the relationship between radiation and thyroid disease is the fact that radiation damage may occur several years after exposure and, as a consequence, many patients may be unaware of, or uncertain about, prior radiation exposure. This phenomenon is known as "referral bias".

Hypothyroidism after exposure to external sources of irradiation

External radiotherapy for benign and malignant diseases

Irradiation to the head and neck has been performed in children since 1920 for the treatment of benign conditions such as enlargement of the thymus, tonsils, adenoids or neck lymph nodes, skin angioma, acne, otitis, or tinea capitis (13 ,19, 21, 22). In the past this modality of treatment was particular popular in the U.S.A, while it was less frequently used in Europe. After 1970, external radiation for benign disorders was virtually abandoned in most countries.

While this modality of treatment has been recognized as a major risk for the subsequent development of thyroid carcinoma, hypothyroidism has seldom been observed. This is probably due to the relatively low doses of radiation delivered to the thyroid, which are sufficient to trigger genetic alterations but are insufficient to cause significant cell death.

External irradiation to the head and neck for malignant diseases

In the case of external radiation to the head and neck for malignant disease, the dose delivered to the thyroid may be very high, and is usually greater than that delivered for the treatment of benign conditions. Animal experiments have shown that, for doses larger than 15–20 Gy, the risk of hypothyroidism per gray increases while the risk of thyroid tumor decreases. This finding has been attributed to cell killing, which decreases the number of viable cells that may become neoplastic while increasing the rate of hypothyroidism.

External beam radiotherapy for lymphoma or head and neck cancer is usually given at dosages of more than 20 Gy (2000 rad). Thyroid exposure is sufficient to produce hypothyroidism, and the risk of hypothyroidism increases with higher doses.

External radiotherapy to the neck for Hodgkin's or non-Hodgkin's lymphomas causes hypothyroidism in 20–50 % of patients (1, 2, 18). Subclinical hypothyroidism may be present for many years before disease becomes symptomatic, but in other cases overt hypothyroidism appears rapidly (4, 8, 20). Transient thyrotoxicosis may precede the development of both transient and permanent hypothyroidism (8). Higher doses of radiation are associated with a higher frequency of hypothyroidism (4, 5, 10). The combination of radiotherapy with chemotherapy increases the risk of developing hypothyroidism (8, 17, 6).

External radiotherapy for tumors of the head and neck results in hypothyroidism in approximately 10–50 % of patients (11, 20, 23, 24). The hypothyroidism is subclinical in about two-thirds. Most cases of hypothyroidism develop within one year.

Another condition frequently associated with hypothyroidism is total body irradiation followed by bone marrow transplantation for acute leukemia or aplastic anemia (3, 12, 23, 26). The median onset is one year after transplantation and in half of the cases hypothyroidism is transient. Total body irradiation delivered in a single dose is much more likely to cause hypothyroidism than irradiation given in 6–8 fractions (12, 26).

The outcome of thyroid damage is probably related not only to radiation dose but also to the distance between the thyroid gland and the radiation field. If this is far from the thyroid, as in case of thoracic or abdominal radiation fields in children, the thyroid gland may receive radiation doses of some hundred mGy, not enough to produce hypothyroidism but sufficient to trigger thyroid cancer (9, 28). By contrast, upper thoracic and neck irradiation is more likely to produce hypothyroidism.

Hypothyroidism after accidental exposure to nuclear explosion or nuclear accidents

Atomic bombs in Hiroshima and Nagasaki

After the atomic bombing in Hiroshima and Nagasaki in 1945, the body dose was mainly due to external irradiation (X-rays and neutrons). The amount of contamination by radioactive isotopes of iodine is not precisely known. The health consequences were studied in a cohort of 94,000 survivors and 26,000 individuals who resided in Hiroshima and Nagasaki shortly after the bombing (27).

While thyroid cancer and benign thyroid nodules occur as stochastic effects after thyroid radiation exposure, hypothyroidism and acute thyroiditis occur as deterministic effects, depending upon the radiation dose.

Primary "spontaneous" hypothyroidism (or subclinical hypothyroidism) has been reported among survivors of the atomic bomb in Nagasaki (14). Among 2587 subjects, hypothyroidism was diagnosed in 43 subjects, 27 of whom were thyroid antibody positive and 16 antibody negative, with no gender difference. Since an association was observed between thyroid dose and prevalence of antibody positive, but not antibody negative, primary hypothyroidism, the latter condition may conceivably stem from an underlying autoimmune thyroid disorder. This concept is supported by the finding of Tamura et al. (25), who found that the frequency of radiation-associated hypothyroidism among patients treated for malignant lymphoma decreased significantly when radiation therapy was combined with chemotherapy and immunosuppressive agents.

Exposure to radioactive iodine after nuclear disasters

Iodine, being physiologically accumulated in the thyroid by an active mechanism, has been widely used for several decades in diagnostic evaluation of the thyroid gland and in treatment of patients with hyperthyroidism and differentiated thyroid cancer. The radiation dose delivered by 131-iodine to the thyroid is 1,000 to 10,000-fold higher than that delivered to other tissues. Thus, even a relatively small amount of 131-iodine may deliver a significant, potentially carcinogenic, radiation dose to the thyroid gland. Increasing the radiation dose above a few hundred MBq increases the likelihood of obtaining cell killing and decreases the probability of tumoral changes.

Hypothyroidism has been reported after exposure to internal radiation (radioactive iodine). Among subjects exposed to the fall-out of the Marshall Islands accident (7), hypothyroidism was noted within 10 years from the accident. On this occasion, most cases were not associated with autoimmune thyroid reaction.

By contrast, an increased prevalence of thyroid auto-antibodies (19.5 %) without hypothyroidism has been reported in children living in a Belarus village heavily contaminated by the post-Chernobyl radioactive fall out compared with children living in a non-contaminated village (prevalence 3.8 %) (16). Susceptibility for developing thyroid autoimmunity increased with age at the time of exposure and, among females, peaked at puberty, suggesting that puberty (estrogen) has an additive effect on radiation in the development of thyroid antibodies in females. The study was conducted only 6–8 years after the Chernobyl accident, which may be the reason why cases of overt hypothyroidism were not found. However, later development of thyroid failure is a possibility in this population.

References

1. Behar RA, Hoppe RT. Radiation therapy in the management of bulky mediastinal Hodgkin's disease. Cancer 1990; 66; 75.
2. Brusamolino E, Lazzarino M, Orlandi E et al. Early-stage Hodgkin's disease: long-term results with radiotherapy alone or combined radiotherapy and chemotherapy. Ann Oncol 1994; 5 (Suppl 2); 101.
3. Carlson K, Lonnerholm G, Smedmyr B, Oberg G, Simonsson B. Thyroid function after autologous bone marrow transplantation. Bone Marrow Transplant 1992; 10; 123.
4. Constine LS, Donaldson SS, McDougall IR, Cox RS, Link MP, Kaplan HS. Thyroid dysfunction after radiotherapy in children with Hodgkin's disease. Cancer 1984; 53; 878.
5. DeVathaire F, Fragu P, Francois P et al. Long-term effects on the thyroid of irradiation for skin angiomas in childhood. Radiat Res 1993; 133; 381.
6. Devney RB, Sklar CA, Nesbit ME Jr et al. Serial thyroid function measurements in children with Hodgkin disease. J Pediatr 1984; 105; 223.
7. Dobyns BM, Hyrmer BA. The surgical management of benign and malignant thyroid neoplasms in Marshall islanders exposed to hydrogen bomb fallout. World J Surg 1992; 16; 126–140.
8. Hancock SL, Cox RS, McDougall IR. Thyroid disease after treatment of Hodgkin's disease. N Engl J Med 1991; 325; 599–605.

9. Hawkins MM, Draper GJ, Kingston JE. Incidence of second primary tumours among childhood cancer survivors. Br J Cancer, 1987; 56; 339–47.
10. Kaplan MM, Garnick MB, Gelber R, et al. Risk factors for thyroid abnormalities after neck irradiation for childhood cancer. Am J Med 1983; 74; 272.
11. Livesey EA, Brook CGD. Thyroid dysfunction after radiotherapy and chemotherapy of brain tumours. Arch Dis Child 1989; 64; 593.
12. Locatelli F, Giorgiani G, Pession A, Bozzola M. Late effects in children after bone marrow transplantation: a review. Haematologica 1993; 78; 319.
13. Lundell M, Hakulinen T, Holm LE. Thyroid cancer after radiotherapy for skin hemangioma in infancy. Rad Res, 1994; 40; 334–9.
14. Nagataki S, Shibata Y, Inoue S, Yokoyama N, Izumi M, Shimaoka K. Thyroid disease among atomic bomb survivors in Nagasaki. JAMA, 1994; 272; 364–70.
15. Pacini F, Vorontsova T, Demidchik E et al. Post-Chernobyl thyroid carcinoma in Belarus children and adolescents: comparison with naturally occurring thyroid carcinoma in Italy and France. J Clin Endocrinol Metab 1997; 82; 3563–9.
16. Pacini F, Vorontsova T, Molinaro E et al. Prevalence of thyroid autoantibodies in children and adolescents from Belarus exposed to the Chernobyl radioactive fallout. Lancet, 1998; 352; 763–6.
17. Pasqualini T, Iorcansky S, Gruneiro L, et al. Thyroid dysfunction in Hodgkin's disease. Cancer 1989; 63; 335.
18. Peerboom PF, Hassink EA, Melkert R, De Wit L, Nooijen WJ, Bruning PF. Thyroid function 10–18 years after mantle field irradiation for Hodgkin's disease. Eur J Cancer 1992; 28A; 1716.
19. Pottern LM, Kaplan MM, Larsen PR, Silva JE, Koining RJ, Lubin JH, Stovall M, Boice JD. Thyroid nodularity after childhood irradiation for lymphoid hyperplasia: a comparison of questionnaire and clinical findings. J Clin Epidemiol, 1990; 43; 449–60.
20. Shafer RB, Nuttall FQ, Pollak K, Kuisk H. Thyroid function after radiation and surgery for head and neck cancer. Arch Intern Med 1975; 135; 843.
21. Shore RE. Issues and epidemiological evidence regarding radiation-induced thyroid cancer. Rad Res 1992; 131; 98–111.
22. Shore RE, Labert RE, Pasternack BS. Follow-up study of patients treated by X-ray epilation for tinea capitis. Arch Environ Health, 1976; 31; 17–24.
23. Sklar CA, Kim TH, Ramsay NKC. Thyroid dysfunction among long-term survivors of bone marrow transplantation. Am J Med 1982; 73; 688.
24. Tami TA, Gomez P, Parker GS, Gupta MB, Frassica DA. Thyroid dysfunction after radiation therapy in head and neck cancer patients. Am J Otolaryngol 1992; 13; 357.
25. Tamura K, Shimaoka K, Friedman M. Thyroid abnormalities associated with treatment of malignant lymphoma. Cancer, 1981; 47:2704–9.
26. Thomas BC, Stanhope R, Plowman PN, Leiper AD. Endocrine function following single fraction and fractionated total body irradiation for bone marrow transplantation in childhood. Acta Endocrinol 1993; 128; 508.
27. Thompson DE, et al. Cancer incidence in atomic bomb survivors – Part II: solid tumors, 1958–1987. Rad Res 1994; 137; S17-S67.
28. Tucker MA, et al. Therapeutic radiation at a young age is linked to second thyroid cancer. Cancer Res, 1991; 51; 2885–8.

Bacterial infections of the thyroid

A. P. Farwell

Division of Endocrinology and Metabolism, Department of Medicine, University of Massachusetts Medical School, 55 Lake Ave, North Worcester, MA 01655, USA

Abstract

Infectious thyroiditis, also known as acute suppurative thyroiditis, bacterial thyroiditis and pyogenic thyroiditis, is a rare disorder. However, thyroidal infections are potentially life threatening and the prognosis is often dependent on the prompt recognition and treatment of this disorder. Acute bacterial thyroiditis is the most common cause of infectious thyroiditis and over 90 % of patients will present with thyroidal pain, tenderness, fever and local compression resulting in dysphagia and dysphonia. Transmission of infective organisms via a pyriform sinus fistula appears to be the most common route of thyroidal infection. In the adult, *S. aureus* and *S. pyogenes* are the offending pathogens in more than ~ 80 % of patients and are the sole pathogen in over 70 % of cases. In children, alpha- and beta-hemolytic *Streptococcus* and a variety of anerobes account for ~ 70 % of cases, while mixed pathogens are identified in > 50 % of cases. Fine needle aspiration biopsy with gram stain and culture will reveal the causative organism in over 90 % of cases and is the diagnostic test of choice. Treatment of acute bacterial thyroiditis requires admission to hospital, drainage of any abscess, and parenteral antimicrobial therapy aimed at the causative agent. Complete recovery is the rule; however, the mortality is close to 100 % if the diagnosis is delayed and antimicrobial therapy is not initiated. Other, less frequent, causes of infectious thyroiditis include fungal, mycobacterial and parasitic organisms. These infections are more likely to have a more chronic and insidious onset.

Introduction

Bacterial infections of the thyroid are rare, with only 224 cases having been reported in the literature from 1900 to 1980 (1) and only 60 cases reported in the pediatric literature (2). However, thyroidal infections are potentially life threatening, with an overall mortality of up to 8.6 % for acute bacterial thyroiditis (1). Patients with the acquired immunodeficiency syndrome (AIDS) are a patient population particularly at risk for bacterial thyroiditis, especially with the advent of protease-inhibitor drugs which have markedly increased the lifespan of these individuals. As with other opportunistic infections with AIDS patients, infections of the thyroid gland often are more chronic and insidious in onset. The prognosis of bacterial thyroiditis is often dependent on the prompt recognition and treatment of this disorder, as mortality may approach 100 % if the diagnosis is delayed and appropriate antimicrobial therapy is not instituted.

Pathogenesis

Infectious thyroiditis is a rare disorder due, in large part, to the resistance of the thyroid gland to infection. Indeed, experimental models of infectious thyroiditis are difficult to develop, as shown by the observation in the 1940's that direct injection of either staphylococci or streptococci into the carotid arteries of dogs rarely produced thyroidal infection (3). The resistance of the thyroid to infection is due to protective mechanisms that include: 1) the rich blood supply to and lymphatic drainage from the thyroid; 2) the high glandular content of iodine, which may be bactericidal; and 3) the separation of the thyroid from other structures of the neck by fascial planes and the complete, protective fibrous capsule surrounding the gland. The most common pre-disposing factor to infections of the thyroid appears to be pre-existing thyroid disease, as simple goiter, nodular goiter, Hashimoto's thyroiditis or thyroid carcinoma has been observed in up to two-thirds of women and one half of men with infectious thyroiditis (1, 4, 5).

Bacterial infections are the most common cause of infectious thyroiditis, comprising 68 % of cases reported up to 1980 (6). Bacterial thyroiditis may occur either via spread from a distant focus through the bloodstream or lymphatics or by direct inoculation from a contiguous focus, either in the setting of thyroid surgery or from communication with other head and neck infections (7). The route of infection was rarely documented in the early literature. Case reports of hematogenous spread from infections of the skin (8), lower respiratory tract, urinary tract and gastrointestinal tract have been described (1). This occurs more often in adults than children, usually in the presence of other underlying illnesses (5, 9). Only one case of infectious thyroiditis has been reported as a complication of thyroid surgery (4), despite an incidence of wound infections of 0.5–1 % (10). Infectious thyroiditis has been reported to occur as a result of direct spread of pathogenic organisms via patent thyroglossal duct fistulae (11). Infections of the retropharyngeal space (pharyngitis and tonsillitis) or the lateral pharyngeal spaces (pharyngitis, tonsillitis, parotitis, otitis and mastoiditis) may rarely spread down posterior and lateral fascial planes into the neck and communicate with the structures in the pretracheal space (12). Infection may also arise directly from the pretracheal space through perforations in the esophagus (1).

The seminal observation regarding the pathogenesis of bacterial thyroiditis was made in 1979 when Takai et al. reported seven cases of infectious thyroiditis due to a fistula originating from the left pyriform sinus (13). Subsequently, studies involving over 100 patients with infectious thyroiditis have identified pyriform sinus fistulae, primarily left-sided, in up to 90 % of these patients, especially in those with recurrent episodes (2, 4, 14–16). Additional reports identified infected embryonic cysts from the third and fourth brachial pouches as routes of thyroidal infection (15, 17–21). However, transmission of infective organisms via a pyriform sinus fistula appears to be the most common route of thyroidal infection.

Clinical presentation and diagnosis

Bacterial thyroiditis is often preceded by an upper respiratory infection, which may induce inflammation of the fistula and promote the transmission of pathogens to the thyroid. Consistent with these observations, bacterial thyroiditis is more common in the late fall and late spring months (2, 4, 14). Over 90 % of patients will present with thyroidal pain, tenderness, fever and local compression resulting in dysphagia and dysphonia (5, 7, 14, 22). The pain may radiate to the ear or mandible on the side of the infection (23) and signs and symptoms of systemic toxicity may be present. The thyroid is tender to palpation, with unilateral or bilateral lobar enlargement, and is associated with erythema and warmth of the skin. Abscess formation is indicated by fluctuance, which may develop over the course of one to three days, so repeated physical examinations are often necessary. Cervical lymphadenopathy is not a prominent feature unless there is a predisposing pharyngitis.

The differential diagnosis of bacterial thyroiditis can be divided into non-thyroidal and thyroidal causes (Table 1). Essentially all of the non-thyroidal causes are infectious in origin and present as discrete painful masses (12, 22). Most often the non-thyroidal nature of these lesions can be ascertained by physical exam alone. Identification of infected thyroglossal duct and brachial cleft cysts may be more problematic due to their close approximation to the thyroid. In these cases, radionuclide, computed tomography and/or ultrasonographic imaging will assist in making the diagnosis.

The most common cause of the painful thyroid is subacute granulomatous thyroiditis, which often results in both local and systemic symptoms similar to those with bacterial thyroiditis (6, 14, 22). In general, patients with bacterial thyroiditis have a greater febrile response that those with subacute granulomatous thyroiditis. Acute hemorrhage into either a cyst or a nodule usually presents with the sudden onset of unilateral neck pain associated with a marked increase in the size of a preexisting nodule (22). The pain associated with a rapidly enlarging carcinoma, usually anaplastic, is often more chronic in nature (24, 25), as is painful Hashimoto's thyroiditis (22, 26). Radiation thyroiditis occurs in the setting of radioactive iodine treatment for hyperthyroidism (22) or following supravoltage external radiation of the an-

Table 1 Differential diagnosis of the painful neck mass

Nonthyroidal
Infected thyroglossal duct cyst
Infected branchial cleft cyst
Infected cystic hygroma
Cervical adenitis
Cellulitis of the anterior neck
Thyroidal
Subacute granulomatous thyroiditis
Infectious thyroiditis
Acute hemorrhage into a cyst
Acute hemorrhage into a benign or malignant nodule
Rapidly enlarging thyroid carcinoma
Painful Hashimoto's thyroiditis
Radiation thyroiditis
Globus hystericus

terior neck for thyroid cancer or lymphoma (27, 28). Globus hystericus, an anxiety reaction that is characterized by a constrictive feeling in the throat, is a diagnosis of exclusion.

Thyroid function tests in the normal range are the most common finding in patients with bacterial thyroiditis (1, 2, 14), although thyrotoxicosis and hypothyroidism have been reported (14, 22, 29). In contrast, overt thyroid dysfunction is a frequent occurrence in patients with subacute granulomatous thyroiditis (22, 30). Leukocytosis and an elevated erythrocyte sedimentation rate are not discriminatory tests as they are commonly observed in both subacute granulomatous thyroiditis and infectious thyroiditis (Table 2).

Fine needle aspiration biopsy is the best single laboratory test in the evaluation of infectious thyroiditis and will be diagnostic in most cases (Table 2 (1, 31, 32)), especially when the tenderness is limited to a solitary nodule or a localized area and subacute granulomatous thyroiditis has been ruled out. In addition to obtaining samples for cytology and gram stain and culture, provision should be made to obtain samples for special studies in the appropriate setting, such as Gomori's silver methenamine stain to identify *Pneumocystis carinii* in the immunocompromised patient (33, 34). Other diagnostic studies include: 1) radionuclide imaging, preferably with radioiodine, in the setting of a solitary painful nodule as a radioactive iodine uptake will provide information on the overall function of the gland (22); 2) radiograph

Table 2 Diagnostic tests in the evaluation of the painful thyroid

Test	Comment
Thyroid function tests	Usually normal, rare case reports of hypothyroidism and thyrotoxicosis
Erythrocyte sedimentation rate	Usually elevated, nonspecific test
Leukocyte count	Usually elevated, nonspecific test
Fine needle aspiration biopsy	Diagnostic in 90 % of cases, test of choice, special stains considered as necessary
Radionuclide imaging	Adjunctive test, radioiodine best, provides information regarding overall gland function
Neck radiograph	Adjunctive test, gas present indicates abscess with anerobic organisms
Magnetic resonance imaging	Adjunctive test, helpful in identifying pyriform sinus fistulae
Ultrasonography	Adjunctive test, helpful in identifying pyriform sinus fistulae
Computed tomography	Adjunctive test, helpful in identifying pyriform sinus fistulae
Barium swallow	Adjunctive test, helpful in identifying pyriform sinus fistulae

of the neck to reveal soft tissue gas, indicating infection with anaerobic, gas-forming organisms; and 3) magnetic resonance imaging, ultrasonography, barium swallow and computed tomography to identify pyriform sinus fistulae or parathyroid abscesses (35–39). These imaging studies are all adjunctive studies and are best reserved for patients in which the diagnosis is unclear (11).

In the adult, *Staphylococcus aureus* and *Streptococcus pyogenes* are the offending pathogens in more than 80 % of patients and are the sole pathogen in over 70 % of cases (1). In children, alpha- and beta-hemolytic *Streptococcus* and a variety of anerobes account for ~ 70 % of cases, while mixed pathogens are identified in > 50 % of cases (2). While no longer common, *Salmonella typhii* was an important cause of infectious thyroiditis historically, with 40 cases reported by 1951 (1). Other thyroidal bacterial pathogens that have been shown to cause infectious thyroiditis include *Salmonella brandenberg, Salmonella enteriditis, Actinomyces naeslund, Actinobacillus actinomycetemcomitans, Brucella melitensis, Clostridium septicum, Eikenella corrodens*, *Enterobacter*, *Escherichia coli, Hemophilus influenzae, Klebsiella* sp., *Pseudomonas aeruginosa*, *Serratia marcescens*, *Acinetobacter baumanii* and *Staphylococcus non-aureus (7)*.

Management and prognosis

Treatment of acute bacterial thyroiditis requires admission to the hospital, drainage of any abscess, and parenteral antimicrobial therapy aimed at the causative agent. Gram stain and culture of the fine needle aspirate will reveal the causative organism in over 90 % of cases. If no organisms are seen on the gram stain, nafcillin and gentamycin or a third generation cephalosporin is appropriate initial therapy in adults while a second generation cephalosporin or clindamicin is reasonable in children. Since a pyriform sinus fistula is the most common route of infection in bacterial thyroiditis (2, 4, 15), a barium swallow (19), computed tomography (36, 39) or magnetic resonance imaging (38) of the neck should be performed to look for communicating fistulae in most patients with the first episode and all patients with recurrent episodes. Such fistulae must be surgically excised for definitive cure and prevention of recurrent infection (4, 15, 21, 40).

Mortality from acute bacterial thyroiditis has markedly improved from the 20–25 % reported in the early 1900s, with the extensive review by Berger estimating an overall mortality of 8.6 % (1). Recent reviews involving over 100 patients failed to list mortality as a complication of acute bacterial thyroiditis (2, 4, 5). However, the mortality is close to 100 % if the diagnosis is delayed and antimicrobial therapy is not initiated (1). In survivors, complete recovery is the rule, although there have been reports of transient hypothyroidism, vocal cord paralysis (which may also be transient (4, 41)), and recurrence of infection as sequelae of acute bacterial thyroiditis (1, 2, 4, 5).

Non-bacterial infections

Fungal infections

Fungal infections of the thyroid, while rare, are the next most common cause of infectious thyroiditis, comprising 15 % of cases reported through 1980 (1). The predominant offending organism is *Aspergillus* species, with at least twenty-six documented cases (1). Virtually all of the affected patients were immunocompromised and had disseminated disease; most cases of thyroidal infection were made at postmortem. Case reports of fungal infections of the thyroid have included *Coccidioides immitis*, *Histoplasma capsulatum*, *Candida albicans*, *Allescheria boydii* and *Nocardia asteroides* (7).

The thyroid is a site of extrapulmonary infection with *Pneumocystis carinii* in patients with AIDS, with asymptomatic infection of the thyroid found in up to 20 % of patients with disseminated *Pneumocystis* infection at autopsy (42). Symptomatic thyroidal infection was first reported in 1988 (43) and followed by numerous other case reports (7). The typical presentation is as a painless thyroid nodule that is increasing in size, occasionally associated with hypothyroidism. The diagnosis of *Pneumocystis carinii* infection is made by performing Gomori's silver methenamine stain on specimens obtained by fine needle aspiration biopsy. Since this is not a routine staining procedure, it must be requested when performing a biopsy on patients who have AIDS or are otherwise immunocompromised. Treatment with parenteral trimethoprim-sulfamethoxazole followed by prolonged oral administration (up to two months) is curative and may result in the restoration of normal thyroid function in regions that were previously "cold" by radioiodine scanning (33).

Mycobacterial infections

The true incidence of infection of the thyroid with *Mycobacterium tuberculosis* is difficult to determine. Using strict pathological criteria, only 19 cases have been reported in the literature (1). Thyroidal tuberculosis is associated with disseminated or miliary disease and symptoms are usually present for months (44). While at least three of the reported patients with tuberculous thyroiditis died (1) and recurrent laryngeal nerve paralysis has been described (45), resolution without sequelae usually follows appropriate antituberculous therapy. Infections with atypical mycobacteria, including *M. cheloni*, *M. intracellulare* and *Mycobacterium avian-intracellulare*, have also been described (1), the latter in patients with AIDS in the setting of widely disseminated disease (46). While acid fast organisms have been found in the thyroid of individuals with disseminated *Mycobacterium leprae* (47), symptomatic thyroid infection has not been described.

Parasitic infections

Several parasitic agents have involved the thyroid on rare occasions. *Echinococcus granulosus*, or tapeworm, has been reported (1) in the setting of a chronic goiter, with the diagnosis is being made at the time of surgery. If echinococcal infection is suspected, biopsy of the lesion is contraindicated due to spillage and rupture of the cyst contents and specific serologic testing should be obtained (7). Surgical removal is the preferred mode of treatment, with antiparasitic agents useful as adjunctive therapy and for inoperable cases. Complications of echinococcal thyroiditis include death, vocal cord paralysis and tracheal perforation (1). Involvement of the thyroid with *Strongyloides stercoralis*, or roundworm, has been described only in the setting of disseminated disease in immunocompromised patients (48). Mortality with disseminated *Strongyloides* infection is high due to both the infection and the immunocompromised status of the patient (7). A single patient with cysticercosis of the thyroid, acquired from ingestion of the eggs of the pork tapeworm *Taenia solium*, has been described (49). This patient died after a two year illness with bilateral thyroid involvement.

Syphilitic infections

Historically, secondary syphilis was frequently associated with pain and swelling of the thyroid that responded to anti-syphilitic therapy, which commonly included iodides (50). However, microbiologic evidence of syphilitic infection of the thyroid is lacking in most of these cases, thus, a direct relationship between treponemal infection and thyroid dysfunction cannot be determined. Indeed, only seven cases of gummata of the thyroid, presenting as painless nodules, have been reported in the world literature (1).

Thyroidal infections in patients with AIDS

With the increasing incidence of infection by human immunodeficiency virus leading to AIDS, several novel opportunistic pathogens have involved the thyroid. The most common infectious organism found in the thyroid at postmortem examination in patients with AIDS is cytomegalovirus (CMV), occurring in the setting of disseminated CMV infection (42, 51). However, symptomatic thyroidal infection with CMV has not been reported. As mentioned above, thyroidal involvement with *Mycobacterium avian-intracellulare* has been reported in the setting of widely disseminated disease (46). The most common pathogen producing symptomatic thyroidal infection is *Pneumocystis carinii*, discussed above.

Conclusions

Bacterial infections of the thyroid gland are uncommon and diagnosis often requires a high index of suspicion. A rational approach to such patients, including history, physical examination, laboratory evaluation, radionuclide or ultrasonographic imaging and fine needle aspiration biopsy, will allow the appropriate diagnosis to be made in the vast majority of cases.

References

1. Berger SA, Zonszein J, Villamena P, Mittman N. Infectious diseases of the thyroid gland. [Review]. Rev Infect Dis 1983;5(1); 108–22.
2. Rich EJ, Mendelman PM. Acute suppurative thyroiditis in pediatric patients. [Review]. Pediatr Infect Dis J 1987;6(10); 936–40.
3. Womack NA. Thyroiditis. Surgery 1944;16; 770–782.
4. Miyauchi A, Matsuzuka F, Kuma K, Takai S. Piriform sinus fistula: an underlying abnormality common in patients with acute suppurative thyroiditis. World J Surg 1990;14(3); 400–5.
5. Jeng LB, Lin JD, Chen MF. Acute suppurative thyroiditis: a ten-year review in a Taiwanese hospital. Scand J Infect Dis 1994;26(3); 297–300.
6. Farwell AP, Braverman LE. Inflammatory thyroid disorders. Otolaryngol Clin North Am 1996;29(4); 541–56.
7. Farwell AP. Infectious thyroiditis. In: Braverman LE, Utiger RD, editors. The Thyroid. Philadelphia: Lippincott-William & Wilkins; 2000. p. 1044–1050.
8. Agarwal A, Mishra SK, Sharma AK. Acute suppurative thyroiditis with demonstrable distant primary focus: a report of two cases. Thyroid 1998;8(5); 399–401.
9. Poelman M, Benoit Y, Laureys G, Craen M, Leroy J. Acute suppurative thyroiditis complicating second allogeneic transplant for juvenile CMML. Bone Marrow Transplantation 1992;10(6); 547–8.
10. Foster RS. Morbidity and mortality after thyroidectomy. Surg Gyn Ob 1978;146; 423–429.
11. Kawanaka M, Sugimoto Y, Suehiro M, Fukuchi M. Thyroid imaging in a typical case of acute suppurative thyroiditis with abscess formation due to infection from a persistent thyroglossal duct. Ann Nucl Med 1994;8(2); 159–62.
12. Brook I. The swollen neck. Cervical lymphadenitis, parotitis, thyroiditis, and infected cysts. [Review]. Infect Dis North Am 1988;2(1); 221–36.
13. Takai S-I, Miyauchi A, Matsuzuka F, Kuma K, Kosaki G. Internal fistula as a route of infection in acute suppurative thyroiditis. Lancet 1979;1; 751–752.
14. Szabo SM, Allen DB. Thyroiditis. Differentiation of acute suppurative and subacute thyroiditis. Case report and review of the literature. [Review]. Clin Pediatr 1989;28(4); 171–4.
15. Har-el G, Sasaki CT, Prager D, Krespi YP. Acute suppurative thyroiditis and the branchial apparatus. Am J Otolaryngol 1991;12(1); 6–11.
16. Skuza K, Rapaport R, Fieldman R, Goldstein S, Marquis J. Recurrent acute suppurative thyroiditis. [Review]. J Otolaryngol 1991;20(2); 126–9.
17. Katz R, Bar-Ziv J, Preminger-Shapiro R, Ben-Tovim R, Rechnic Y. Pyogenic thyroiditis due to branchial pouch sinus. Isr J Med Sci 1989;25(11); 641–4.
18. Tovi F, Gatot A, Bar-Ziv J, Yanay I. Recurrent suppurative thyroiditis due to fourth branchial pouch sinus. Int J Ped Otorhinolaryngol 1985;9(1); 89–96.
19. Ueda J, Kobayashi Y, Hara K, Kishino B, Fushimi H, Sawada S. Routes of infection of acute suppurative thyroiditis diagnosed by barium examination. Acta Radiologica 1986;27(2); 209–11.
20. Yamashita J, Ogawa M, Yamashita S, Saishoji T, Nomura K, Tsuruta J. Acute suppurative thyroiditis in an asymptomatic woman: an atypical presentation simulating thyroid carcinoma. Clin Endocrinol (Oxf) 1994;40(1); 145–9.
21. Ozaki O, Sugimoto T, Suzuki A, Yashiro T, Ito K, Hosoda Y. Cervical thymic cyst as a cause of acute suppurative thyroiditis. Jap J Surg 1990;20(5); 593–6.
22. Singer PA. Thyroiditis. Acute, subacute, and chronic. [Review]. Med Clin North Am 1991;75(1); 61–77.
23. Stevenson J. Acute bacterial thyroiditis presenting as otalgia. J Laryngol Otol 1991;105(9); 788–9.
24. van der Sluis RF, Wobbes T, Schoots FJ. Thyroid cancer mimicking thyroiditis. J Surg Oncol 1986;33(1); 66–8.
25. Walfish PG, Chan JY, Ing HD, Rosen IB. Esophageal carcinoma masquerading as recurrent acute suppurative thyroiditis. Arch Intern Med 1985;145(2); 346–7.
26. Leung AK, Hegde K. Hashimoto's thyroiditis simulating De Quervain's thyroiditis. J Adolesc Health Care 1988;9(5); 434–5.

27. Pottern LM, Kaplan MM, Larsen PR, Silva JE, Koenig RJ, Lubin JH, et al. Thyroid nodularity after childhood irradiation for lymphoid hyperplasia: a comparison of questionnaire and clinical findings. J Clin Epidemiol 1990;43(5); 449–60.
28. Feyerabend T, Kapp B, Richter E, Becker W, Reiners C. Incidence of hypothyroidism after irradiation of the neck with special reference to lymphoma patients. A retrospective and prospective analysis. Acta Oncol 1990;29(5); 597–602.
29. Walsh CH, Dunne C. Hyperthyroidism associated with acute suppurative thyroiditis. Irish Journal of Medical Science 1992;161(5); 137.
30. Kitchener MI, Chapman IM. Subacute thyroiditis: a review of 105 cases. Clin Nucl Med 1989;14(6); 439–42.
31. Lin JD, Huang BY, Huang HS, Juang JH, Jeng LB. Ultrasonography and fine needle aspiration cytology of acute suppurative thyroiditis. Chang Gung Med J 1993;16(2); 93–8.
32. Singh SK, Agrawal JK, Kumar M, Shukla HS. Fine needle aspiration cytology in the management of acute suppurative thyroiditis. ENT J 1994;73(6); 415–7.
33. Battan R, Mariuz P, Raviglione MC, Sabatini MT, Mullen MP, Poretsky L. Pneumocystis carinii infection of the thyroid in a hypothyroid patient with AIDS: Diagnosis by fine needle aspiration biopsy. J Clin Endocrinol Metab 1991;72; 724–726.
34. Guttler R, Singer PA, Axline SG, Greaves TS, McGill JJ. Pneumocystis carinii thyroiditis. Report of three cases and review of the literature [published erratum appears in Arch Intern Med 1993 Apr 26;153(8):1002]. [Review]. Arch Intern Med 1993;153(3); 393–6.
35. Ahuja AT, Griffiths JF, Roebuck DJ, Loftus WK, Lau KY, Yeung CK, et al. The role of ultrasound and oesophagography in the management of acute suppurative thyroiditis in children associated with congenital pyriform fossa sinus. Clin Radiol 1998;53(3); 209–11.
36. Bar-Ziv J, Slasky BS, Sichel JY, Lieberman A, Katz R. Branchial pouch sinus tract from the piriform fossa causing acute suppurative thyroiditis, neck abscess, or both: CT appearance and the use of air as a contrast agent. Am J Roentgenol 1996;167(6); 1569–72.
37. Bernard PJ, Som PM, Urken ML, Lawson W, Biller HF. The CT findings of acute thyroiditis and acute suppurative thyroiditis. Otolaryngology Head & Neck Surgery 1988;99(5); 489–93.
38. Hatakenaka M, Murakami J, Murayama S, Sakai S, Hashiguchi N, Zaizen Y, et al. Acute suppurative perithyroiditis: MR findings. Pediatr Radiol 1997;27(4); 353–5.
39. Kinoshita T, Ishii K, Naganuma H, Mori Y, Nakagawa H. Acute suppurative thyroiditis arising from a piriform sinus fistula: CT diagnosis. Radiat Med 1998;16(3); 217–9.
40. Nonomura N, Ikarashi F, Fujisaki T, Nakano Y. Surgical approach to pyriform sinus fistula. Am J Otolaryngol 1993;14(2); 111–5.
41. Boyd CM, Esclamado RM, Telian SA. Impaired vocal cord mobility in the setting of acute suppurative thyroiditis. Head Neck 1997;19(3); 235–7.
42. Reichert CM, O'Leary TJ, Levens DL, Simrell CR, Macher AM. Autopsy pathology in the acquired immunodeficiency syndrome. Am J Pathol 1983;112; 357–382.
43. Gallant JE, Enriquez RE, Cohen KL, Hammers LW. Pneumocystis carinii thyroiditis. Am J Med 1988;84(2); 303–6.
44. Das DK, Pant CS, Chachra KL, Gupta AK. Fine needle aspiration cytology diagnosis of tuberculous thyroiditis. A report of eight cases. Acta Cytologica 1992;36(4); 517–22.
45. Emery P. Tuberculous abscess of the thyroid with recurrent laryngeal nerve palsy: a case report and review of the literature. J. Laryngol. Otol. 1980;94; 553–558.
46. Horsburgh CR. *Mycobacterium avium* complex infection in the acquired immunodeficiency syndrome. N Engl J Med 1991;324; 1332–1338.
47. Hastings RC, Gillis TP, Krahenbuhl JL, Franzblau SG. Leprosy. Clin Microbiol Rev 1988;1; 330-.
48. Scowden EB, Schaffner W, Stone WJ. Overwelming strongyloidias: An unappreciated opportunistic infection. Medicine 1978;57; 527–544.
49. Leelachaikul P, Chuahirun S. Cysticercosis of the thyroid gland in severe cerebral cysticercosis. Report of a case. J Med Assoc Thai 1977;60; 405.
50. Netherton EN. Syphilis and thyroid disease with special reference to hyperthyroidism. Amer J Syph 1932;16; 479–510.
51. Frank TS, LiVolsi VA, Connor AM. Cytomegalovirus infection of the thyroid in immunocompromised adults. Yale J Biol Med 1987;60; 1–8.

HIV infection and the thyroid

G. J. Kahaly

Department of Medicine, Endocrinology and Metabolism, Gutenberg University Hospital, Mainz, Germany

Introduction

Endocrine dysfunction is not uncommon in human immunodeficiency virus (HIV) disease. Gonadal dysfunction is highly prevalent, affecting nearly half of all men with acquired immunodeficiency syndrome (AIDS) and is most often associated with low gonadotropin levels. Women with HIV disease also have altered gonadal function and an associated loss of muscle mass. Furthermore, acquired growth hormone resistance, related in part to undernutrition, is also seen in HIV-infected patients. Clinical adrenal disease is seen primarily among patients with disseminated cytomegalovirus or those who take medications that predispose to adrenal insufficiency. In addition to adrenalopathy, organ-specific disease secondary to opportunistic infection can result in testicular, thyroid, pituitary, and hypothalamic destruction. When acutely ill, HIV patients can develop the metabolic derangements that accompany any severe systemic disorder (1, 2).

Thyroid function

During infection with HIV, overt clinical or biochemical thyroid dysfunction is rare. When present, thyroid failure generally results from the destruction of the thyroid gland by opportunistic infections such as Pneumocystis carinii, or tumoral processes such as Kaposi sarcoma (1–3). Less frequently, hypothalamic-pituitary failure due to central nervous system infections is involved. Some cases of thyroiditis with thyrotoxicosis or hypothyroidism due to Pneumocystis carinii have been reported. Subtle alterations of thyroid function tests are more common in HIV infection and are sometimes already detectable in the early phase of the disease. Contrary to what is observed in severe non-thyroidal illnesses, the low T_3 syndrome and the sick euthyroid syndrome are less marked; these changes are mainly present in the final stage of the disease, when anorexia and weight loss occur, and indicate a poor outcome. Unique abnormalities of thyroid function indices have been documented. A progressive elevation in serum thyroxin binding globulin (TBG), but not in other binding proteins such as CBG and SHBG, accompanying the decline of the CD4 lymphocyte count, and associated with a concomitant increase in the serum T_4 value, has been reported. An unusual prolonged maintenance of normal T_3 levels with a paradoxical decrease in serum rT_3 values has also been recognized. Finally, hypothyroid-like regulation of the pituitary-thyroid-axis, possibly directed to limit hypermetabolism in HIV infection, has been observed. The recognition of these particular thyroid profiles is of clinical importance as serum TBG appears to be a specific marker of the progression of HIV infection and serum T_3 a reliable prognostic indicator for AIDS.

During the asymptomatic phases of HIV infection, patients usually display elevated serum T_4, normal T_3 and decreased rT_3 while maintaining normal serum TSH. However, in HIV-positive patients who are either asymptomatic or have less severe disease, mean 24-hour TSH levels are higher, owing to an increase in TSH pulse amplitude that is associated with an increased TSH responsiveness to TRH and a normal nocturnal TSH surge (3). A progressive elevation of serum TBG, accompanying the decline of CD4 lymphocyte count and associated with a concomitant increase in the serum T_4 values, has been noted. Even in the most severely ill HIV-infected patient, thc low T_4 state is rarely observed (4). Patients who have substantial weight loss often have similar values although low serum T_3 concentrations would be expected (5). Whether this failure of serum T_3 concentrations to fall in response to weight loss contributes to the wasting that occurs in these patients is not known (6). Serum TSH concentrations remain within the normal range, but they are often in the upper portion of that range. As the HIV infection progresses these alterations tend to become more prominent until AIDS-defining illnesses, such as pneumocystis pneumonia, occur, when a typical low T_3 state usually develops (7). The causes of the alterations in the asymptomatic phases of HIV infection is unknown but may be related to changes in the cytokine signaling pattern associated with the disease.

In AIDS patients, during the terminal phase of the disease, serum thyroid hormone concentrations are reduced and serum TSH is normal or low, similar to patients with other causes of severe nonthyroidal illness (8). Studies of thyroid function tests emphasize that the presence of acute secondary infection must be analyzed when evaluating such patients. In addition to euthyroid sick syndrome other hormonal axes are affected by severe illness. These alterations may be cytokine mediated. As with seronegative patients, these changes may be transient and resolve with successful treatment of the intervening illness (2).

Clinical studies

Thyroid function and regulation were studied in 14 consecutive male outpatients with asymptomatic HIV infection (CDC II/III) or AIDS (CDC IV) who were free of concomitant infections and hepatic dysfunction, and in eight healthy, age- and weight matched male controls. Blood was sampled every 10 minutes over 24 hours for measurement of TSH. T_3 and T_4 did not differ between HIV-infected patients and controls, but HIV patients had lower thyroid hormone-binding index, FT_4 index, FT_4, and rT_3 values and higher TBG values. Mean 24-hour TSH levels were increased among HIV patients, associated with increased mean TSH pulse amplitude and TSH responsiveness to TRH. No differences were observed between asymptomatic HIV-seropositive and AIDS patients. In conclusion, there was hypothyroid-like regulation of the pituitary-thyroid axis in stable HIV infection, which differs distinctly from the euthyroid sick syndrome in non-HIV-nonthyroidal illness (9). In another study (10), FT_4 was at or below the lower limit of normal in 18 % of 167 children with HIV infection (mean age 9 years). TSH and TBG levels were above the normal range in 31 % and 30 % of the children, respectively. There was an inverse correlation between CD4+ cell count and TSH, and between CD4+ and TBG. These findings indicate that thyroid abnormalities occur frequently in children with HIV infection, have a different profile from the thyroid abnormalities associated with other chronic disease conditions, and correlate with disease progression.

Anti-thyroid autoantibodies detected in adult patients represent the only type of organ-specific autoantibodies reported in HIV infection. In a study investigating vertically HIV infected children, 34 % showed anti-thyroglobulin (Tg) antibodies (11). Asymptomatic patients, seroreverted and healthy controls did not show any anti-thyroid antibodies. High Tg levels were observed in 38 % of the 40 HIV infected patients and high TSH concentrations were found in 27.5 % of the HIV children. High TSH values were observed more frequently among infected children with moderate or severe immunocompromised status. TBG levels were high in 68 % of the HIV children and in 22 % of the seroreverted.

Thyroiditis and lymphoma of the thyroid gland

Pneumocystis carinii pneumonia is the most common opportunistic infection among patients with HIV infection, occurring in over 80 % of patients not receiving prophylaxis (12). Because pneumocystis infection is common, it may be useful to review in some detail the presentation of thyroidal infection with this organism. Infection of the thyroid is found in up to 20 % of patients with disseminated pneumocystis infection at autopsy. However, symptomatic infection of the thyroid is rare. Most AIDS patients with thyroid involvement present with an enlarging diffuse or nodular goiter, which is often tender, and may contain calcifications. The infectious agent or Kaposi's sarcoma is almost always present in many other organs. However, isolated pneumocystis thyroiditis has been reported. Fine-needle aspiration of the thyroid gland has been positive for pneumocystis in 10 cases, for cryptococcus in 1 case, for aspergillus in 1 case, and for Kaposi's sarcoma in 2 cases (13). Pneumocystis carinii has been shown to cause a syndrome of painful thyroiditis in which hyperthyroidism is followed by hypothyroidism in association with decreased uptake on scanning and a firm tender gland, much like that associated with subacute painful autoimmune thyroiditis. The increasing incidence of Pneumocystis thyroiditis may be related to the increased use of inhaled pentamidine, which is associated with extrapulmonary pneumocystis infections. In addition, clinically apparent thyroid masses from aspergillus have been reported but are not associated with a thyroiditis-like picture. Intrathyroidal foci of cytomegalovirus, mycobacterium avium-intracellulare, cryptococcus, and Kaposi's sarcoma have also been demonstrated at autopsy but have not yet been implicated in clinical thyroid disease among patients with AIDS.

Gallant et al. reported an intravenous drug user with AIDS, receiving no prophylaxis, who presented with 2 weeks of left-sided neck swelling and dysphagia (14). Physical examination revealed a diffusely enlarged (5 x 10 cm), mildly tender left lobe of the thyroid, and a 3 x 5 cm right lobe that was more tender. On ultrasound examination of the neck, an enlarged left thyroid lobe with heterogeneous echogenicity was seen. Calcification, reported in another cases of extrapulmonary pneumocystosis was not observed. On thyroid radionuclide imaging, the left lobe of the thyroid was not visualized; thyroid function was normal. Fine needle aspiration of the thyroid revealed the presence of Pneumocystis carinii organisms. With trimethoprim-sulfamethoxazole therapy, the size of the thyroid decreased rapidly, and a repeat aspiration of the gland after 3 weeks of therapy revealed a smaller number of organisms. A third biopsy specimen after 7 weeks of therapy revealed no organisms. A subsequent series of patients with extrapulmonary pneumocystosis included a brief report of a 49-year-old homosexual man with a prior episode of Pneumocystis carinii pneumonia and maintained on aerosol pentamidine secondary prophylaxis, and who developed a left-sided neck mass; a cold nodule was found on thyroid radionuclide imaging (15). Fine needle aspiration yielded pneumocystis organisms. In contrast to the previous patient, there was no biochemical evidence of hypothyroidism. Finally, hyperthyroidism due to lymphoma involving the thyroid gland in a patient with AIDS has been recently reported (16). Most lymphomas that develop in AIDS patients are B-cell lymphomas; T-cell lymphomas are uncommon.

References

1. Grinspoon SK, Bilezikian JB. HIV disease and the endocrine system. N Engl J Med 1992; 327: 1360.
2. Sellmeyer DE, Grunfeld C. Endocrine and metabolic disturbances in human immuno-deficiency virus infection and the acquired immune deficiency syndrome. Endocr Rev 1996; 17: 518.
3. Lambert M. Thyroid dysfunction in HIV infection. Bailliere's Clin Endocrinol Metab 1994; 8: 825.
4. LoPresti, JS, Fried JC, Spencer CA, Nicoloff JT. Unique alterations of thyroid hormone indices in the acquired immunodeficiency syndrome. Ann Intern Med 1989; 110: 970.
5. Coodley GO, Loveless MO, Nelson HD, Coodley MK. Endocrine function in the HIV wasting syndrome. J Acquir Immune Defic Syndr 1994; 7: 46.
6. Hommes MJT, Romijn JA, Goodfried MH, et al. Increased resting energy expenditure in human immunodeficiency virus-infected men. Metabolism 1990; 39: 1186.
7. Fried JC, LoPresti JS, Micon M, et al. Serum triiodothyronine values. Prognostic indicators of acute

mortality due to Pneumocystis carinii pneumonia associated with acquired immunodeficiency syndrome. Arch Intern Med 1990; 150: 406.

8. Merenich JA. Hypothalamic and pituitary function in AIDS. Bailliere's Clin Endocrinol Metab 1994; 8: 757.
9. Hommes MJT, Romijn JA, Endert E, et al. Hypothyroid-like regulation of the pituitary thyroid axis in stable human immunodeficiency virus infection. Metabolism 1993; 42: 556.
10. Hirschfeld S, Laue L, Cutler GB, Pizzo PA. Thyroid abnormalities in children infected with human immunodeficiency virus. J Pediatr 1996; 128: 70.
11. Fundaro C, Olivieri A, Rendeli C et al. Occurrence of anti-thyroid autoantibodies in children vertically infected with HIV-1. J Pediatr Endocrinol Metab 1998; 11: 745.
12. Northfelt DW, Clement MJ, Safrin S. Extrapulmonary pneumocystis: clinical features in human immunodeficiency virus infection. Medicine 1990; 69: 392.
13. Guttler R, Singer PA. Pneumocystis carinii thyroiditis. Report of three cases and review of the literature. Arch Intern Med 1993; 153: 393.
14. Gallant JE, Enriquez RE, Cohen KL, Hammers LW. Pneumocystis carinii thyroiditis. Am J Med 1988; 85: 250.
15. Battan R, Mariuz P, Raviglone ML, et al. Pneumocystis carinii infection of the thyroid in a hypothyroid patient with AIDS: diagnosis by fine needle aspiration biopsy. J Clin Endocrinol Metab 1991; 72: 724.
16. Samuels MH, Launder T. Hyperthyroidism due to lymphoma involving the thyroid gland in a patient with acquired immunodeficiency syndrome: case report and review of the literature. Thyroid 1998; 8: 673.

Posters

Iodine deficiency evaluated in schoolchildren from two deficient parts of Romania using the Rapid Urinary Iodide Test

A. Dalea, [1]Gh. Dragatoiu, [1]G. Hazi, M. Purice, [2]M. Cojocaru, [2]C. Culpoi, [1]L. Gozariu, [2]E. Zbranca

Institute of Endocrinology C.I. Parhon, Bucharest; [1] Dept. of Endocrinology UMF Cluj; [2] Dept. of Endocrinology UMF Iasi, Romania

Aim of the study: To evaluate iodine deficiency in schoolchildren in two representative deficient regions of Romania – Cluj and Iasi – and surroundings, using a rapid, simple and cost effective method for determination of urinary iodide concentration – the Rapid Urinary Iodide Test.

Material and method: The study was performed in two main representative regions of Romania, Cluj and Iasi. 260 children from Cluj and 59 from Iasi were studied. Equal numbers of girls and boys were included, and the age range was 7–16 years. Urinary iodide concentration was determined in fresh urine samples by a rapid urinary test (Rapid Urinary Iodide Test), a method based on catalytic oxidation of tetramethylbenzidine and peracetic acid/H_2O_2 giving rise to colored products. Prior to analysis, interfering substances were removed using a purified activated charcoal column. Results were classified as <10, 10–30, or >30 μg/dl.

Results:
Cluj: Out of 260 children, 79 children without goiter had urinary iodide concentrations <10 μg/dl, and 11 between 10–30μg/dl; 138 children with goiter had urinary iodide concentrations <10 μg/dl and 32 between 10–30 μg/dl. In the age groups 7–9.5 and 12–13.5 years >60 % of children had urinary iodide concentrations <10 μg/dl. Among children aged 10–11.5 and 14–16 years, >50% had urinary iodide concentrations of 10–30 μg/dl. Iodine deficiency (urinary iodine concentration < 10 μg/dl) was found in 47 % of the boys and in 62 % of the girls.
Iasi: 68 % of the children investigated had urinary iodide concentrations <10 μg/dl (50 % with goiter) and 32 % 10–30 μg/dl. None of the children screened had a urinary iodide concentration >30 μg/dl.

Conclusions:

1. The Rapid Urinary Iodide Test confirmed low iodide excretion in 80,5 % of the screened children, confirming low iodine intake in the regions previous known to be deficient.
2. These determinations are easy and rapid to perform and are sufficiently accurate to determine iodine intake. They permit differential evaluation of iodine requirements.

Determination of urinary iodine – a diagnostic criterion for iodine deficiency

M. Adam, [1]J.P. Bourguignon, [1]J. Giellen, [1]T. Gougnard, [1]J. Rigo, A. Dalea

Children's Hospital, University of Medicine and Pharmacy, Cluj-Napoca, Romania, and [1]Centre Hospitalier Universitaire, Liège, Belgium

Iodine deficiency is a major public health problem, the most important cause of mental deficiency in the world. Iodine constitutes an essential factor in the synthesis of thyroid hormones, which play a decisive role in cell metabolism, in the growth and development especially of the brain. The major proportion of iodine is excreted in the urine, urinary iodine being a good indicator of iodine ingestion. Urinary iodine excretion shows day-to-day variation within individuals, and correct evaluation requires measurement of iodine in a representative number of cases. We determined urinary iodine in 5 ml urine samples obtained from 100 newborn infants born in Cluj-Napoca, and compared the values with those from 100 newborn infants born in Liège-Belgium. The determinations were performed using one of the methods approved by the International Council for Control of Iodine Deficiency Disorders in the Laboratories of Centre Hospitalière Universitaire in Liège. Urine iodine levels reflected mild iodine deficiency among infants born in Liège and moderate or severe deficiency among those born in Cluj-Napoca. We recommend that greater publicity should be given on the effects of iodine deficit in order to heighten awareness among medical and paramedical professions and to stimulate concrete measures for prophylaxis against iodine deficiency.

Urinary iodine excretion during normal pregnancy in healthy women living in the seaside region of Bulgaria

M. Petrova, L. Koeva, [1]P. Chankova

Clinic of Endocrinology, [1]Clinic of Nephrology, Haematology and Haemodialysis, Medical University of Varna, Varna, Bulgaria

The National program for the elimination of iodine deficiency reports that Bulgaria is a country with mild to moderate iodine deficiency: a goiter prevalence of 29 %, iodine excretion 20–60 μg/dl. One-third of the country is mountainous or semimountainous. Varna and the Black Sea region are situated on a plain. A continuous increase in thyroid disease has been observed among young adults and pregnant women.

Aim: A prospective study was undertaken to evaluate urinary iodine excretion and changes in maternal thyroid function during pregnancy among healthy women in the seaside region of Bulgaria. The cohort included a total of 1100 pregnant women (mean age 28.0 ± 3.5 years). Iodine concentration in a random urine sample, thyroid tests FT_4, TSH, T_3/T_4 ratio and thyroid volume were measured at initial presentation, during the first and third trimesters, and after delivery.

Results: Urinary iodine levels were: mean 77.5 ± 29.23, median 80.0; mean 45.11 ± 25.34, median 45.54; mean 45.26 ± 30.84, median 39.44 during the first and third trimesters and after delivery respectively. 35.59 % manifested urinary iodine levels characteristic of mild, and 14 % of moderate iodine deficiency. Total T_3 was 1.83 ± 0.54 before and 2.118 ± 0.80 nmol/l (normal range: 0.5–2) after delivery; total T_4 was 115.7 ± 36.69; 125.6 ± 54.07 nmol/l (normal range: 50–150). T_3/T_4 ratio was 15.64 ± 4.89 and 18.37 ± 6.26; TSH was 1.64 ± 0.97 and 3.95 ± 5.612 (normal range: 0.2–0.4 mU/l, p<0.0001) TV was 19.95 ± 2.38 and 24.49 ± 5.03 ml; FT_4 was 13.7 ± 1.9 and13.1 ± 1.2. 17 % of healthy pregnant women had goiter.

Conclusion: In the seaside region of Bulgaria pregnant women manifest mild to moderate ID.

Silent iodine prophylaxis in Western Europe only partly corrects iodine deficiency: the case of Belgium

F. Delange, A. Van Onderbergen, W. Shabana, E. Vandemeulebroucke, F. Vertongen, D. Gnat, M. Dramaix

International Council for Control of Iodine Deficiency Disorders (ICCIDD), Free Universities of Brussels, Brussels, Belgium

Belgium is one of the Western European countries in which no program of correction of iodine deficiency using iodized salt has been implemented despite having well documented mild iodine deficiency. In 1995, the median urinary iodine concentration was 55 µg/l (normal: 100–200 µg/l) and the prevalence of goiter based on thyroid ultrasonography was 11 % (normal: below 5 %) in representatives samples of schoolchildren aged 6–12 years. This paper reports the results of a national survey of iodine nutrition in Belgium performed three years later, based again on the measurements of thyroid volume by ultrasonography and urinary iodine concentrations. A "ThyroMobil" van equipped with ultrasound, deep freezer and computer visited 23 selected sites in the ten provinces of the country. The survey included 2,855 schoolchildren aged 6 to 12 years (1,365 boys and 1,490 girls; 37–286 per site). The results show an homogeneous situation in the whole country with a median urinary iodine of 80 µg/l (range in the 10 provinces: 73–90 µg/l) and a prevalence of goiter of 5.7 % (range: 3.9–7.7 %). Urinary iodine slightly decreases with age in girls and reaches a critical value of 59 µg/L at the age of 12 years, associated with a prevalence of goiter of 18.4 %.

We conclude from our data that iodine nutrition has slightly improved in Belgium but remains characteristic of mild iodine deficiency with public health consequences. The recent improvement indicates silent iodine prophylaxis as there have been no official measures of salt iodization. Silent iodine prophylaxis only partly corrects iodine deficiency in Western Europe. Active measures including the implementation of a program of salt iodization and iodine supplementation of target groups are urgently required.

Situation analysis on the total goiter rate (TGR) in Armenia

E.N. Toromanyan, S.E. Bagdasaryan

Republican Endocrinology Center, Yerevan, Armenia

The Republic of Armenia (RA) is a mountainous country at high risk of IDD. Moderate IDD has been reported from different mountain regions for decades. Cretins have been observed.

In 1995 UNICEF and Ministry of Health decided to conduct a program of IDD elimination in Armenia. Two target groups were examined: 3200 school-aged children (6–12 years) and 633 pregnant women. The survey method used was "lot quality assurance sampling" (LQAS).

TGR among school-aged children was 39.9 % (Ia: 26.4 %; Ib: 6,9 %; II: 5.8 %; III: 0.8 %). TGR among pregnant women was 50.4 % (Ia: 26.4 %; Ib: 11.2 %; II: 10.6 %; III: 2.2 %). More than 30 cases of cretinism were discovered in different regions of RA.

Since 1997 all salt manufactured in Armenia has been iodized.

In 1999 the survey was repeated at the same schools and among pregnant women. The results of this survey suggest an insignificant decrease in the TGR levels. Drug treatment of target groups of school-aged children (6–12 years of age) and pregnant women with iodine (Jodid 100 and Jodid 200) and thyroid hormones is required to eliminate the IDD.

Environmental factors and endemic goiter in Crete (Greece)

D.A. Koutras, M.A. Boukis, G. Pavlides, E. Mamalaki, M. Alevizaki, J. Mantzos, E. Mantzos, M. Chalkiadaki, E. Choustoulakis, M. Zampoulakis, E. Papavasiliou

Athens University Endocrine Unit, "Evgendion" Hospital, Dept. of Clinical Therapeutics, "Alexandra" Hospital, and Heraklion University Dept. of Endocrinology, Athens, Greece

We previously studied endemic iodine deficiency goiter in the island of Crete. Iodine intake is now normal, but goiter is still frequent. We therefore studied all the schoolchildren in 4 primary and 2 secondary schools in the Heraklion prefecture, Crete, by a) palpation, b) ultrasound (US), c) questionnaire, d) estimation of serum thyroid hormones (T_4, T_3 and autoantibodies by RIA, and TSH by IRMA) and e) estimation of urinary iodine (Benotti and Benotti 1963), thiocyanate (Pettigrew and Fell 1972) and creatinine (Jaffé 1986). Of 534 schoolchildren examined clinically, 172 (32 %) had a palpable thyroid, but only 72 (13 %) a goiter by the PAHO criteria (Delange et al. 1986). 179 schoolchildren were examined by US. 40 (22 %) had an increased volume for age and sex according to the criteria of Delange et al. 1997, but in only 5 (3 %) was this more than 50 % above the upper limit of normal. The urinary I/Cr was 140 ± 75.1 µg I/g Cr in those with enlarged thyroids and 131 ± 67.6 in those without ($t = 1.97$, $p = 0.41$ N.S.). Urinary thiocyanate was 10.37 ± 3.44 among those with enlarged thyroids and 9.65 ±: 3.56 µg I/g Cr among those without ($t = 1.99$, $p = 0,40$ N.S.). Urinary thiocyanate was increased among children with thyroid enlargement compared to those without in only one village ($p < 0.02$). T_4, T_3, TSH and autoantibodies were normal. In summary, although definite clinical goiter is rare, subclinical thyroid enlargement is still common in Crete, in spite of adequate iodine intake. The role of environmental goitrogens will be discussed.

Thyroid volume and urinary iodine in Hungarian school children

F. Péter, [1]J. Podoba, [2]P.P. Bourdoux, Á. Muzsnai, I. Szécsényi Nagy

Buda Children's Hospital, Budapest, Hungary; [1]Postgraduate Medical School, Bratislava, Slovakia; [2]Laboratorie de Pédiatrie, Univ. Libre de Bruxelles, Brussels, Belgium

The aim of this study is to analyze the working of ThyroMobil (TM) system in an area, where the localization of iodine deficient settlements is "island-like" and there is no general iodine prevention. – Recently the Swiss TM-results were published, reporting thyroid volume and urinary iodine of school children from two cities with previously determined adequate iodide supply. Iodine intake was found appropriate in comparison with WHO reference values. – In this presentation Hungarian thyroid volume data of the TM study (three settlements) were processed in the form of the Swiss publication:

Age	7	8	9	10	11	12	13 years
No. of boys/girls	19/13	41/32	50/46	38/44	19/15	20/14	13/17
Volume (median)	3.9/3.6	5.2/4.1	4.4/4.4	4.7/4.7	5.3/5.8	5.8/5.8	7.1/6.8 ml
WHO reference	3.4/3.4	3.7/3.9	4.1/4.4	4.5/5.0	5.1/5.7	5.7/6.3	6.5/7.0 ml
No. of cases >P_{97}	1/-	4/-	6/2	-/1	-/-	-/1	-/- (Total:15)

While these results suggest similar conclusions, considering the urinary iodine median values of the three settlements (11.5, 7.3, and 5.2 μg/dl) leads to different conclusions. Different results were also obtained when thyroid volume was measured by ultrasound among the same children by another examiner and using different equipment:

Age of boys	7	8	9	10	13 age (years)
Volume (median) TM	3.9	4.4	3.7	4.6	8.4 (few cases aged 11–12 yrs)
Szécsényi Nagy et al.	4.9	4.9	5.4	6.1	8.7 (Vol.TM(SzN = cca 0.8)

A *representative* national survey was organized measuring urinary iodine (3100 samples from school children from 55 settlements), not uncommonly with extremely different results between neighboring settlements (map will be presented).

In conclusion:

1. *Measuring urinary iodine could be the first act in a mass survey* because it is much more useful (mare easily organized and standardized, much cheaper, probably more sensitive etc) than thyroid volumetry by ultrasound. The latter would be more appropriate for goitrous areas or where low urinary iodine is frequent, especially in regions characterized by "island-like" iodine deficiency;
2. General iodine prevention (roughly similar iodine intake) may be a prerequisite for use of a representative survey testing the status of iodine nutrition in an iodine deficient country.

Continuous rise of urinary iodide excretion and drop in thyroid gland volume among adolescents in Mecklenburg-Vorpommern from 1993–1997

R. Hampel, A. Gordalla, H. Zöllner, D. Klinke, M. Demuth

Dept. of Endocrinology and Metabolic Diseases, Clinic of Internal Medicine, University of Rostock, Germany

Improved legislation (1989, 1993) and as well as public education are likely to improve the iodide intake of the German population. Children and adolescents should be the first to benefit. We investigated thyroid volumes and urinary iodide excretion among 2906 pupils aged 10 to 18 years in MV in 1993, 1995, and 1997. Median urinary iodide excretion rose from 73 µg/g creatinine in 1993 to 133 in 1997. Over the same period, the prevalence of goiter, according to the reference range of Gutekunst, dropped from 33 % to 10 % and median thyroid volume fell from 11 ml to 6 ml. While only 6 % of subjects excreted more than 150 µg iodide/g creatinine in 1993, this figure rose to 33 % in 1997. Improved dietary iodide is due to increased use of iodide fortified salt in the food industry.

In spring 1999 we measured the urinary iodide excretion of 3058 healthy children aged 6 to 12 years in 75 regions of Germany using the Cer-Arsenit method (Wawschinek). The median urinary iodide excretion was 13.9 µg/dl.

IDD in Uzbekistan

S.I. Ismailov, L.B. Nugmanova, T.K. Ibragimov, S.F. Rasulov, L.Z. Ashurova,

Institute of Endocrinology Academy of Science of Uzbekistan, Tashkent, Uzbekistan

Uzbekistan is considered to be an endemic zone for iodine deficiency disorders. Since USSR collapsed this problem has increased in importance because most of CIS countries started to produce and consume their own salt, which was not iodized. To evaluate IDD in Uzbekistan in 1998, we carried out an epidemiological investigation in all the regions of the country. The population from newborns up to 30 years of age were chosen for surveillance of IDD. 22.000 people of both sexes have been investigated, using palpation, ultrasonography, urinary iodine concentration and iodine concentration in the salt, T_3, T_4, TSH in blood serum, anthropometry. The investigation was sponsored by Merck KGaA. The data collected have proven that IDD is severe, with a goiter prevalence of 50–60 %, urinary iodine concentration less then 10 μg/dl in 97.4 % of the population, and hypothyroidism in 30 % of those investigated.

At present, 5 installations for iodization of salt and 15 tons of potassium iodate have been brought to mining plants in Uzbekistan by UNICEF. By November 1999, 23 % of salt in the city of Tashkent was iodized, mostly through private enterprises.

At the present time, progress is being made and many effective steps are being taken for eradication of IDD in Uzbekistan.

Reproducibility of determination on thyroid volume by 3D-ultrasound in comparison to the ellipsoid method

E. Werner, **J. Rendl**, S. Schlögl, J. Terekhova, M. Laßmann, Chr. Reiners

Clinic for Nuclear Medicine, University of Würzburg, Würzburg, Germany

Determination of thyroid volume by 3D-ultrasound is more exact than the conventional ellipsoid method. However, 3D-ultrasound is time consuming. For clinical requirements, detection of changes on follow-up is more important than absolute accuracy. The aim of this study was to compare reproducibility of thyroid volume determination by 3D-ultrasound and the conventional method.

Methods: 25 patients had two ultrasound scans performed by two experienced investigators with an interval of approximately 3 months (109 ± 28 days). 24 patients had the second scan as part of their follow up after radioiodine treatment. One patient had the second ultrasound scan for follow up of nodular goiter. Baseline and follow up thyroid volumes were determined by the same physician using both the ellipsoid and 3D method. For the ellipsoid method, 3 diameters of a thyroid lobe were determined and the volume of the lobe was calculated by the product of these diameters and the factor 0.5. For the 3D-method, 6 sagittal slices rotated around the longest axis of the lobe were generated. The investigator drew the outline of the thyroid in each slice, and the outline of the remaining thyroid was completed by the computer using spline interpolation. The volume was calculated by adding the voxels within the thyroid lobe.

Results: Because of the radioiodine treatment, the volume between the measurements decreased about 27 % ± 19 % and 20 % ± 25 % calculated by the ellipsoid method and the 3D-method respectively. The mean values did not differ significantly (t-test). The coefficient of variation (percent standard deviation) of the second measurement is an estimate of reproducibility, and was 25 % for the 3D and 19 % for the conventional method (difference not significant in the F-Test).

Discussion and conclusions: Although 3D-ultrasound provides a more exact measure of thyroid volume than the conventional method, its reproducibility is equal to or worse than the conventional method. Since the systematic errors involved in the ellipsoid method are the same for the first and the repeated measurements, the fact that it is not as exact as 3D-method does not affect the reproducibility.

Thyroid functional disorders and prevalence of diffuse non-toxic goiter (DNTG) in iodine deficiency in pregnant woman (PW) in the Moscow region

A.V. Dreval, T.S. Kamynina, **O.A. Netchaeva**, I.D. Chikh

Department of Endocrinology of Moscow Regional Clinical Scientific Research Institute, Moscow, Russia

The Moscow region has recently been reported as an area of mild iodine deficiency (data from epidemiological study of prevalence of endemic goiter, 1997–99). PW are the primary target group in an iodine deficient population. However there are no data concerning the prevalence of functional disorders and DNTG among PW in this region.

Material and methods: We studied 23 PW with palpable goiter, aged 19–35 years at their first antenatal visit (at 13–16 weeks of gestation, second trimester) and at 13–16 weeks after starting iodine and L-thyroxine treatment. Median urinary iodine excretion was 9.17 μg/dl, confirming mild iodine deficiency. Thyroid gland size was assessed by palpation and ultrasound. Based on WHO criteria, the degree of thyroid enlargement by palpation was grade I in 18, and II in 5 PW. Mean thyroid volume by ultrasonography was 13.4 ± 5.4 ml. DNTG was confirmed by ultrasound alone in 15 out of 23 PW (thyroid volume >18 ml). We observed following thyroid abnormalities: hyperechoic changes in 2, both hyperechoic and hypoechoic areas in 4, hypoechoic nodules (8 and 12 mm in diameter) in 2. We measured TSH and FT_4 to exclude subclinical and overt hypothyroidism. The mean TSH was 1.6 ± 1.1 (reference range 2.2 ± 1.2 mU/l), and the mean FT_4 was 13.1 ± 2.6 (13.3 ± 3.7 pmol/l.) With these data from the second trimester (with thyroid hypofunction resulting from iodine deficiency), we aimed to restore the normal functional state using the following treatment: 1) iodine supplementation as an iodized salt at a daily dosage of 6 g salt (18 PW); 2) L-thyroxine for patients with DNTG at a daily dosage of 25 μg per day (5 PW). This resulted in a reduction in thyroid volume and an increase in FT_4 in the 5 PW with DTNG in the third trimester compared with the second trimester.

Conclusion: Iodine deficiency is associated with adaptive functional abnormalities in the majority of PW and the development of DNTG with more significant changes in thyroid status in some. This condition should be corrected with iodine supplementation or thyroxine therapy.

Frequency and evolution of subclinical hypothyroidism amongst healthy pregnant women from the Bulgarian Black Sea region

L. Koeva, M. Petrova

Clinic of Endocrinology, Medical University of Varna, Varna, Bulgaria

Subclinical hypothyroidism during pregnancy increases the risk to both the mother and the newborn. The frequency amongst pregnant women in another seaboard country, Japan, is 0.11 % for transient disease and 0.19 % for permanent disease. Bulgaria is a country with mild to moderate iodine deficiency, with legally determined iodine supplementation of target age groups.

Aims: Prospective study of frequency and evolution of subclinical hypothyroidism in healthy pregnant women from the seaside region with positive antithyroid antibodies.

Materials and methods: Screening of 1100 pregnant women for thyroid diseases revealed diffuse goiter and positive antibodies in 167. Hormonal status, thyroid volume and iodine concentration in a random urine sample were determined during the first trimester of pregnancy and at the end of the first year after delivery.

Results: Before delivery 6 of the 167 subjects had TSH values of 4–6 mU/l (mean TSH 4.35 ± 0.54, mean TV 19.28 ± 2.2 ml).

The hormonal status after delivery defines three groups:

1. TSH 4–6 mU/l, n = 15, with mean TSH 5.12 ± 0.67 and TV 21.74 ml.
2. TSH 6–10 mU/l, n = 17, with mean TSH 6.86 ± 0.99 and TV 20.45 ± 2.96 ml.
3. TSH >10 mU/l, n = 17, with mean TSH 19.99 ± 5.93 and TV 20.81 ± 2.39.

Two pregnant women with TSH >100mU/l had still births.
The median iodine concentration among the 167 women during the first trimester was 80.0, compared with 39.4 after delivery.

Conclusion: It is difficult to define precisely whether iodine deficiency or autoimmune mechanisms prevail in the progression of subclinical hypothyroidism after delivery but the monitored frequency of 29 % (49 out of 167 women) suggests that mass screening and monitoring of thyroid function in pregnant women is worthwhile.

The ecological ill-being of territories and endemic goiter

L. A. Scheplyangina

Research Center of Children's Health, Moscow, Russia

In Russia, about 70 % of territories, all with a high density of industrial enterprises, are iodine deficient.

In the present study, we examined groups of 500 children 4–14 years old from territories with similar iodine contents and different levels of industrial pollution.

The median urinary iodine excretion was 6.1 μg/dl in the first region and 5.8 μg/dl in the second region, with anthropogenic loads of 14.7 and 7.2 points, respectively, and goiter frequencies 57.6 % and 28.4 %, respectively. The contribution of xenobiotics to goiter prevalence among children has been established. The estimate of the attributive risk (AR) and relative risk (RR) values indicated that industrial pollution increases the frequency of goiter by 22.3 % ($r = 0.975$), with an RR value of 4.5 (confidence interval 1.0–1.6).

Besides its goitrogenic effects, industrial pollution has toxic effects on the thyroid, as evidenced by the higher frequency of subclinical hypothyroidism among children from the first region (54 %) compared with those from the second region (26.5 %).

Thus, industrial pollution increases the intensity of endemic goiter, and should be taken into consideration for iodine prophylaxis and treatment of endemic goiter.

Effects of mass preventive iodine administration on the results of congenital hypothyroidism screening in Moscow

E.P. Kasatkina, D.E. Shilin, E.I. Osmanova, A.D. Baikov, A.P. Andreitschenko, L.K. Krivskaya

Dept. of Pediatric and Adolescent Endocrinology, Russian Medical Academy of Postgraduate Education; Federal Neonatal Screening Center, Moscow, Russia

In 1994–96 years mild iodine deficiency was revealed in Moscow. The median renal iodine excretion in 1680 children aged 9–12 years was 72 μg/l (range 41–87) [Dedov et al., 1999]. Massive preventive measures aimed at elimination of the iodine deficiency-related disorders with the use of iodized table salt (potassium iodine 40 ± 15 mg/kg of salt) were initiated in 1997 in the Russian capital. To evaluate the effectiveness of preventive iodine administration (PIA), the results of neonatal hypothyroidism screening in 344,604 children born in Moscow in 1995–99 years were analyzed in accordance with WHO recommendations (1994). The incidence of neonatal hyperthyrotropinemia (NHT; TSH – Neonatal DELFIA, Wallak, Finland) was calculated annually during the 5-year period. Before PIA was introduced, the frequency of NHT >5 mU/l was 38.3 ± 0.2 %, i. e. moderate [20–39.9%] in 1995, dropping to 31.6 ± 0.2 % ($p<10^{-6}$) and maintaining the same level in 1997. The incidence fell sharply reduced after introduction of PIA to 14.2 ± 0.1 % by 1999 ($p<10^{-6}$) becoming mild [3–19.9%]. At the same time, the frequency of NHT ≥20 mU/l decreased from 3.69 ± 0.04 % in 1995 to 2.89 ± 0.06 % in 1996, 1.85 ± 0.05 % in 1997, 0.85 ± 0.04 % in 1998 and 0.51 ± 0.04 % in 1999 (for each succeeding year $p<10^{-6}$). Thus, after the introduction of PIA, the frequency of NHT in Moscow fell significantly: the incidence of TSH >5 mU/l – fell by 24 % to less than 1/3, and the incidence of TSH >20 mU/l fell by 3 % to 1/7.

Conclusion: Introduction of iodized table salt into the diet of a major city population with mild iodine deficiency results in a significant positive effect on thyroid status among newborns, signifying improved maternal and fetal iodine status. Nevertheless, the frequency of NHT of more than 5 mU/l still exceeds the sporadic rate by almost 5 times (14 % versus 3 %), and confirms the continuing iodine deficiency. This suggests that improved awareness among the population through increased media coverage is necessary to promote dietary intake of iodized food products and the introduction of group prophylaxis among pregnant women throughout gestation.

Efficiency of long term iodine prophylaxis estimated by biological monitoring

A.V. Dreval, T.S. Kamynina, O.A. Netchaeva, [1]G.A. Gerasimov, [1]N.Y. Sviridenko

Endocrinology Department, Moscow Regional Research Clinical Institute; [1]The Research Centre of Endocrinology, Moscow, Russia

We studied schoolboys from the Moscow Region, among whom moderate iodine deficiency was found 5 years previously, and in whom prophylaxis measures were attempted. The efficiency of these measures was studied using 2 groups. The first group of 46 pupils had not received regular iodine prophylaxis; The second group of 41 pupils received regular iodine prophylaxis consisting of: 1) inclusion in the diet of iodized salt (150 µg iodine/day); 2) some courses of KI, one tablet/day, containing 200 µg iodine per tablet; 3) in some cases, iodized bread (150 µg iodine/day). Five years ago, children from the second group had also received a single dose of iodine in a prolonged oral iodide containing drug , which was completely eliminated over 12 months – with a return of urinary iodine excretion to baseline values. We estimated median urinary iodine excretion, volume of the thyroid gland by ultrasound, and serum TSH. In the first group median urinary iodine excretion has not changed significantly (6.2 µg/dl in 1993, 7.4 µg/dl in 1998). The frequency of goiter increased from 22.6% to 30.4%. The mean volume of the thyroid gland also increased from 5.2 ± 0.2 to 12.9 ± 1.4 ml; the mean TSH was within normal limits (1.6 ± 0.5 and 1.8 ± 1.0 µU/ml). In the second group the median urinary iodine excretion increased more than 2-fold (from 6.2 to 16.3 µg/dl)), the frequency of goiter has decreased considerably from 22.6 % to 7.3 %, and the mean volume of the thyroid gland has increased from 5.2 ± 0.2 to 7.6 ± 3.0 ml; the mean TSH was normal (1.6 ± 0.5 and 1.3 ± 0.7 µU/ml).

Conclusion: Regular iodine deficiency prophylaxis among children reduced the frequency of goiter and prevented pathological growth of thyroid volume during puberty.

Treatment of iodine deficiency goiter with iodine or iodine and levo-thyroxine combination

Z.S. Bencsik, P. Mezei, C. Komora

Saint George's Hospital, Székesfehérvár, Hungary

Objective: We assessed the effect of iodine or iodine plus levothyroxine on thyroid size in endemic goiter patients.

Design: Iodine (200 µg) or iodine and levothyroxine (200 µg + 75 µg per day) were given orally for 12 months in a prospective study.

Patients: One hundred euthyroid patients, 89 females and 11 males, median age 37 (range 18–71) with diffuse iodine deficiency goiters were studied.

Measurements: TSH, free T_4, antibody to thyroid peroxidase (aTPO), thyroid size by ultrasonography.

Results: After three months of therapy, TSH levels were suppressed in six patients. After 12 months of therapy, a reduction in goiter size was documented (1.1–31.7 %, median 15.3) in 85 cases, and thyroid size was within the normal range in 45 patients. The goiter size increased in four cases and was unchanged in five cases. Therapy was the most effective among patients 18–30 years old, if the echotexture of the thyroid gland was normal, and among those with goiter for 5–9 years.

Conclusions: These data indicate that the risk of oral administration of 200 µg iodine or 75 µg T_4 and 200 µg iodine is low. We found this therapeutic approach is less effective than previously reported. The best prognostic factors for effectiveness of therapy are patient age and the echotexture of the thyroid gland.

Screening for hypothyroidism in the elderly

J.M.F. Adam, M. Ayub, H. Sanusi

Diabetes and Endocrinology Section, Faculty of Medicine, Hasanuddin University, Makassar, Indonesia

Background: Several studies have confirmed that the prevalence of hypothyroidism is high among elderly people. Until now there are no data concerning the prevalence of hypothyroidism among elderly people in our country. In the year 2000, the elderly population in our country will be around 16 million or 15 % of the whole population. The aim of this study was to determine the prevalence of hypothyroidism among elderly people in the city of Makassar.

Subjects and methods: Five hundred subjects, age > 60 years old were invited to participate in this study. These 500 persons were chosen from 10 separate areas in the city of Makassar. They consisted of 182 males and 318 females. All subjects were active. History taking and physical examinations were performed on all subjects. Venous plasma was obtained for a TSH test. For the determination of TSH we used ThyroChek. 0.1 ml of plasma was added to the ThyroChek glass fiber filter. The test was positive for hypothyroidism, if the TSH > 5 μIU/ml.

Results: Twenty-five subjects gave a positive test for hypothyroidism (prevalence of 5 %). More males than females, 5.5 % among males and 4.7 % in females. The prevalence of hypothyroidism increased with age, being highest in the age > 80 years old. The most common presenting symptoms were fatigue, muscle cramp, arthralgia, and cold intolerance. There were no specific clinical signs, around 72 % having no symptoms.

Conclusions: The prevalence of hypothyroidism among the elderly in this study is similar to that reported in other studies. Most hypothyroid elderly patients are subclinical, and therefore screening among the elderly is important. ThyroChek is a very simple test for the detection of hypothyroidism and is a valuable method for screening in the population.

Reevaluation of diagnosis and further details of congenital hypothyroidism screened in neonatal period

Á. Muzsnai, L. Kovács, I. Szécsényi-Nagy, E. Hegedüs, F. Péter

Buda Children's Hospital, Budapest, Hungary

Nationwide screening for congenital hypothyroidism was introduced more than 17 years ago using TSH measurement. Two laboratories are responsible for testing the whole population, where the incidence is around 1:3,800. Data from the screening center located in the capital city are presented. We studied patients discovered on screening to have congenital hypothyroidism and on replacement, using the T_4-T_3 withdrawal test (change L-T_4 to T_3 for 3 weeks plus 1 week total withdrawal before hormone measurement) then radionuclide imaging (Tc99m) and ultrasound scan. Laboratory and imaging results were analyzed together with the neonatal thyroglobulin-level to determine the underlying etiology among 54 patients. The T_4-T_3 withdrawal test revealed 4 transient cases, all with normally localized thyroid glands. Agenesis was diagnosed in 8 cases, ectopic lingual thyroid in 8, hypoplasia or destructive processes resulting in hypothyroidism in 14 children. Na/I symporter defect is presumed in 12 patients, and other inborn errors of thyroxine synthesis in 9 cases. To enable more accurate classification of etiology, and to discover more about the pathogenesis of congenital hypothyroidism, genetic and DNA analyses are proposed.

Relation between thyroid function and skeletal muscle involvement in hypothyroidism

C. Grossegger, [1]E. Hartl, A. Kroiss, [2]J. Finsterer, [1]C. Stöllberger

Dept. of Nuclear Medicine, Krankenanstalt Rudolfstiftung; [1]2nd Internal Dept., Krankenanstalt Rudolfstiftung; [2]Ludwig Boltzmann Institute for Research in Neuromuscular Disorders, Vienna, Austria

Though hypothyroidism is a common endocrinological condition, it is not known how often skeletal muscle is involved and if there is a relation between the severity of hypothyroidism and the skeletal muscle involvement. In this prospective study, we investigated the frequency of muscle symptoms, symptoms of hypothyroidism, high serum CK, and the relation between CK and thyroid function tests. During a 6-month period, 69 patients, aged 16–87 years, with newly diagnosed hypothyroidism were included. Sixty-one of these patients had subclinical and 8 overt hypothyroidism. Twenty-five percent of the patients complained of muscle symptoms. Muscle symptoms were observed in 16 patients with subclinical and one patient with overt hypothyroidism. Symptoms of hypothyroidism were equally frequent among patients with and without muscle symptoms (82 and 88 % respectively). The frequency of a raised CK among patients with hypothyroidism was 3 %. CK was not significantly correlated with any of the thyroid function tests.

In conclusion, there seems to be only a poor relationship between the severity of the skeletal muscle involvement and the severity of hypothyroidism. Skeletal muscle seems to be less frequently involved in patients with hypothyroidism than previously reported.

Increased rate of hypothyroidism in the elderly by (super)sufficient alimentary iodine intake

P. Bottermann, [1]I. Zosin, [2]E. Zbranca

[1]2nd Medical Clinic, Faculty of Medicine, Technical University of Munich, Munich, Germany; [1] Clinic of Endocrinology, University of Medicine and Pharmacy, Timisoara; [2]UMF Iasi, Iasi, Romania

Purpose: Are there differences in (mild) hypothyroidism among the elderly depending upon dietary iodine intake? To answer this, TSH determinations were performed in clinically healthy persons in senior homes in two different regions of Romania, one with mild alimentary iodine deficiency (Iasi), the other one with a mild excess of dietary iodine intake (Timisoara).

Material and methods: Iasi N = 68, mean age 72.3 (57–87) years. Timisoara N = 78, mean age 70.5 (55–97) years. TSH by IRMA: normal range: 0.24–3.4 mU/L.

Results: In Iasi in 8 of 68 persons (11.8 %) the TSH was >3.4 mU/L (4.68 ± 2.14 mU/l; mean ± SD). In Timisoara in 22 of 78 persons (28.2 %) the TSH was >3.4 mU/L (4.68 ± 2.14 mU/l; mean ± SD).

Discussion: There were no differences in the mean age or age range or in others circumstances of the inhabitants of the senior homes in the two regions. Nearly all persons have lived all their lives in their region. The higher iodine intake in Timisoara could be acting through a higher rate of clinically inapparent chronic thyroiditis with destruction of thyroid tissue and explain the higher frequency of elevated TSH values in this region.

Conclusion: The rate of (mild) hypothyroidism in older persons may depend on the amount of (life-long) dietary iodine intake.

Kinetics and effects of selenium administration in grade 1 hypothyroidism

L.H. Duntas, E. Mantzou, P. Marafelia, G.R. Piperingos, D.A. Koutras

Endocrine Unit, "Evgenidion Hospital", University of Athens, Athens, Greece

Background: Selenium (Se) is an essential component of type I deiodinase, a key enzyme of thyroid hormone metabolism, and is also involved in the pathophysiology of thyroid gland. Currently, the effect of Se on thyroid is a matter of dispute. The aim of this study was to determine the bioavailability and kinetic profile of orally administered Se (Seleno-1-Methionine) and to follow the effects of 4 weeks' treatment with Se on thyroid function.

Methods: Six euthyroid volunteers (V) and 8 patients with grade I hypothyroidism (HYPO) (TSH 4–6 μU/ml) were studied. All V and HYPO had normal urinary iodine excretion. The V received orally 200 μg Se and blood samples were drawn at 0, 2, 4, 6 and 24 h to determine serum concentrations of FT_4, T_3, T_4, TSH and Se. The HYPO patients were treated with Se 200 μg/daily for 4 weeks. Blood samples were collected at 0, 1 and 4 weeks of treatment. Se was measured by atomic absorption (normal range: 71–125 μg/l).

Results: Se increased after 2 h (140 ± 15 μg/l), peaked at 4 h (150 ± 17 μg/l) and was at the upper limit at 24 h (125 ± 11 μg/l). T_4 increased slowly from 8.5 ± 0.7 μg/dl to 9.1 ± 0.8 μg/dl at 24 h. In HYPO T_4 increased after 4 weeks of treatment by 37.8 % (7.4 ± 0.7 vs 10.2 ± 1.0 μg/dl; $p<0.001$), T_3 fell by 30.4 % (115 ± 12 vs 80 ± 9 ng/dl; $p<0.001$) and TSH remained unaltered. Se increased significantly compared to basal levels (124 ± 13 vs 78 ± 9 μg/l; $p<0.001$). The linear regression analysis did not reveal any statistical significant correlation between Se and T_3 ($r = 0.2551$; $p = 0.5421$) or between Se and T_4 ($r = 0.3383$; $p = 0.4125$).

Conclusions: Orally administered Se is slowly and effectively absorbed. A dose up to 200 μg/daily does not lead to toxic levels in blood. Se enhances T_4 and inhibits T_3 without affecting TSH. These effects were observed in a non iodine and Se deficient area and therefore, may differ in deficient populations. Finally, Se might be therapeutically helpful in certain thyroid diseases.

Pathogenesis of ovarian hypofunction in primary hypothyroidism

V.V. Potine, N.N. Tkatchenko, I.O. Kriheli, A.B. Loginov

Dept of Reproduction Endocrinology, The D.O. Ott Research Institute of Obstetrics and Gynecology, RAMS, Saint Petersburg, Russia

39 patients with primary hypothyroidism at the age of 18–40 years were examined to study the influence of the thyroid hypofunction on the hypothalamus-hypophysis-ovary axis. The diagnosis was confirmed by decreased blood levels of triiodothyronine (0.3 ± 0.1 nmol/l) and thyroxine (32.4 ± 6.5 nmol/l) and high TSH level (60.4 ± 13.6 mIU/l). Anovulation was observed in all women. Basal LH (8.8 ± 1.3 IU/l) and FSH (5.4 ± 0.5 IU/l) level did not differ significantly from those in serum from healthy women of reproductive age (8.6 ± 0.5 IU/l and 4.7 ± 0.6 IU/l, respectively). Hyperprolactinemia was noted in half the patients (range 938 mIU/l to 3324 mIU/I). The metoclopromide test (10 mg intravenously) showed a reduction in dopaminergic inhibition of hypophyseal lactotrophic function among patients with hyperprolactinemia. Modulation of the preovulatory increase of estradiol by parenteral administration resulted in the expected decrease in gonadotropins on the second day of estradiol test (negative feed-back mechanism). The LH increase on the fifth test day (7.4 ± 2.5 IU/l) was considerably lower in comparison to that in euthyroid women with normogonadotropic amenorrhea (25.9 ± 2.5 IU/l) and to the periovulatory LH level in healthy women (20 IU/l-60 IU/l). These results show that the main cause of anovulation in women with primary hypothyroidism is a disorder in the positive feedback mechanism between the ovaries and hypophysis.

Influence of thyroid medicines on neuromuscular disorder in hypothyroidism

N.E. Dribinskaya, I.A. Strokov, **A.S. Ametov**

Dept. of Endocrinology, Russian Medical Academy Postgraduate Education, Moscow, Russia

Neuromuscular dysfunction is found in 70% of cases of hypothyroidism, however treatment of hypothyroidism does not always result in clinical amelioration. The purpose of the present study was to assess effect of treatment for thyroid dysfunction on neuromuscular symptoms using a scoring system for assessment of neuromuscular dysfunction. Evaluation of neurological status (assessment of muscular weakness on a scale from 5 to 1, of deep reflexes patterns, various sensory modalities), the serum creatine kinase (CPK), electromyography studies of the peroneal, sural, median nerves and quadriceps femoris muscle were performed in 80 patients with overt primary hypothyroidism due to autoimmune thyroiditis (46 patients) or thyroidectomy (34 patients). The mean duration of the disease was 7.26 ± 1.85 years, mean TSH was 30.07 ± 6.48 mIU/l (normal range 0.3–4.5 mIU/l), the mean free T_4 8.51 ± 1.00 pmol/l (11–26 pmol/l), free T_3 1.83 ± 0.37 pmol/l (2.5–5.8 pmol/l). The interval between the first and the second examination was 12 months after starting replacement therapy. Nerve involvement was established in 75 cases, with concurrent muscle lesions in 14 cases.

With normalization of thyroid function (TSH 3.43 ± 0.50 mIU/l ($p<0,01$), free T_4 14.05 ± 0.75 pmol/l ($p<0.01$), free T_3 2.13 ± 0.28 pmol/l ($p<0.01$)) in 87% of patients we observed restoration of muscular strength, relaxation time and amplitude of deep reflexes, of sensory modalities, CPK and also the electrophysiological changes. 13% of cases experienced no improvement in the neuromuscular disorder.

These findings confirm the reversibility of neuromuscular dysfunction after normalization of thyroid function. The scoring system for neuromuscular disorder in hypothyroidism allows objective evaluation of the severity of these abnormalities. For the remaining 13% of patients with neuromuscular complications, the issue of the necessity of additional therapy requires further clarification.

In conclusion, thyroid treatment leads to restoration of neuromuscular function in most cases.

Treatment of hypothyroidism requires a long term hormonal therapy with Euthyrox

A.V. Shcherbak, **D.V. Kirienko**, P.N. Bodnar

Dept. of Endocrinology, State Medical University, City Clinical Endocrinological Hospital, Kiev, Ukraine

Levothyroxine is a reliable and commonly prescribed drug for treating thyroid disease, but excessive dosage may have adverse effects. Among patients with hypothyroidism, levothyroxine is used as replacement therapy. Euthyrox® (Levothyroxine, Merck KGaA) has been present in the pharmaceutical market in Ukraine for more than two years. The effects of Euthyrox® were studied among 42 adults (30 women and 12 men), mean age 46.6 years (range 28 to 70 years), with clinical hypothyroidism. Hypothyroidism was diagnosed when a TSH was greater than 6,0 μU/ml or if a history of hypothyroidism requiring replacement therapy was documented. 21 % of patients had thyroglobulin antibodies and 29 % had thyroid microsomal antibodies with titers ranging from 1:200 to 1:3200. The Euthyrox® dosage varied between individuals from 0.6 to 3.2 μg/kg. For most patients, therapy was initiated with a full replacement dosage (1.6 μg/kg body weight), which is usually 75 to 100 μg/day for women and 100 to 150 μg/day for men; the duration was six months. As endpoints of this study, we used thyroid volume reduction, thyroid hormones, TSH and thyroid histograms. The goal was to normalize the serum TSH. There was a negative linear relation between the equilibrium dose and the TSH value ($r = 0.82$; $p<0,001$), and a positive relation with the L-T_4 concentration ($r = 0,72$; $p<0,001$). No adverse reactions were noted. We conclude that Euthyrox® replacement therapy is effective, inexpensive, and free of complications with proper patient monitoring. The Euthyrox® maintenance dosage depends on the cause of hypothyroidism, on the degree of biochemical abnormality and the patient's age, sex and weight.

Triiodothyronine enhances vitamin concentrations in hypothyroid thyroid cancer patients previously treated with thyroxine alone

R. Bunevičius, L.R. Černiauskienė, [1]A.J. Prange Jr.

Kaunas Medical University, Kaunas, Lithuania; [1]University of North Carolina, Chapel Hill, North Carolina, USA

In a previous report (Bunevicius et al, 1999) our group described the results of treating 33 hypothyroid patients with thyroxine (T_4) alone or with a reduced amount of T_4 combined with a small amount of triiodothyronine (T_3). Improvements in mental function and an increase in concentration of sex hormone-binding globulin (SH-BG) occurred after combined treatment. The present report focuses on thyroid cancer patients. It presents findings of changes in antioxidant activity and lipid peroxidation that may be of special relevance for cancer patients.

We treated seventeen hypothyroid patients (15 women and two men) with their usual dose of T_4 or with a regimen in which 50 µg of T_4 had been replaced by 12.5 µg of T_3. Patients were randomly assigned to first one regimen for five weeks and then to the other regimen for an additional five weeks.

Concentrations of free T_4 and total T_4 diminished while the concentrations of total T_3 and thyrotropin increased under combined treatment. The changes in concentration of triglycerides and cholesterol were trivial. However, the increase in the concentration of malondialdehyde (MDA) approached statistical significance. After combined treatment, the increase in concentration of vitamin E, though small, was statistically significant (0.85 ± 0.15 mg/dl vs. 0.93 ± 0.20 mg/dl, $p<0.05$) while an increase in vitamin A concentration was insignificant. Changes in T_3 concentration were correlated positively and significantly with changes in vitamin A concentration ($r = 0.64$; $p = 0.006$). Changes in cholesterol levels were correlated positively with vitamin E and MDA concentrations ($r = 0.83$, $p<0.001$ and $r = 0.54$, $p = 0.03$, respectively).

The present data demonstrate that combined replacement with T_4 and T_3 stimulates antioxidant activity, in comparison to treatment with T_4 alone. Changes in vitamin A concentration is directly related to change in T_3 level and changes in vitamin E concentration to cholesterol concentration.

Thyroid status and blood level of polychlorinated biphenyls and pesticides in exposed and control population

P. Langer, [1]M. Tajtáková, [2]A. Kočan, [2]J. Petrík, [2]J. Chovancová, [2]B. Drobná, [2]S. Jursa, [2]M. Pavúk, P. Bohov, I. Klimeš

Institute of Experimental Endocrinology, Slovak Academy of Sciences, Bratislava; [1]1st Clinic of Internal Medicine, P. J. Šafárik University, Košice; [2]Institute of Preventive and Clinical Medicine, Bratislava, Slovakia

Objective: To compare the thyroid status of the employees (EMPL) of formerly polychlorinated biphenyls (PCB) producing factory with that of control population (CONT) with respect to the blood levels of PCB and other organochlorinated pollutants.

Subjects and methods: In 101 EMPL (59 males and 42 females) and 360 CONT (181 males and 179 females) the thyroid volume (ThV) was measured by ultrasound and the level of TSH and antithyroperoxidase antibodies (anti-TPO) was estimated. The plasma level of PCB, hexachlorobenzene (HCB), hexachlorocyclohexane (HCH), DDT and DDE was estimated by congener specific analysis with the aid of microcapillary gas chromatography/mass spectrometry.

Results and conclusions: Both ThV and PCB level in 101 EMPL (16.3±0.73 ml and 7300 ± 871 ng/g lipids) were significantly higher ($p<0.001$) than in 360 CONT (14.0 ± 0.32 ml and 2045 ± 147 ng/g). As shown in the Table, among 59 male EMPL the frequency of several measures (ThV >20.0 ml, hypoechogenicity, solitary nodules, positive anti-TPO and abnormal TSH) was significantly higher ($p<0.001$) than among 181 male CONT. The same Table shows that there was no difference in the frequency of such measures between 42 female EMPL and 179 female CONT. Moreover, the frequency of hypoechogenicity, solitary nodules, anti-TPO and abnormal TSH among 179 female CONT was about 4–8 times higher than that among 181 male CONT, which is usual female/male ratio. In contrast, the frequency of those measures (except ThV >20.0 ml and abnormal TSH) in male EMPL and female EMPL was the same.

Although increased ThV results from various causes, it appeared that it is partly related to the increased plasma levels of all individual organochlorines estimated.

However, the most remarkable interrelation was found between ThV and the sum (total level) of PCB+HCB+HCH+DDT+DDE. Thus, in the 10% of subjects with the highest total organochlorines level (15,643–64,376 ng/g) the frequency of ThV >20.0 ml (15/46 = 32.6%) was significantly higher (p<0.001) than that in the 80% of subjects (31/368 = 8.4%) with low total levels (1,016–11,664 ng/g). From this appears that all organochlorines measured may participate in the increase of ThV, although PCB was the most abundant.

Measure	**Male EPL (N = 59)**	**Male CONT (N = 181)**	**P[2]**	**Female EMPL (N = 42)**	**Female CONT (N = 179)**
ThV >20.0ml	30.5%[1]	19.9%	<9,991	14.2%[1]	10.6%
Hypoechogenicity	44.1%	11.6%	<9,991	42.8%	46.4%
Solit. nodules >10mm	10.2%	2.7%	<0.025	11.9%	10.6%
Anti-TPO positive	20.3%	2.2%	<0.001	16.6%	20.7%
TSH <0.3 and >4.5mU/l	30.5%[1]	3.8%	<0.001	11.9%[1]	13.4%

[1] = P <0.05 in the same line; [2] = P shows the difference between "Male EMPL" and "Male CONT"

Increased thyroid volume and prevalence of high TSH level in schoolchildren from the area contaminated by nitrates

M. Tajtáková, [1]**P. Langer**, Z. Semanová, Z. Tomková, [1]P. Bohov, [2]E. Szökeová, [2]J. Majoros, [1]E. Šeböková, J. Petrovičová

1st Clinic of Internal Medicine, Faculty of Medicine, P. J. Šafárik University of Košice, Košice; [1]Institute of Experimental Endocrinology, Slovak Academy of Sciences, Bratislava; [2]State Institute of Hygiene and Epidemiology, Košice, Slovakia

Objective: This study was a part of extensive field surveys of the possible effects of environmental pollution on the thyroid status of iodine replete population and related to the previously published observation on possible effects of polychlorinated biphenyls on the thyroid of the employees of chemical factory (Langer P., Tajtáková M. et al.: Eur. J. Endocrinol. 139: 402–9, 1998) and was designed to search for possible differences in thyroid volume (ThV) and prevalence of subclinical signs of thyroid disorders in schoolchildren from the area heavily contaminated by nitrates as compared to controls.

Subjects and methods: ThV was estimated by ultrasound in 10 and 13 year old children from nitrate contaminated (NIT; n = 244, 107 boys and 137 girls) and control areas (CON; n = 248, 127 boys and 121 girls). The distances between the 3 examined villages in each area were 3-10 km, the nutrition profile and urinary iodine being the same. Both examined areas are highly agricultural and with large amounts of nitrate fertilizers in use and penetration to superficial underground water. In the NIT area, the drinking water (which is used also for the preparation of all food) comes from superficial wells and contains high level of nitrates (among 64 samples of water the level of nitrate (NO_3^-) was >50 mg/l in 46, >100 mg/l in 30, and >200 mg/l in 14), while that in CON comes by water pipe from mountain spring and appears to be virtually nitrate free (15 samples had <2.0 mg/l). Serum level of TSH (supersensitive IRMA method) and thyroperoxidase antibodies (anti-TPO) by RIA was estimated in 230 NIT and 188 CON children. Urinary iodine was estimated by mild acid digestion method followed by the Sandell-Kolthoff colorimetric reaction. For statistical evaluation the chi-square test was used.

Results: ThV in NIT area was significantly increased in both age groups. Thus, the prevalence of ThV greater than 7.0 ml/m^2 body surface area in 10 year old children was 25/90 (27.7%) in NIT versus 11/92 (11.9%) in CON ($p < 0.0l$) and that in 13 year old children was 33/154 (21.4%) in NIT versus 16/156 (10.2%) in CON ($p < 0.01$). The prevalence of TSH levels >5.0 mU/l was significantly higher in NIT (13/230 = 5.6% vs. 2/188 = 1.1%; $p < 0.01$). In NIT area the prevalence of TSH level >3.5 mU/l (40/230 = 17.4% in NIT vs. 28/188 = 14.9% in CON), positive anti-TPO (6/230 = 2.6% in NIT vs. 2/188 = 1.1% in CON) and of thyroid ultrasound hypoechogenicity (27/230 = 11.7% in NIT vs. 19/188 = 10.1% in CON) was slightly but not significantly increased. The median values of urinary iodine from both areas were in the range of 11–15 µg/l, indicating satisfactory iodine intake.

Conclusions: Increased thyroid volume and prevalence of high TSH level was found in children from the area heavily contaminated by nitrates in drinking water from superficial wells as compared to controls from a neighboring area supplied by nitrate free drinking water from mountain spring. Since the urinary iodine was in satisfactory range, it is suggested that the increased prevalence of thyroid disorders may result from the increased nitrate intake.

Development of Graves' disease after radioiodine treatment for a toxic nodule. Is the hyperthyroidism always triggered by 131-I therapy?

H. Niepomniszcze, F. Pitoia, C. Goodall, M. Manavela, O.D. Bruno

Division of Endocrinology, Hospital de Clínicas, University of Buenos Aires, Buenos Aires, Argentina

Recently, the transition from nodular toxic goiter to autoimmune hyperthyroidism triggered by 131-I therapy has been given much prominence (Thyroid 1999, 9:477). However, de novo development of hyperthyroidism is not always a consequence of such therapy. We present two cases of patients who developed Graves' hyperthyroidism after treatment with radioactive iodine for solitary autonomously functioning toxic nodule (AFTN). Both patients had relatives with autoimmune thyroid diseases.

Case 1 is a woman who received 20 mCi of 131-I as treatment of a 3cm hot nodule at the age of 33 yrs. At that time she had undetectable TSH with T_3 = 145 ng/dl, T_4 = 8.4 µg/dl and MCHA = 1/6400. 6 months later she had normal thyroid scintigraphy, TSH = 1.6 µU/ml, T_3 = 120 ng/dl, T_4 = 8.5 µg/dl, MCHA = 1/6400 and TGHA negative. She remained euthyroid for 10 years until 1 month after delivery of her second child, developing Graves' hyperthyroidism (T_3 = 313 ng/dl, T_4 = 20.7 µg/dl, TSH <0.05 µU/ml, MCHA = 1/102400 and TRAb = 59U/L [normal <15]. Scintigraphy showed homogeneous distribution of radioiodine uptake in a diffusely enlarged thyroid gland. She was treated once more with 8mCi of 131-I.

Case 2, a 58 year-old woman, received 25 mCi of 131-I as treatment of an AFTN. She had T_3 = 317 ng/dl, T_4 = 13 µg/dl, FT_4 = 2.7 ng/dl, TPO-Ab = 40 U/ml (normal <0.5), TRAb negative. 5 months later she was clinically euthyroid with TSH = 3.5 µU/ml and T_3 = 115 ng/dl. She remained euthyroid for a further 11 months, then developing hyperthyroidism with diffuse thyroid radioiodine uptake, apart from a 1 cm cold area in the same location as the previous toxic nodule. She did not take antithyroid treatment despite her clinically mild hyperthyroidism, remaining toxic for, at least, another 8 months: T_3 = 210 ng/dl, T_4 = 16.2 μg/dl, TSH <<0.1 μU/ml, TPO-Ab = 45 U/ml and TRAb negative. 5 months after these last assays she became spontaneously euthyroid, with TSH = 4.5 μU/ml, T_3 = 146 ng/dl and T_4 = 10.2 μg/dl.

In these patients, hyperthyroidism developed 10 years (Case 1) and 16 months (Case 2) after 131-I therapy. We think that such prolonged time lag argues against a direct relationship between the 131-I therapy and the development of Graves' disease in these women, at least in Case 1.

Immune response in anti-TPO +ve pregnant women antenatally and during postpartum period

A. Kokandi, A.B. Parkes, L.D.K.E. Premawardhana, **J.H. Lazarus**

Department of Medicine, University of Wales College of Medicine, Cardiff, Wales, United Kingdom

Postpartum thyroiditis characterized by thyroid dysfunction occurring usually between 6 and 24 weeks postpartum is seen in up to 50% of antiTPO +ve women as ascertained at 16 weeks gestation. Although known to be immune mediated the precise changes in the immune system are unclear. In this preliminary study we report an analysis of the Th1 (reflected by IFNγ secretion) and Th2 status (IL-4) evaluated by fluorescence activated cell sorter (FACS) analysis of peripheral blood lymphocytes (PBL) obtained from 8 anti-TPO Ab +ve women at 36 weeks gestation and 6, 12 and 24 weeks postpartum. PBL were stimulated with PMA and ionomycin with monensin for 4 hours before staining with appropriate monoclonal antibodies for intracellular cytokines and FACS analysis.

CD4/CD8 ratios ranged from 2.4 to 5.2 (mean 3.92) before delivery and fell to 3.17, 2.04 and 1.93 at 6, 12 and 24 weeks postnatal (PN). IL-4 (expressed as % CD4+CD3+cells) rose from 0.97% at 36 weeks AN to 3.88%, 4.57% and 5.01% at 6, 12 and 24 weeks PN respectively. In contrast % IFNγ rose from zero at 36 weeks AN to a maximum of 2.0 at 12 weeks and declined to 0.22% at 24 weeks with the result that the IL-4/IFN ratio declined from 2–5 at 36 weeks AN to 0.03 at 24 weeks PN.

These data suggest while both cytokines are suppressed in late pregnancy the relative changes postpartum show a return to Th1 status in TPO Ab+ve women. The relationship of these changes to the development of thyroid dysfunction is as yet unclear.

TSH, free T_4 and anti-TPO levels in pregnant women

D. Hauerová, R. Pikner, D. Mrazová, **O. Topolcan**, L. Pecen

2nd Dept. of Internal Medicine, Charles University Hospital, Plzen, Czech Republic

The frequency of thyroid gland disorders in pregnancy is approximately 10% (0.4–25%). Untreated thyroid diseases in pregnancy represent a serious risk for both mother and fetus (post-natal thyroiditis in mothers and low birth weight, or neonatal thyroid disease in children). In our study, we assessed 650 serum samples obtained from pregnant women during routine blood sampling for Down syndrome screening in the second trimester. In all women, we assessed TSH (IRMA, Immunotech, Czech Republic), anti TPO (RIA, Brahms, Germany) and free T_4 (RIA, Immunotech, Czech Republic), with reference values of 0.3 to 4.5 mlU/L for TSH, <40 mU/l for anti TPO and 10 to 25 pmol/l for free T_4. 2.3 % of TSH levels in pregnant women were lower than 0.3 mlU/L and 1.5 % were above 4.5 mlU/L. Elevated anti-TPO levels were found in 9.4% of women. 2.9% of women had free T_4 lower than 10 pmol/l and none had higher value than 25 pmol/l. The authors will discuss the correlation of these results with clinical status of examined women and potential role of TSH, free T_4 and anti TPO as screening tools of thyroid gland disorders in pregnancy.

This work was supported by grant of IGA MH CR.

Tobacco and Graves' (Basedow) disease

E. Zbranca, D.D. Branisteanu, V. Mogos, C. Vulpoi, C. Cristea, B. Galusca, B. Scurtu, A. Toma

Dept. of Endocrinology, University of Medicine and Pharmacy "GrT Popa", Iasi, Romania

Both thyroid dysfunction and smoking are frequent in the general population, with prevalence of around 10% and over 30%, respectively. Many studies have suggested that tobacco interferes with normal thyroid function, as well as with the evolution of thyroid pathology. Some of these studies suggest a significant correlation of Graves' Basedow disease and Graves' ophthalmopathy with smoking.

In order to investigate the connection between Graves' disease, its associated ophthalmopathy and smoking, we retrospectively studied a group of 270 patients with Graves' disease (233 females and 37 males). The incidence of smoking in this group was compared to that found in a control, thyroid disease-free group of 120 patients. The incidence of smokers was significantly higher in the group with Graves' disease (145 out of 270, 54%) than in the control group (42 out of 120, 35%) ($p < 0.01$). The 143 patients with Graves' ophthalmopathy included a higher percentage of smokers than those without ophthalmopathy (63% compared to 43%, $p < 0.01$). This difference was due mainly to female patients (76 smokers out of 123 female patients with ophthalmopathy, 62%, compared with only 44 smoking ophthalmopathy-free Graves' patients out of 109, 40%, $p < 0.001$). Forty-four out of 90 (49%) tobacco users with ophthalmopathy were heavy smokers (i. e. over one pack per day for over 20 years), an incidence significantly higher than that of heavy smokers found among smoking Graves' patients without ophthalmopathy (19 out of 55, 35%), or among smoking patients in the control group (13 out of 42, 31%) ($p < 0.05$, and $p < 0.01$, respectively).

The data obtained support the hypothesis of tobacco influence upon Graves' disease evolution. Smoking seems to trigger both thyroid disease and ophthalmopathy appearance, especially in females. The risk of ophthalmopathy development may depend upon the amount of cigarettes smoked.

Smoking and severity of thyroid eye disease

I. Duncea, C. Blendea, A. Dalea, C. Gruiţă

Endocrinology Department, University of Medicine and Pharmacy, Cluj – Napoca, Romania

Smoking is an important risk factor for developing several orbital disease, with proptosis and diplopia. In order to evaluate the relationship between smoking and thyroid eye disease, we studied two groups of patients with Basedow-Graves' disease, in-patients of the Endocrinology Department between November 1998 and September 1999. All patients were treated with oral cortisone therapy. We compared smokers group-S (37 patients: 10 males, 27 females, mean age of the group 38.8 years) with non-smokers group non-S (75 patients: 16 males, 59 females – mean age 42.1 years). The severity of thyroid eye disease was evaluated using the Werner scale (NO SPECS); edematous orbitopathy (Werner ≥ 2) was present in 86.8 % of patients in group-S and 65.2 % of patients in group non-S; the difference was statistically significant, $p<0.001$. Among female patients, 85.1 % of smokers had edematous orbitopathy, compared with only 62.7 % of the non-smokers, $p < 0.001$. Ten of the female smokers (37 %) needed also radiotherapy, compared with 9 of the non-smokers (15.3 %). In males, the percentage with edematous disease was 90 % in group S and 75 % in non-S, $p<0.001$. Six of the male smokers (60 %) were also treated with conventional radiotherapy, compared with only two of the non-smokers (12.5 %). Our study underlines the importance of smoking as a risk factor for development of edematous eye disease, in both male and female patients.

Evaluation of osteoporotic fracture risk with quantitative ultrasound bone densitometry (QUS) in post-menopausal women with hyper-thyroidism and with suppressive treatment with thyroid hormones

C. Poiana, I. Virtej

Institute of Endocrinology, "C.I.Parhon", Bucharest, Romania

The primary effect of thyroid hormone excess due to hyperthyroidism or suppressive treatment with thyroid hormones on bone metabolism is the stimulation of bone resorption, increasing bone turnover and the ratio of osteoresorbing surfaces to osteoforming surfaces, and decreasing the duration of the bone remodeling cycle.

The result is a net decrease in bone mineral density (BMD) and increased risk of osteoporotic fractures.

Our study aimed to evaluate the influence of thyrotoxicosis on fracture risk in postmenopausal women. We investigated 25 women with Graves' disease and 25 women with subclinical thyrotoxicosis due to suppressive treatment with thyroid hormones for thyroid carcinoma (after thyroidectomy and radioiodine treatment), and compared them with a control group of 100 healthy postmenopausal women.

Quantitative ultrasound (QUS) bone densitometry was performed in all women, at the calcaneum with an Achilles Lunar Plus device. The parameters measured by QUS were BUA (broadband ultrasound attenuation), SOS (speed of sound) and the clinical Stiffness index.

Conclusions: Osteoporotic fracture risk was significantly increased ($p<0.05$) among all patients with thyrotoxicosis, the greater risk being among patients receiving suppressive treatment with thyroid hormones for thyroid carcinoma. The fracture risk increased with the duration of the therapy. Among postmenopausal women, thyrotoxicosis is an additional risk factor for osteoporosis, the risk for osteoporotic fractures increasing with the number of years post-menopause.

Functional, immunological and ultrasonographical aspects in different forms of autoimmune thyroiditis (AIT) in an iodine sufficient area

I. Zosin, [1]P. Bottermann, C. Crista, M. Vlad, A. Milos

Clinic of Endocrinology, University of Medicine and Pharmacy, Timisoara, Romania, [1]2nd Medical Clinic, Faculty of Medicine, Technical University of Munich, Munich, Germany

Autoimmune thyroiditis (AIT) comprises several entities, with different age distributions, clinico-functional presentation, immunological profile and histopathological picture. We studied 160 patients with AIT from an iodine sufficient area (age range 10–72 years, mean 40.48 years, 157 females, 3 males). The diagnosis was established on clinico-functional parameters, thyroid-specific antibodies levels (TPO-Abs, Tg-Abs) and ultrasonographic data. Hashimoto's disease accounted for 40.63 % of cases, atrophic thyroiditis for 36.25 %, and asymptomatic thyroiditis for 13.13 %. The juvenile variant (10 % of cases) comprised mainly asymptomatic subjects. From the functional point of view, the presentation of Hashimoto's disease was heterogeneous (euthyroidism, clinical and subclinical hypothyroidism and thyrotoxicosis). Atrophic AIT presented as subclinical hypothyroidism (30 % of cases) and clinical hypothyroidism (70 % of patients). None of the patients presenting with the asymptomatic form of the disease had evidence of thyroid dysfunction. Regarding the antithyroid antibodies, both (TPO-Abs, Tg-Abs) were detected in all described forms. The distribution of antibodies (both, TPO-Abs alone, Tg-Abs alone) and the titers differed between AIT forms. The classical ultrasonographic pattern of the disease was observed in 96.98 % patients. Unusual patterns, such as nonhypoechoic inhomogeneous parenchyma, pseudo- and nodular forms led to additional in vivo investigations (RAIU, fine-needle biopsy). The diagnostic value of Doppler ultrasonography performed in this group of patients is thus still dubious.

In summary, different forms of AIT may represent distinct entities with a common pathogenesis or different stages of a single disorder. While the diagnosis of AIT is easy in the majority of cases, the underlying mechanisms of the disease and its course are not yet completely elucidated.

Use of the oral TRH Test to detect subclinical thyroid dysfunction in patients with chronic autoimmune thyroiditis

[1]R. Villaseca, **C. Liberman**

Dept. of Endocrinology, Hospital Clinico de la Universidad de Chile, [1]Clinica Alemana, Santiago de Chile, Chile

Chronic autoimmune thyroiditis (CAT) is a frequent cause of hypothyroidism in iodine sufficient areas. However, there is no current method of predicting which patients will become hypothyroid and which will remain euthyroid. This is an important consideration before using thyroid hormone therapy in early stages of the disease.

The oral TRH test has been used for the diagnosis of subclinical hypothyroidism. Oral TRH produces greater and longer lasting TSH response than parenteral TRH. This difference may improve the detection of thyroid dysfunction.

Objective: To evaluate prospectively whether the oral TRH test predicts development of hypothyroidism among patients with CAT.

Methods: Nine female patients with CAT from an iodine sufficient area were included in the study (age range 28–75 years, mean: 52 years). Diagnosis of CAT was confirmed by positive antimicrosomal antibodies (l/400 or greater). All patients had normal basal TSH (1.51 ± 0.76 μU/ml) and a normal TSH response at 30 minutes in the i.v. TRH test (13.16 ± 4.99 μU/ml). An oral TRH test was performed (40 mg; Roche) and TSH was measured at 0, 120, 180 and 240 minutes. According to standard criteria a response of 40 μUI/ml or less at 120 min was considered normal. After 7 years of follow up all patients were analyzed with T_4, TSH and anti-TPO levels, apart from one subject who was studied at 5 years. This patient was started on thyroid hormone therapy because of an elevated basal TSH. Hypothyroidism was diagnosed if the TSH level was 10 μU/ml or greater. Subclinical hypothyroidism was diagnosed if the basal TSH was between 5 and 10 μU/ml.

Results: In four of the nine patients the oral TRH test was normal and in five it was abnormal . Three of those with abnormal oral tests (60 %) developed hypothyroidism during follow up compared with only one among those with normal oral tests (25 %). After 7 years all patients had positive TPO antibodies (mean 450.77 ± 192.35 U/ml), but there was no significant difference in antibody concentrations (388.0 ± 202.19 vs. 501 ± 190.38 U/ml; $p > 0.01$).

Conclusion: An abnormal oral TRH test may detect early thyroid dysfunction among patients with CAT. This test may help to predict development of subclinical hypothyroidism.

Influence of levothyroxine on the circulation in thyroid gland of children with autoimmune thyroiditis

V. Matyushenko, **P. Bodnar**

Dept. of Endocrinology, National Medical University, Kiev, Ukraine

94 children with autoimmune thyroiditis (AIT) aged from 5 to 15 (76 (81 %) girls and 18 (19 %) boys) were examined. 82 children (87 %) had the hypertrophic form of disease (68 girls and 14 boys) and 12 children (13 %) the atrophic form of disease. 79 children with the hypertrophic form and 4 children with the atrophic form were euthyroid, while 8 children with the atrophic form and 3 children with the hypertrophic form were hypothyroid.

All children received monotherapy with L-thyroxine "Euthyrox®". Patients were classified according to the amount of thyroxine they received. Group I (n = 25) received a minimal dose of preparation 1 μg/kg body weight daily. Group II (n = 28, euthyroid) received a mean therapeutic dose of 1.6 μg/kg body weight daily. Group III (n = 28, euthyroid) received a dose causing maximum TSH suppression, mean dosage 2.22 ± 0.63 μg/kg body weight daily. Group IV (n = 11, hypothyroid) received a suppressive dose of thyroxine. The mean duration of treatment was 5.58 ± 2.3 months.

For evaluation of circulation in thyroid gland (TG), both qualitative (presence of circulation, direction, form of Doppler curve) and quantitative (V_{max}, V_{min}, tamx, PI, RI) indices of circulation by echodopplergraphy were used.

Our results suggest that, in hypertrophic AIT with euthyroidism, there is pronounced compensatory TG hypervascularization. L-thyroxine considerably influences the TG circulation indices among children with AIT, enhancing blood flow velocities (V_{max}, tamx) and normalizing peripheral resistance indices (PI, RI). Taking into account the known immunosuppressive effect of the preparation, L-thyroxine may improve the state of intraorganic TG arteries and normalize peripheral resistance. This leads to a reduction in the number of blood vessels operating at any one time, giving rise to qualitative changes and a reduction in color on the blood flow cartogram. This effect is maximized when suppressive L-thyroxine doses are given in euthyroid AIT.

Incidence of thyroid carcinoma in Varna region (North Eastern Bulgaria) for the period 1995–1999

K. Hristozov, L. Koeva, [1]R. Nenkov, [1]Y. Kouzmanov, [2]S. Vitcheva, [3]V. Hristova, [4]S. Alexandrov

Department of Endocrinology and Gastroenterology; [1]Department of Surgical Diseases; [2]Department of General and Clinical Pathology, Medical University: [3]Pathology Ward, Regional Hospital; [4]Pathology Ward, Naval Hospital, Varna, Bulgaria

The increase in thyroid carcinoma following the Chernobyl disaster is a topical problem in thyroid disease. It is well known that North Eastern Bulgaria is one of the regions subject to ionizing radiation in May 1986. The purpose of the present study was to establish using histological material the incidence, type and stage of thyroid carcinoma patients for the period 1995–1999. Surgery was performed on 961 patients with nodular pathology of the thyroid gland (M/F 1:5.3). Thyroid carcinoma was found in 73 (7.5 %) patients (10 men, 63 women, mean age 47.3, 34 under 45 years and 39 above 45 years).

On histology, 53 carcinomas were papillary (72.6 %), 10 were follicular (13.6 %), 2 were medullary (2.7 %), and 6 were undifferentiated (8.2 %).

The carcinoma was found in a solitary node in 56 patients (76.7 %), in nodular goiter in 15 (20.6 %), and was multifocal in 2 patients (2.7 %). Thyrotoxicosis (diffuse toxic goiter in the surrounding parenchyma) was found in 4 (5.4 %) patients, while concomitant Hashimoto's thyroiditis was found in 5 (6.8 %) patients, of whom 3 had papillary, 1 follicular and 1 undifferentiated carcinoma.

37 patients (50.6 %) had stage 1 disease, 15 (20,5 %) stage 2 disease, 14 (9,5 %) stage 3 disease, and 14 (19.4 %) stage 4 disease. Patients under 45 years had predominantly stage 1 differentiated thyroid carcinoma (apart from 1 case with stage 1 medullary carcinoma and 2 with stage 4 undifferentiated carcinoma). The incidence of thyroid carcinoma is compared before the Chernobyl disaster, and after 5 and 10 years. Objective and subjective factors influencing its incidence are discussed.

Histological profile of thyroid cancer in an area of mild endemic goiter

V. Mogos, E. Zbranca, C. Vulpoi, C. Cristea, [1]V. Strat, [1]E. Cotea, [1]D. Niculescu, [1]M.R. Diaconescu, [2]N. Florea, [2]G. Costachescu, [3]M. Rusu

1st Department of Endocrinology; [1]1st Department of Surgery; [2]Department of Pathology; [3]Department of Nuclear Medicine, University of Medicine and Pharmacy, Iasi, Romania

Iodine supply can influence the incidence of different histological forms of thyroid cancer. We have evaluated the prevalence of different histological forms of cancer in an area with mild endemic goiter proven by ultrasonographic studies and determination of urinary iodine. Among 270 cases of thyroid cancer (208 women and 62 men) hospitalized during a 25 years period (1975–1999) we found the following forms: papillary 47.40 %, follicular 22.59 %, folliculo-papillary cancer with areas of undifferentiated thyroid cancer 8.5 %, undifferentiated cancer 5.62 %, medullary 6.29 %, other forms (lymphoma, sarcoma) 5.55 %. The percentage of papillary form is higher than that of other forms but remains lower than that reported from iodine sufficient areas. Conversely, the incidence of follicular and undifferentiated form is higher in our region than that reported from iodine sufficient areas. We noted a large number of cases with undifferentiated cancer developing within differentiated forms. The proportion of papillary cancer has increased from 39.70 % (during 1975–1980) to 49 % (during 1991–1999) and the proportion of follicular cancer has decreased from 43.8 % to 22 % over the same period, probably because of a slight improvement in iodine intake. The mean ages of patients with different forms of thyroid cancer were 44.6 years for papillary forms, 43.3 years for follicular cancer, 56.7 years for less differentiated follicular cancers, 53.3 years for mixed forms, and 55.7 years for undifferentiated cancer. There was a trend to develop more aggressive forms in younger patients than in other reported series.

Conclusion: Even mild iodine deficiency may be associated with a decreased incidence of papillary thyroid cancer with an excellent prognosis and an increased incidence of follicular cancer with a poorer prognosis, and mixed form with undifferentiated foci and a poor prognosis.

Sodium iodide transporter (NIS) expression in thyroid, gastro-esophageal and breast tumors

O. Dohan, M. Paroder, [1]S. Fineberg, [2]I. Wapnir, N. Carrasco, [3]A. Altorjay

Dept. of Molecular Pharmacology, Albert Einstein College of Medicine, New York, NY; [1]Dept. of Pathology, Montefiori Medical Center, Bronx, NY; [2]Dept of Surgery, UMDNJ Medical School, New Brunswick, NJ, USA; [3]Dept. of Surgery, HIETE, Budapest, Hungary

The active transport of iodide into the thyroid is mediated by the sodium iodide symporter (NIS). The activity of this molecule has been widely used in the diagnosis of thyroid cancer, which is partly based on decreased iodide transport into tumoral relative to surrounding tissue. Much less is known about the physiological and pathophysiological role of NIS in other iodide transporting tissues, such as salivary glands, lactating mammary glands and gastric mucosa. Therefore, we investigated NIS expression in thyroid, gastroesophageal and breast tumors by immunoblot analysis, immunohistochemistry and flow cytometry, using site-directed polyclonal antibodies against the C terminus of NIS. Twenty differentiated thyroid carcinomas were analyzed by immunohistochemistry. One medullary carcinoma was negative. 7 out of 14 papillary carcinomas were positive, and 4 out of 5 follicular carcinomas were also positive for NIS staining. Interestingly, the localization of the staining was mostly intracellular, in contrast to the basolateral staining observed in the surrounding normal tissue. We have investigated 28 gastroesophageal tumors by immunoblot analysis: 16 cardia tumors (3 lymphomas, 13 adenocarcinomas) and 12 planocellular carcinomas of the esophagus. Only 9 out of 16 cardia tumors and 3 from 12 esophagus exhibited NIS expression. Even when NIS expression was observed in tumoral tissue, it was consistently decreased with respect to normal tissue. Ten out of the 16 "normal" mucosa samples adjacent to the cardia tumor tissues expressed NIS, whereas the other 6 samples exhibited no NIS expression. Four out of 12 "normal" mucosa samples adjacent to the esophagus tumors showed NIS expression. Sixteen breast tumors (14 carcinomas, 2 fibroadenomas) were investigated by flow cytometry. Eight cases were positive, seven negative. 14 out of 16 samples were positive for NIS staining by immunohistochemistry. However, by flow cytometry 8 cases were positive, and 7 negative suggesting that the aspirated cells came from a different area of the tumor. Two cases were negative by both methods. Assessing NIS expression in thyroid, breast and gastroesophageal tumors may provide additional diagnostic, prognostic and therapeutic information in these lethal diseases.

Value of the repeat fine-needle aspiration biopsy in the follow up of thyroid disease

J. Čap, [1]A. Ryška, [1]E. Hovorková, P. Řehořková, [1]Z. Kerekes

2nd Dept. of Internal Medicine and [1]Institute of Pathology, University Hospital, Hradec Králové, Czech Republic

Among more than 3000 fine needle aspiration biopsies (FNAB) performed in last 7 years, we found 303 patients (36 men and 267 women) with uninodular (70 cases) and multinodular goiter (194 cases) or Hashimoto's thyroiditis (39 cases) in whom the same nodule was investigated repeatedly over an interval of 28 ± 21 months (median 24 months). In 29 instances (9.6 %) one of the aspirate was non-diagnostic, leaving 274 patients for evaluation (two FNABs were performed in 197, three in 56 and four in 21 cases). Ninety-three patients were operated on and correlation with pathological examination was possible.

FNAB	**Number**	**Histology**	
		benign	**malignant**
Benign – repeatedly	226	61	1
Benign – suspicious	27	15	7
Suspicious – benign	12	1	0
Suspicious – repeatedly	9	5	4

In 27 cases (10.7 % of benign first FNABs) the repeated aspirate was suspicious of malignancy. Twenty two of these patients underwent surgery and histopathological examination confirmed malignancy in seven. In 5 patients the carcinoma did not increase in size by more than 25 % over a period of 24–55 months. On re-evaluation, the first FNAB result should have been considered suspicious in 6 cases. Four of them were obtained in the first 2 years, when the experience of cytopathologist was limited (2 follicular, 1 papillary, and 1 poorly differentiated carcinomas were interpreted as microfollicular or oncocytic nodules). Over the last five years, 1 lymphoma was misinterpreted as Hashimoto's thyroiditis and 1 medullary carcinoma as inflammation. In one case only the first FNAB result was that of typical colloidal nodular goiter probably because of the sampling error.

Conclusion: Repeated FNAB corrected false negative results in 7 of 253 (2,8 %) patients. It is warranted if the FNAB result is not typical for colloidal goiter and/or the adequacy of sampling is in doubt. The frequency of false FNABs decreases with the cytopathologist's experience.

Limited value of (18)FDG-PET among patients with clinically occult medullary thyroid carcinoma (MTC)

A. Kurtaran, A. Becherer, Ch. Pötzi, S. Ofluoglu, A. Kroiss, H. Vierhapper, R Dudczak, B. Niederle, K. Kletter, I. Virgolini

Dept. of Nuclear Medicine, University of Vienna, Austria

The localization of recurrent and metastatic tumor sites among patients with medullary thyroid carcinoma (MTC) is still difficult. The present study evaluates the clinical value of [18F]FDG-PET in localizing clinically occult recurrent/metastatic MTC.

Methods: 20 patients (11 male, 9 female, mean age 56.6 ± 13.7) with elevated calcitonin levels after primary surgery were included in this study. After intravenous injection of 300–370 MBq [18F]FDG, whole body images were performed with a dedicated PET tomograph (GE Advance, GE Medical Systems, Wukesha, WI). Abnormal [18F]FDG foci were compared to radiological methods (RM) including ultrasound, computed tomography, and/or magnetic resonance imaging. In one patient histological confirmation was available.

Results: In 65% (13/20) of the patients [18F]FDG images showed a normal [18F]FDG distribution (false negative study). [18F]FDG whole body images identified abnormal accumulation in only 35% (7/20) of the patients. In one of these patients with abnormal [18F]FDG uptake in thyroid region histological evaluation revealed, however, normal thyroid remnant (false positive study).

Conclusion: We conclude that [18F]FDG whole body imaging has a very low sensitivity for localizing recurrent and/or metastatic MTC lesions and has no clinical benefits. [18F]FDG should not be performed routinely in patients with recurrent/metastatic MTC.

FDG-PET, radioiodine, and imaging in a patient with poorly differentiated "insular" thyroid carcinoma

G. Zettinig, Th. Leitha, [1]B. Niederle, [2]K. Kaserer, A. Becherer, K. Kletter, R. Dudczak

Dept of Nuclear Medicine, [1]Dept of Surgery and [2]Dept of Pathology, University of Vienna, Vienna, Austria

Poorly differentiated "insular" thyroid carcinoma has been recognized as a separate entity from other tumors of the thyroid gland over the past few years. It is regarded as being intermediate between well differentiated and anaplastic thyroid cancer in its histological pattern as well as in its clinical course. Insular carcinoma is known to enhance 131-I but there are no data about FDG-PET imaging features of histologically proven insular tumors.

We report FDG-PET, Tc99m-MIBI, and radioiodine imaging features in a 63-year-old patient with metastatic insular thyroid carcinoma. After total thyroidectomy (histology: poorly differentiated "insular" carcinoma pT3) performed in another hospital, the patient was admitted to our department for radioiodine treatment. No signs of recurrence were present until sixteen months, when the thyroglobulin level increased. A 131-I scan demonstrated a single lesion in the right lung and further radioiodine treatment was performed (cumulative dose 26,860 MBq 131-I).

Two years after initial diagnosis, FDG-PET and a Tc99m-MIBI scan were performed within one week under thyroxine treatment. Thyroxine replacement was then withdrawn and six weeks later, a 131-I whole body scan was done. Both radioiodine and MIBI imaging demonstrated increased tracer uptake in the known lung lesion. However, FDG-PET showed a normal tracer distribution. MRI and CT confirmed a 12-mm lesion in the right upper lobe.

These preliminary findings support the concept of the "flip-flop phenomenon" also in insular thyroid carcinoma. It is noteworthy that, despite a poorly differentiated tumor on histology, glucose metabolism was not increased in our patient with an insular tumor.

Suppressive L-thyroxine therapy of patients operated on for a differentiated thyroid cancer

E.V. Epshtein, V.A. Oleinik, T.K. Sovenko

Institute of Endocrinology and Metabolism, Kiev, Ukraine

Patients who have been operated on for a differentiated thyroid cancer receive lifelong suppressive L-thyroxine therapy in order to suppress pituitary secretion of thyrotropin (TSH) which stimulates growth and development both of normal and metastatic thyroid cells. At the same time, suppressive L-thyroxine therapy supplies the body with the amounts of thyroid hormones needed for compensation of hypothyroidism after thyroidectomy. Short-term cessation of suppressive therapy is used for preparation for whole body scintigraphy, radioiodine therapy, and for measurement of serum thyroglobulin (a marker of appearance and development of differentiated thyroid cancer). The L-thyroxine dose is adjusted individually to provide the minimum amount required to suppress the TSH to below 0.1 mIU/l. We have estimated efficacy of suppressive L-thyroxine therapy in 173 patients with differentiated thyroid cancer after thyroidectomy.

Among patients aged 12 to 14 years, suppression of pituitary TSH production was achieved using a mean L-thyroxine dosage of 3.02 ± 0.10 µg/kg body weight. Among patients aged 15 to 18, the required dosage was 3.04 ± 0.12 µg/kg, while patients aged 19 to 30 years required 2.69 ± 0.05 µg/kg (significantly lower than in the first two groups).

Opposite effects of p53 and mdm2 on the radiation response of human medullary thyroid carcinoma cells

[1]J.A. Velasco, T. Dilla, **P. Santisteban**

Instituto de Investigaciones Biomédicas Alberto Sols, CSIC-UAM, and [1]Centro Nacional de Investigaciones Oncológicas Carlos III, Madrid, Spain

External radiation treatment, alone or in combination with chemotherapy, may be an alternative to surgical intervention in the clinical management of medullary thyroid carcinoma (MTC) tumors. Rational use of radiotherapy would be supported with the knowledge of how different oncogenes and tumor suppressors may contribute to the behavior of tumor cells upon radiation treatment. We have previously characterized the participation of p53 and mdm2 in the growth control properties of MTT cells, a MTC derived cell line naturally devoid of both cell cycle regulators. Exogenous expression of p53 causes significant growth retardation due to a transient G1 arrest of the cell cycle (Velasco et al., Int. J. Cancer 73, 449–455, 1997). Likewise, mdm2 overexpression has a negative effect on cell growth, as demonstrated by colony formation assays, cell number determination and flow cytometry. These experiments allowed us to conclude that in MTT cells, mdm2 mediates cell death by an apoptotic pathway that involves down-regulation of bcl2 (Dilla et al, Endocrinology 141, 420–429, 2000).

Since the p53-mdm2 pathway is involved in the cellular response to radiation-induced DNA damage, we have evaluated radiation survival of MTT cells expressing p53 or mdm2 by clonogenic assays. Cells were plated at low density and exposed to a ^{60}Co source at a dose of 1.5 Gy/min. Colonies containing at least 50 cells were counted and data from triplicate experiments were fitted using the single hit-multitarget and the linear quadratic models.

Results showed that p53 confers cellular radioresistance to MTT cells, presumably due to the ability of p53 to activate specific repair mechanism, as determined by dose fractionation experiments. On the other hand, cell killing was significantly higher in mdm2 expressing cells, indicating that the oncoprotein sensitizes MTT cells to ionizing radiation. Cell cycle distribution of MTT and MTT-mdm2 cells at different times after radiation and the participation of cell cycle regulatory proteins are currently under investigation, and the results will be presented in the meeting.

We conclude that p53 and mdm2 exert antagonistic effects on radiation response in MTT cells. Of special interest is the fact that mdm2 may confer radiation sensitivity on medullary thyroid carcinoma cell lines devoid of p53, thus making them more amenable to radiation treatment.

Supported by Grants CAM 08.1/0025/97 and 08.1/0025.1/99 (Spain)

Our experience in the postoperative follow-up of the medullary thyroid carcinoma

M. Ghemigian, A. Ghemigian, D. Păun, S. Păun

"C.I. Parhon" Institute of Endocrinology, Bucharest, Romania

Medullary thyroid carcinoma (MTC), which results from neoplastic transformation of the parafollicular C cells that secrete the peptide hormone calcitonin, differs from other thyroid carcinomas because of the embryological origin of C cells, as well as in its clinical, histopathological and therapeutic characteristics.

The aim of this study was to evaluate serum calcitonin as a marker of MTC evolution after surgery. We retrospectively evaluated 49 patients with MCT and treated by total thyroidectomy in the Surgery Department of the Institute of Endocrinology "C.I. Parhon" in the period 1991–1998. The MCT was sporadic in 46 patients and familial in 3 patients, being a component of MEN 2A.

All patients had elevated preoperative basal plasma calcitonin levels. After surgery the patients were followed-up by periodic clinical examination, measurement of serum calcitonin concentration, and imaging techniques (ultrasonography, CT studies and in one case Octreoscan).

Local neck recurrence of tumor as well as recurrences in the cervical and mediastinal lymph nodes occurred in 10 patients; surgical reintervention (1–4 times) was performed in all the cases. We found positive correlation levels and aggressive evolution of MCT in 9 patients.

In conclusion, serum calcitonin cannot be used as the only test for accurate postoperative follow up of MCT, of its recurrences and metastases, and needs to be construed in the context of the clinical examination and imaging techniques.

Expression of the MET/Hepatocyte Growth Factor Receptor in papillary thyroid carcinomas

E.A. Troshina, N.V. Mazurina, [1]A. Belfiore

Russian Endocrinology Center, Moscow, Russia; [1]Instituto di Medicina Interna, Cattedra di Endocrinologia, Catania, Italy

To investigate the clinical impact of Met/hepatocyte growth factor receptor (HGF-R) expression in thyroid cancer, we studied 121 thyroid papillary carcinomas from patients followed-up for 25–50 months post-thyroidectomy. Met/HGF-R expression was evaluated by semiquantitative immunohistochemistry, measuring both the proportion (on a scale of 0–5) and the intensity (0–5) of stained cells and calculating a total score (scale of 0–10). Met/HGF-R was absent from normal thyroid tissue and was expressed at various levels in most papillary carcinomas. Papillary carcinomas were categorized as having negative/low Met/HGF-R ($n = 42$) or high Met/HGF-R expression ($n = 56$). High Met/HGF-R was inversely associated with vascular invasion ($p = 0.0308$), but not with other prognostic factors. Negative/low Met/HGF-R expression was the most effective predictor of distant metastases ($p = 0.0037$), better than extrathyroidal invasion ($p = 0.0190$), and age >45 years ($p = 0.0098$). These findings suggest a role for Met/HGF-R in papillary thyroid cancer and its clinical use to select patients with a high risk of distant metastases.

In conclusion, our study indicates that 1) overexpression of Met/HGF-R is an early phenomenon in thyroid carcinogenesis and is restricted to the papillary histotype; and 2) in papillary thyroid cancer, negative/low Met/GHF-R expression is the most important predictor of development of hematogenous metastases.

A new germline mutation in the TSH receptor (TSHR) gene causing non-autoimmune autosomal dominant hyperthyroidism

L. Persani, [1]M.C. Proverbio, L. Alberti, [1]G. Weber, [1]G. Chiumello

Institute of Endocrine Sciences, [1]Istituto Auxologico Italiano IRCCS; III Pediatric Clinic, University of Milan, Istituto Scientifico S. Raffaele, Milan, Italy

Constitutively active germline mutations of TSHR have been so far reported in 8 European families affected with familial non-autoimmune hyperthyroidism and goiter. We now report the case of a new Italian family with three members affected with juvenile hyperthyroidism. The proband is a 5 years old female, who came to our attention because of accelerated growth, accompanied recently with progressive worsening of symptoms such as nervousness, sweating and palpitations. Bone age advanced by about 2 years, with normal GH/IGF1 axis. Thyroid function tests were indicative of hyperthyroidism (TSH <0.01 mU/l (0.3–0.4); FT_4 3.55 ng/l (0.9–1.9); FT_3 10.2 ng/L (1.8–4.6)), in the absence of anti-thyroid autoantibodies (anti-TSHR, anti-Tg and anti-TPO) and any other signs of specific or nonspecific autoimmune diseases. Orbital ultrasound excluded thyroid-associated ophthalmopathy. Thyroid volume was modestly, but diffusely increased on ultrasound. ^{99}Tc uptake was also diffuse. Ovarian ultrasound was normal and beta-hCG was undetectable. The clinical history revealed that the patient's father and elder half-sister (child of father's first marriage) had both undergone total thyroidectomy for non-autoimmune hyperthyroidism and goiter at 18 and 9 years, respectively. Genomic DNA from peripheral lymphocytes was obtained from all family members. In the 3 affected cases, automatic sequencing of TSHR gene revealed the presence of a new point mutation at codon 597 (GTC to TTC), resulting in the substitution V597F in the fifth transmembrane domain. A different substitution at this codon (V597L) has been recently reported to cause sporadic hyperthyroidism in one infant aged 9 months. The V597L mutant exhibited a 3-fold increase in constitutive activity in transient expression experiments. Preliminary studies of the V597F mutant indicate a modest increase in constitutive activity and enhanced responsiveness to TSH. These results are consistent with the later onset of the phenotypic expression of the mutation V597F. Differences in the clinical onset of non-autoimmune autosomal dominant hyperthyroidism within one family may also be influenced by environmental factors, such as iodine intake.

Some considerations regarding thyroid morphology and function among amiodarone-treated patients

I. Zosin, L. Jurj, A. Milos, C. Crista, M. Vlad

Clinic of Endocrinology, University of Medicine and Pharmacy, Timisoara, Romania

We studied 24 subjects from an iodine replete area (median urinary iodine >100 µg/l) treated with amiodarone for supraventricular or ventricular arrhythmias. The age of cases ranged from 19–74 years (mean 59.2 years) and the F/M ratio was 16/8. The duration of treatment with amiodarone ranged from 3 months to 9 years, and was not continuous in some cases.

Treatment was stopped in 9 cases for different reasons (such as adequate therapeutic response, occurrence of thyroid dysfunction). We divided cases into 3 subgroups depending upon length of treatment (3 months – 1 year, >1 year – 3 years, more than 3 years). Before beginning treatment, 4 cases had known thyroid pathology (nodular or diffuse euthyroid goiters). Investigations comprised thyroid ultrasonography, functional determinations (TSH, FT_4) and immunological parameters (TPO-Abs, Tg-Abs). Among the first group (9 patients, mean age 58.66 years, F/M 7/2), 2 subjects had normal thyroid morphology and function, 2 patients had asymptomatic AIT, and 5 cases were hypothyroid (1 clinical, 4 subclinical – 3 with significant antibody levels), and 1 patient had nodular thyrotoxicosis. In the second subgroup (11 subjects, mean age 59.63 years, F/M 6/5), thyroid function was normal in 4 patients. Despite being euthyroid, 2 had goiters (one diffuse, one multinodular). Hypothyroidism was diagnosed in 3 cases (2 clinical, 1 subclinical). These cases presented none but all significant antibody titers. 2 patients developed thyrotoxicosis (probably of destructive-type). Among the third subgroup (4 subjects, mean age 59.25 years, F/M 3/l) 2 developed autoimmune hypothyroidism and 1 developed thyrotoxicosis with diffuse goiter, but no antibodies. These data do not support a correlation between the duration of amiodarone administration and the occurrence of thyroid disease. The main thyroid pathology was autoimmune hypothyroidism. The incidence and the type of amiodarone induced thyroid disease may be correlated with iodine intake, previous subclinical thyroid disease, and the age of the patient. These results suggest the need for careful thyroid investigation prior to amiodarone administration.

Amiodarone-associated thyroid dysfunction: long-term follow-up

G.J. Kahaly, [1]E. Himmrich, [1]O. Przibille, A. Helms, [2]G. Rippin, J. Beyer, [1]S. Mohr-Kahaly

Depts. of Endocrinology/Metabolism, [1]Cardiology, and [2]Medical Statistics, Gutenberg-University Hospital, Mainz, Germany

Although amiodarone is an effective antiarrhythmic agent, long-term therapy may be associated with unwanted effects. In the University outpatient clinic of cardiology, a retrospective analysis was performed to examine the frequency of amiodarone-associated thyroid dysfunction among adults with ischemic heart disease and/or dilated cardiomyopathy. We report our experience in 88 patients (median age 56 years, 52 males) who had been taking amiodarone for an average of 5 years, the longest follow up was 9 years. An initial loading dose of 0.6–1.2 g/day was given for 1 week, followed by 0.2–0.4 g/day for 1 month; thereafter, the maintenance dose was determined by balancing control of arrhythmia against side effects. All patients were evaluated for thyroid status (thyroid related hormones and autoantibodies, as well as ultrasound) and cardiac complications. Sixty nine subjects (78 %) were taking the drug for primary arrhythmias, including the Wolff-Parkinson-White syndrome. Drug levels of amiodarone and desethyl amiodarone correlated with dosage ($r = 0.6$, $p<0.001$ and $r = 0.67$, $p<0.001$, respectively). Of the 88 subjects, 32 (36 %) developed thyroid dysfunction: 19 (21 %) became hyperthyroid (12 subclinical) and 13 hypothyroid (15 %, 7 subclinical). Thyroglobulin-, thyroid peroxidase-, and TSH receptor autoantibodies were present in 33 (38 %), 29 (33 %) and 4 (5 %) amiodarone patients, respectively. A heterogeneous echostructure of the thyroid gland was observed in all cases, and thyroid nodules and cysts were noted in 40 (45 %) subjects. Fine needle biopsies of the thyroid in the antibody positive subjects revealed diffuse lymphocytic infiltration. Female sex (odds ratio 3.0, $p = 0.01$), and amiodarone >0.2 g/day (odds ratio 4.0, $p = 0.005$) were significant risk factors for thyroid dysfunction. Thus, amiodarone-associated thyroid dysfunction is common in adults with ischemic heart disease and/or cardiomyopathy. Women and subjects taking high doses are at particular risk. Amiodarone should be used only when other antiarrhythmics are ineffective or contraindicated. Vigilance is required to detect and treat thyroid dysfunction.

Thyroid nodules – frequency of detection by ultrasound data and outcomes of conservative treatment

D. Metreveli, K. Mikadze, L. Baghaturia
Center of Endocrinology, Metabolism and Dietology, Tbilisi, Georgia

Nodular thyroid disease is extremely common; a 5 to 10 % lifetime risk exists for developing a palpable thyroid nodule. With sensitive imaging studies, more than a third of all women will be found to have at least one thyroid nodule (S. Feld et al. 1996). How can the less common malignant thyroid nodule be distinguished from the much more common benign nodule? How frequently can a positive medical outcome be achieved with the help of conservative (medical) therapy of nodular thyroid disease?

We have analyzed the data of 3124 patients with various diseases of thyroid gland. On ultrasonography thyroid nodules were detected in 938 (30 %) of patients, with multinodular changes in 466 (49.7 %) patients. Nodule size was defined in 921 patients. Nodules less than 5 mm were present in 11 (1.2 %), 5–10 mm in115 (12.5 %), 10–20 mm in 375 (40.7 %), 20–30 mm in 219 (23.8 %), 30–40 mm in 118 (12.8 %), and more than 40 mm in 83 (9 %). Elevated blood concentration of ABTPO and/or ABTG was detected in 447 (61,4 %) from 725 patients with nodular goiter. Iodine deficiency was discovered in 261 (75.4 %) out of 346 patients. On biochemical testing, 515 (54.9 %) patients were euthyroid, 322 (34.3 %) were hypothyroid (clinical or subclinical), and101 (10.8 %) were hyperthyroid. 69 (7,35 %) out of 938 patients with nodular goiter underwent initial surgery. Of the remaining 869 patients, 221 were not followed up, 38 pregnant patients. The remaining 610 patients with nodular goiter received levothyroxine suppression therapy unless contraindicated, using dosages of 100–200 μg per day. A positive outcome was obtained in 219 (35.9 %) cases. No nodule was seen on repeat ultrasound in 89 cases (14.6 %) at the end of the treatment. Nodule size reduced by 50 % or more in 113 cases (18.5 %). And by 20–50 % in 17 cases (1.8 %). Most of these patients had autoimmune thyroid pathology.

Radioiodine treatment for large multinodular goiter: cure rate of thyrotoxicosis and improvement of the obstructive symptoms

P. Gál, **A. Konrády**

"Jávorszky Ödön" Hospital, Vác, Hungary

Patients with multinodular goiter and tracheal compression are generally referred for surgery. The decision is complicated when:

1. The patient has had goiter resection previously, increasing the risk of serious post-operative complications.
2. The patient is at increased surgical risk because of other severe illness(es) and therefore surgery is contraindicated. In these cases only radioiodine treatment will improve the symptoms.

Between 1996 and 1999 forty-two patients with multinodular goiter were treated with ^{131}I. 62 % (26/42) had tracheal compression and/or dislocation.

A detailed history was taken for subjective symptoms (dyspnea and dysphagia). Thyroid function tests (TSH, FT_4, FT_3) and a scan were performed prior to and after treatment. Compressive signs and symptoms were investigated with x-ray investigation of tracheal region from two directions and the smallest diameter was measured. Thyroid volume was estimated by ultrasound.

Of the 42 patients 38 were female and 4 male. The mean age was 64.5 years (36–78). 33 of them suffered from thyrotoxicosis and 9 had euthyroid multinodular goiter. 26 patients had obstructive symptoms. Mean thyroid volume was 103 g. Radioiodine dose was determined individually, taking into consideration goiter volume and turnover of ^{131}I. Patients received 3.7–5.5 MBq/g (mean dose 1103 MBq, range 530–2050 MBq, radiation dose 150–200 Gy).

In five cases the ^{131}I therapy was repeated. The period of follow-up ranged from . 6 to 25 months.

Thyrotoxicosis was corrected in 73 % (24/33). Five patients remained thyrotoxic and four became hypothyroid (15 and 12 %). Obstructive symptoms improved in

45 % (12/26) measured by x-ray and in 60 % (16/26) subjectively. Goiter size was reduced by a mean of 41 % one year after treatment.

We conclude that large toxic multinodular goiter can be treated effectively with ^{131}I and that improvement of obstructive symptoms can be expected in half of the patients.

Blood suppression induced by antithyroid drugs – imidazole derivatives

T.S. Kaminina, V.A. Gubkina,

Dept. of Endocrinology of Moscow Regional Research Institute, Moscow, Russia

Imidazole derivatives (ID) are very effective antithyroid drugs, but may induce neutropenia (NP). Two basic mechanisms are responsible for drug-induced NP: direct marrow suppression and immune-mediated granulocyte destruction. The mean frequency of NP is 6 %, but only 0.17 % of patients with diffuse toxic goiter (DTG) develop agranulocytosis. NP sometimes may predict agranulocytosis. The risk of agranulocytosis is higher among patients aged more than 40 years. Both NP and agranulocytosis are indications for withdrawal of ID drugs.

We studied 414 patients, aged 20–70 years with DTG receiving Mercasolil (or thiamazole) at an initial daily dosage of 30 mg. We observed reduction of absolute number of circulating neutrophils below $2.0x10^9$ per liter (NP effect), due to marrow suppression, in 15 patients (3.6 %) aged 20–30 years, 5 with severe, and 12 with moderate thyrotoxicosis. NP occurred after 8 weeks of ID intake in 7, after 20 weeks in 4, and after one year or more in 4 patients. In the last group ID were used repeatedly for DTG relapse, and in two others after a short period off therapy. Agranulocytosis occurred after repeated ID therapy in 2 women (0.75 %) both aged 63 years. Following a diagnosis of agranulocytosis or NP, antithyroid drugs were discontinued immediately, and thyrotoxicosis was treated with lithium carbonate (900–1200 mg daily) and cardioselective beta-blockers (in individual daily dose). Treatment of agranulocytosis should include broad spectrum antibiotics and glucocorticoids.

In conclusion: 2 risk factors have significant influence on the development of ID-induced NP: duration of treatment more than 8 weeks and repeated ID intake in connection with DTG relapse. This factor reflects the important role of impaired immunological regulation in formation of ID-induced NP and agranulocytosis.

Effects of hemithyroidectomy on changes of rat thyroid morphology; studies with application of microscopic image computer analysis

W. Koptas, R. Głoskowska-Koptas, D.D. Słowínska-Klencka, E. Sewerynek, A. Zygmunt, **A. Lewiński**

Department of Thyroidology, Institute of Endocrinology, Medical University of Łodź, Łodź, Poland

The aim of the study was to evaluate morphological changes in rat thyroid lobe remaining after hemithyroidectomy (hemiTx), and to assess effects of L-thyroxine (L-T_4) administration on the histological structure of rat thyroid lobe remaining after hemiTx.

108 male Wistar rates were used, weighing 250 ± 20 g at the beginning of the experiment. Left hemiTx was performed in the experimental groups of rats and sham-operation in the control groups. Experimental animals received a solution of L-T_4 (30 µg/kg body weight) and controls 0.9% solution of NaCl only. Morphological studies were performed at "0", and then 2 and 4 weeks after surgery.

The following parameters were studied: The absolute weight of thyroid lobe, the relative volumes of compartments, absolute weights of compartments and changes of the ratio of the relative epithelium weight to colloid. The analysis of microscopic images was performed by means of the "Compartments" computer program, designed for this purpose by Klencki and Lewiński (1994). Statistical analysis was performed by one-way ANOVA and the Newman-Keuls' test.

Results:

1. Hypertrophy of the thyroid lobe remaining after hemiTx was noted 2 weeks after surgery;
2. The observed hypertrophy of the thyroid lobe was the result of an increased absolute weight of the epithelium and colloid;
3. L-T_4 administration decreased the ratio of the relative epithelium volume to colloid;
4. The inhibiting effect of L-T_4 on thyroid lobe hypertrophy was visible after 2 weeks.

Changes in the volumes of the epithelium, colloid, and stroma after hemithyroidectomy in rats following various iodine supplies and L-thyroxine administration

R. Głoskowska-Koptas, W. Koptas, M. Klencki, E. Sewerynek, **A. Lewiński**

Department of Thyroidology, Institute of Endocrinology, Medical University Łodź, Łodź, Poland

The goal of the study was an evaluation of the effectiveness of various iodine diets and of L-thyroxine (L-T_4) administration in inhibiting hypertrophy of rat thyroid lobe remaining after contralateral hemithyroidectomy (hemiTx).

In the study, normal iodine diet (250 μg/kg), as well as high-iodine diets (750 and/or 1500 μg/kg) were applied (Altromin, Germany). 300 male Wistar rats weighing 120 ± 10 g at the beginning of the experiment, were used. Left hemiTx was performed on experimental animals and sham-operation on control animals. L-Thyroxine was administered intraperitonealy to experimental animals (30 μg/kg body weight daily) and a 0.9 % solution of NaCl in control rats. Measurements were carried out at time "0", 3 weeks and 6 weeks from the beginning of experiment.

The following parameters were analyzed; relative thyroid weight, relative volumes of histological compartments, relative weights of histological compartments. Microscopic analysis was performed by means of the "Compartments" computer program, designed for this purpose by Klencki and Lewiński (1994). Statistical analysis was performed by one-way ANOVA and the Newman-Keuls test.

Results:

1. In rats on a normal iodine diet, there was partial inhibition of hypertrophy of the lobe remaining after hemiTx after 6 weeks;
2. L-T_4 administration together with each of applied iodine diets, entirely inhibited hypertrophy of the lobe remaining after hemiTx within 3 weeks of the start of the experiment;
3. No changes in the relative volumes of thyroid histological compartments were observed after any of the applied iodine diets; only in the case of L-T_4 administra-

tion was increased colloid volume observed, while the relative epithelium volume and the epithelium/colloid ratio decreased;

4. The greatest reduction in the relative epithelium weight was noted after normal iodine diet (250 µg/kg);
5. After high-iodine diet (1500 µg/kg) the relative colloid weight increased;
6. The relative weight of the stroma increased as a result of the administration of high-iodine diets (750 and/or 1500 µg/kg).

Dithyron – decision support system for interpretation of laboratory findings

L. Pecen, **O. Topolcan**, D. Hauerová, R. Pikner, D. Mrazová

Institute of Computer Science, Academy of Sciences of Prague, Prague, Czech Republic

The authors have proposed the use of Dithyron software for interpreting laboratory data concerning thyroidal disorders. From the mathematical point of view the system was based on probabilistic network theory. Dithyron software has two functions:

1. If the patient's diagnosis is not defined, then the probable diagnosis is estimated on the basis of laboratory findings, taking into consideration the prevalence of different thyroidal defects given by sex and age.
2. If thyroid dysfunction has been determined, therapy is assessed and the laboratory findings are used to explore whether other diagnoses are possible, if the drug dosage (antithyroid drugs or synthetic hormones) is entered, then the program proposes alterations to optimize the dosage (with the aim of minimizing oscillations between hyperthyroidism and hypothyroidism, which often occur during treatment with antithyroid drugs and thyroid hormones).

Model parameters are estimated on the basis of statistical processing of a suitable reference file of patients, taking into consideration information from the literature and from experts. The model and its software implantation have been in use since 1996.

This work was supported by grant of IGA MH CR.

Index

I

K

L

M

N

T